D1606429

Trauma, Psychopathology, and Violence

Trauma, Psychopathology, and Violence

CAUSES, CONSEQUENCES, OR CORRELATES?

EDITED BY

CATHY SPATZ WIDOM, PhD

Department of Psychology
John Jay College of Criminal Justice
City University of New York
New York, NY

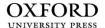

OXFORD
UNIVERSITY PRESS

OXFORD
UNIVERSITY PRESS

Oxford University Press is a department of the University of Oxford.
It furthers the University's objective of excellence in research,
scholarship, and education by publishing worldwide.

Oxford   New York
Auckland   Cape Town   Dar es Salaam   Hong Kong   Karachi
Kuala Lumpur   Madrid   Melbourne   Mexico City   Nairobi
New Delhi   Shanghai   Taipei   Toronto

With offices in
Argentina   Austria   Brazil   Chile   Czech Republic   France   Greece
Guatemala   Hungary   Italy   Japan   Poland   Portugal   Singapore
South Korea   Switzerland   Thailand   Turkey   Ukraine   Vietnam

Copyright © 2012 by Oxford University Press USA

Published in the United States of America by
Oxford University Press
198 Madison Avenue, New York, NY 10016, United States of America
www.oup.com

Oxford is a registered trademark of Oxford University Press in the UK and in certain other countries

Library of Congress Cataloging-in-Publication Data

Trauma, psychopathology, and violence : causes, correlates,
or consequences / edited by Cathy Spatz Widom.
p. ; cm. — (American Psychopathological Association)
Includes bibliographical references and index.
ISBN 978-0-19-978309-0 (hardcover)
I. Widom, Cathy Spatz, II. Series: American Psychopathological Association series.
[DNLM: 1. Stress Disorders, Post-Traumatic—complications. 2. Stress Disorders,
Post-Traumatic—psychology. 3. Personality Disorders—etiology.
4. Violence—psychology. WM 172.5]
618.92'8521—dc23   2011038851

1 3 5 7 9 8 6 4 2
Printed in the United States of America
on acid-free paper

Foreword

For the past 100 years the American Psychopathological Association (APPA) has been hosting scientific meetings annually on topics of current interest to audiences consisting of both established and young investigators, clinicians, students, and others. The design of the meeting is unique in that the APPA Council selects from among nominations by the membership at large a single member to serve as its president and to create, with input from council members, a two-and-a-half-day scientific meeting. Both the topic and the roster of invited speakers are of the president's choosing. Ample time is provided after each presentation for discussion, and there are no parallel sessions; thus attendees come away from the meeting having been updated on the latest research around the chosen topic.

The council chose Cathy Spatz Widom, Distinguished Professor at John Jay College, as the first president for the second 100 years of the APPA because of her high level of scholarly achievement in a topic of ongoing interest. The relationship between trauma and/or severe adversity and subsequent psychopathology continues to be an important area of scientific inquiry with profound implications for mental illness in general. It is apparent that the etiology of virtually all forms of psychopathology is a mixture of genetic and environmental factors. Post-traumatic stress disorder putatively constitutes one end of a genetic/environmental continuum in that it is the only disorder defined in the *Diagnostic and Statistical Manual* for which an environmental event (trauma) is required for the diagnosis. But although trauma might be definitionally necessary to the diagnosis, it is manifestly not a sufficient cause. As reviewed and demonstrated in various presentations at the meeting, the severity of trauma is not necessarily correlated with the severity or even the development of PTSD, and predisposition plays a major role in who among those exposed to a traumatic event will develop PTSD. A clearer understanding of this intriguing genetic/environmental relationship could be a significant source of clues for a better etiological understanding of the psychopathologies in general.

As is typical of the APPA meetings, Dr. Widom selected topics covering a wide range of relevant scientific questions and speakers whose research is on the cutting edge of this challenging area of inquiry. This volume is a valuable resource for anyone interested in etiology in psychopathology, and it is a superb addition to the library of volumes deriving from the APPA annual meetings.

John E. Helzer, MD
Professor of Psychiatry, Emeritus
Member, APPA Council

Preface

The motivation for this book was very personal and selfish. In my own research, I have been struggling with how to tease out causes and consequences of three related phenomena—trauma, psychopathology, and violence—and whether to accept that the best the field can do is describe the relationships among these without being able to say anything about causality. When I was elected president of the American Psychopathological Association, it seemed a natural extension of these concerns for me to choose as the topic of the annual meeting "Trauma, Psychopathology, and Violence: Causes, Consequences, or Correlates?"

The challenge to the authors of the chapters in this book was to think about how to move the field (broadly defined) ahead in order to go beyond descriptive studies. Establishing cause and effect in research is always a difficult endeavor, but this task is especially challenging when it involves complex phenomena such as trauma, psychopathology, and violence. In many cases, as discussed in this volume, even defining these phenomena can be problematic. Several chapters make the point that preexisting personal characteristics that place an individual at risk for trauma and mental health outcomes or violence add complexity to the untangling of these relationships. In addition, these particular topics often involve strongly held beliefs and assumptions and also often receive substantial media attention, with stories based on individual cases or narratives. However, before they accept these characterizations, it is the role of researchers to try to design research to disentangle causes from associations and to attempt to interpret evidence objectively. Indeed, each of the chapters herein offers suggestions of research needed in order to answer remaining critical questions.

In Chapter 1, Naomi Breslau sets the context for the subsequent chapters in this book by dissecting the diagnosis of post-traumatic stress disorder (PTSD) and arguing that its heterogeneity requires different approaches to research. The next two chapters focus on biological and genetic factors that are central to understanding the relationships among trauma, psychopathology, and violence. In this new and exciting research, Chapter 2, by Tania Roth and Frances Champagne, discusses epigenetic pathways and the consequences of adversity and trauma. Chapter 3, by Sara Jaffee ("Teasing Out the Role of Genotype in the Development of Psychopathology in Maltreated Children"), summarizes the current state of knowledge about the role of genotype as a moderator of the relationship between child maltreatment and subsequent development.

As a psychologist with early training in child development and family relationships, I recognize the importance of childhood as having a lasting influence on growth and development. For this reason, this volume contains several chapters that focus on different ways in which childhood might have an impact on exposure to trauma, violence, and the emergence of psychopathology. In Chapter 4, Michael De Bellis describes his ideas about the intergenerational transmission of family violence, including discussion of neurobiological factors. Based on new analyses from the Columbia Children's longitudinal study, Patricia Cohen, Thomas Crawford, Henian Chen, Stephanie Kasen, and Kathy Gordon (Chapter 5) examine "predictors, correlates, and consequences of trajectories of antisocial personality disorder symptoms from early adolescence to the mid-30s." In Chapter 6, Angela Narayan and Ann Masten adopt a different approach and broader focus and synthesize the current state of knowledge regarding children and adolescents in disaster, war, and terrorism.

There has also been increased attention paid to what has been called an "ecological model" of development. This model not only emphasizes the importance of the individual characteristics of the person but argues that it is also important to take into account characteristics of the family, neighborhood, and community in which a person lives. Thus, this volume includes chapters on how culture and community context play a role in potential relationships among trauma, psychopathology, and violence. For example, Fran Norris (Chapter 7) writes about "four meanings of 'community' in disaster," drawing heavily on her own research on disasters. Rosalind Wright (Chapter 8) considers the "epidemiology of violence exposure in the home and community and children's physical health risk" while using the paradigm of the urban asthma/allergy problem. Carol North (Chapter 9) explores "causality in the development and timing of disaster-related PTSD." In Chapter 10 ("Causal Thinking and Complex Systems Approaches for Understanding the Consequences of Trauma"), Melissa Tracy, Magdalena Cerdá, and Sandro Galea argue that the complex systems dynamic might be particularly suitable for the study of trauma and its consequences, given the reciprocal relations between trauma and psychopathology and the influence of other factors on one's risk for trauma and psychopathology.

Trauma, psychopathology, and violence as particular topics (individually or together) often receive substantial media attention. In Chapter 11, "Trauma, Psychopathology, and Violence in Recent Combat Veterans," Deirdre MacManus and Simon Wessely argue that before we accept the views that are often portrayed in the media, there is a need for robust research to enlighten us about the etiological pathways to violence in combat veterans.

In the final chapter (Chapter 12), "Childhood Trauma, Psychopathology, and Violence: Disentangling Causes, Consequences, and Correlates," Sally Czaja and I write about the challenges to conducting research in the field of child maltreatment and present new findings that raise questions about some of the common assumptions in the field.

I want to publicly thank all of the authors who truly rose to the challenge that I posed to them when asking them to speak at the 2011 American Psychopathological Association (APPA) meeting and to prepare their chapters. I know it was a difficult task (and several of the speakers suggested that I was a hard taskmaster), but I hope this volume serves as a worthwhile contribution, and one that will hopefully push these fields ahead in terms of our understanding of causality in these complex relationships. At a minimum, I hope that this volume stimulates and encourages other researchers to debate the issues raised here and to engage in research to address some of the challenges posed.

I also want to acknowledge the help of Kim Fader and Catina Calahan, who worked to make the 2011 APPA conference so successful. I would also like to thank the APPA board members for their feedback on the selection of topics and speakers for the meeting and for this volume. Finally, I would like to acknowledge the editors at Oxford University Press, particularly Craig Panner, for his continued support and enthusiasm for this project.

Contents

Contents

Contents

Contributors

NAOMI BRESLAU, PhD
Department of Epidemiology
Michigan State University
East Lansing, MI

MAGDALENA CERDÁ, MPH, DrPH
Department of Epidemiology
Mailman School of Public Health
Columbia University
New York, NY

FRANCES A. CHAMPAGNE, PhD
Department of Psychology
Columbia University
New York, NY

HENIAN CHEN, MS, PhD
New York State Psychiatric Institute
New York, NY

PATRICIA COHEN, PhD
Mailman School of Public Health
Columbia University
New York, NY

THOMAS CRAWFORD, PhD
New York State Psychiatric Institute
New York, NY

SALLY J. CZAJA, PhD
Psychology Department
John Jay College
City University of New York
New York, NY

MICHAEL D. DE BELLIS, MD, MPH
Director, Healthy Childhood Brain
    Development and Developmental
    Traumatology
Research Program
Department of Psychiatry and
    Behavioral Sciences
Duke University Medical Center
Durham, NC

SANDRO GALEA, MD, DrPH
Department of Epidemiology
Mailman School of Public Health
Columbia University
New York, NY

KATHY GORDON, BA
New York State Psychiatric Institute
New York, NY

Contributors

SARA R. JAFFEE, PhD
Institute of Psychiatry
King's College London
London, UK

STEPHANIE KASEN, PhD
Department of Psychiatry
Columbia University College
   of Physicians and Surgeons
New York, NY

DEIRDRE MACMANUS, MBChB,
   MSc, MRCPsych
Institute of Psychiatry
King's College London
London, UK

ANN S. MASTEN, PhD
Institute of Child Development
University of Minnesota
Minneapolis, MN

ANGELA J. NARAYAN, BA
Institute of Child Development
University of Minnesota
   Twin Cities
Minneapolis, MN

FRAN H. NORRIS, PhD
Dartmouth Medical School
Department of Veterans
   Affairs National Center
   for PTSD
White River Junction, VT

CAROL S. NORTH, MD, MPE
VA North Texas Health Care System
   Departments of Psychiatry and
   Surgery/Division of Emergency
   Medicine
The University of Texas
   Southwestern Medical Center
Dallas, TX

TANIA L. ROTH, PhD
Department of Psychology
University of Delaware
Newark, DE

MELISSA TRACY, PhD
Department of Epidemiology
Mailman School of Public Health
Columbia University
New York, NY

SIMON WESSELY, MSc, MD,
   FRCPsych, FRCP,
   FMedSci, FKC
Institute of Psychiatry
Department of Psychological
   Medicine
King's Centre for Military Health
   Research
King's College London
London, UK

CATHY SPATZ WIDOM, PhD
Department of Psychology
John Jay College
City University of New York
New York, NY

ROSALIND J. WRIGHT, MD, MPH
Channing Laboratory
Brigham & Women's Hospital
Harvard Medical School

Department of Environmental
   Health
Harvard School of Public Health
Boston, MA

PART I

Setting the Context

1

Post-traumatic Syndromes and the Problem of Heterogeneity

NAOMI BRESLAU

A volume of lectures that Paul Hoch presented to the Columbia Psychoanalytic Clinic was published in 1972, eight years after his death. In the preface, the editors wrote, "In the opinion of several contemporary psychiatrists these lectures are the most instructive since Emil Kraepelin and Eugene Bleuler wrote their books many years ago" (Strahl & Lewis, 1972).

Hoch divides the traumatic mental disorders into two groups—traumatic psychoses and traumatic neuroses—and then divides the traumatic neuroses into subgroups: (1) the postconcussion organic reaction syndromes, in which symptoms of encephalopathy are caused directly by a physical trauma, and (2) the post-traumatic neurotic reaction syndromes, in which there are no organic sequelae and symptoms are independent of brain alterations. According to Hoch, it is difficult to differentiate between the organic and the neurotic subgroups. In the majority of cases, the clinical picture is a mixture of organic symptoms—notably, headaches or dizziness—and neurotic symptoms that include irritability, impaired concentration, and withdrawal. Differentiation is further hampered by the fact that clinicians must depend on the patients' self-reports, and no conclusive laboratory tests are available other than sodium amytal interviews.

Indeed, the basis for Hoch's distinction between the organic and the neurotic subgroups is itself unclear. Is the distinctiveness of the neurosis based on its psychological symptoms or psychological pathogenesis? In either event, Hoch wishes to emphasize that the symptoms express the patient's striving for both primary and secondary gains (Strahl & Lewis, p. 188):

> This matter of secondary gains should probably be taken into consideration in many cases, particularly when the compensations involved are quite obvious . . . . For many patients, gains are not financial, but rather a convenient opportunity to withdraw from sexual, social, professional, or other responsibilities with which the patient feels unable to cope. (pp. 189–190)

Hoch does not elaborate on what he means by "primary gain." For an explanation of the term we don't have to look very far; the texts on conversion disorder in the third (American Psychiatric Association [APA], 1980, p. 244) and fourth (APA, 1994, p. 453) editions of the *Diagnostic and Statistical Manual of Mental Disorders* describe how an individual achieves primary gain "by keeping an internal conflict or need out of awareness."

In 1943, Hoch published a paper in the *American Journal of Psychiatry* titled "Psychopathology of the Traumatic War Neuroses" as part of a symposium on psychiatry in the armed forces. Ambivalence about psychogenic trauma is evident here, too. He makes several observations based on case material of merchant marine seamen. (Hock served as a consultant for the U.S. Public Health Service, War Shipping Administration.) The seamen showed a strong tendency to recover from harrowing experiences, and preexisting abnormal personality traits did not influence the rate of breakdown or recovery. Hoch attributes this to several factors that distinguish the merchant marine seamen from other servicemen: their service is voluntary, and they are not entitled to war pensions. The exception Hoch makes for the seamen confirms by implication the general rule that predispositions—abnormal personality traits—do influence breakdown and recovery.

Hoch's uneasiness about a purely psychological etiology of post-traumatic symptoms, except the symptoms that can be attributed to primary or secondary gains and predispositions, reflects the prevailing view of his time. During both World Wars, military psychiatrists diagnosed trauma-related syndromes such as shell shock and battle fatigue. Clinicians believed that in the majority of cases, the reactions gradually dissipated. Persistent reactions were suspected to be the result of predisposition (e.g., personality deficits) or malingering. The possibility of purely psychogenic post-traumatic syndromes affecting normal men (i.e., in the absence of a predisposition) was hotly debated, and Hoch's apparent ambivalence in this regard is characteristic of psychiatrists of his generation.

All this changed in 1980 with the publication of *DSM-III* and its distinctive post-trauma syndrome, post-traumatic stress disorder (PTSD). *DSM-III* created a new syndrome in which the central etiology is the *remembered traumatic event.* It established that experiences such as combat or severe accidents can cause a chronic psychiatric syndrome in persons with no predispositions and who are not driven by secondary gains. PTSD was initially conceived of as a natural response to such experiences. A few skeptics (Goodwin & Guze, 1984) questioned both the validity of a diagnosis based on this etiology (that is, whether PTSD exists as a clinical entity) and the feasibility of distinguishing true cases from false positives, factitious cases, and malingering. Goodwin and Guze describe the political context in which PTSD was adopted and how groups advocating on behalf of Vietnam veterans had vigorously promoted it. They comment, "Rarely before had so many claimants presented themselves to psychiatric examiners having read printed checklists describing the diagnostic feature of the disorder for which they sought compensation." The decision to award compensation to veterans was made even more difficult for clinicians by the "almost total lack of evidence that PTSD, and especially delayed type, exist as a clinical entity" (1984, pp. 95–96).

PTSD: The Stressor Criterion and Traumatic Memory

PTSD was created as the official post-trauma syndrome during the post–Vietnam War period in order to meet the needs of veterans who suffered chronic problems attributed to their war experience. The criterion symptoms that define PTSD in *DSM-III* are not diagnostically specific; most of them characterize other mental disorders (chiefly anxiety and depressive disorders) and are used in the definitions of these disorders. A distinct PTSD category that is different from these other disorders was created in *DSM-III* by connecting the criterion symptoms to an etiology—the remembered traumatic event. The trauma (A) creates a distressing memory that is "reexperienced" (B), and the victim adapts through avoidance and emotional numbing (C) and arousal symptoms (D). PTSD is distinguishable from the other disorders because traumatic memory alters the meaning of its symptoms. It is through this structure that "reexperiences" in PTSD are differentiated from "ruminations" in depression, "avoidance" (of stimuli that trigger traumatic memory) is differentiated from phobic disorders, and so on.

Historical accounts show that this was the model that the *DSM* committee knew when PTSD was written into *DSM-III* (Scott, 1990; Young, 1997). This also was the way that the majority of researchers and clinicians familiar with the literature on PTSD understood it. Another group of researchers and clinicians has interpreted the PTSD definition as strictly consistent with the *DSM-III* editorial position. They have assumed that PTSD, like most other disorders in *DSM-III*, is defined by the presence of the indicated criterion symptoms, and that any presumption about connections among symptoms is not justified. Studies that use "PTSD symptoms" as a continuum, "subthreshold," or "partial" PTSD have understood the *DSM* definition in this way.

Since 1980, controversies about PTSD have focused primarily on the stressor criterion that defines the etiologic event. The planning of *DSM-5* has intensified the controversy and motivated commentary from leading PTSD researchers. In a recent review, North, Suris, Davis, and Smith (2009) stated that "it is still not established whether or not there are specific types of traumatic events . . . that are associated with a syndrome that is cohesive in clinical characteristics . . ." (p. 34). In regard to the PTSD syndrome (Criteria [B]–[D]), North et al. (2009) are reasonably confident that the empirical evidence supports the *DSM* definition as capturing the typical clinical picture in victims of directly experienced severe traumas. The challenge they see is in establishing the true range of stressors responsible for PTSD. They leave open the possibility that stressors other than directly experienced severe traumas might be responsible for syndromes other than PTSD or for post-trauma distress, which is not a psychiatric disorder.

Other researchers have advocated the elimination of the stressor criterion altogether. However, this proposal is not intended to undermine the role of traumatic memory in PTSD. To the contrary, these researchers take PTSD's etiology for granted: "The full PTSD syndrome hardly ever occurs in the absence of an event that reasonably can be described as traumatic. In other words, criterion A simply describes the usual context of PTSD without contributing itself to diagnostic precision" (Brewin, Lanius, Novac, Schnyder, & Galea, 2009, p. 369). What these critics reject is the utility (even the possibility) of bracketing the range of events that can cause the syndrome.

Proposals have also been made for correcting what has been criticized as an over-inclusive stressor criterion in *DSM-IV* (McNally, 2003; Spitzer, First, & Wakefield, 2007), which creates heterogeneity in the population diagnosed with PTSD.

The *DSM-5* committee has posted on its Web site a proposal for a tighter definition. The committee's goal is "to make a better distinction between traumatic and events that are distressing but which do not exceed the 'traumatic' threshold." In other words, what the committee is aiming for is to maintain severe events, that is, those with a high probability of PTSD, and delete events unlikely to be responsible for PTSD.

Risk Factors as Sources of Heterogeneity: Trauma Severity

When PTSD researchers use the term "heterogeneity," it is generally with respect to risk factors. PTSD diagnosis requires an etiologic stressor. Risk factors introduce heterogeneity in the stressor– PTSD relationship by enhancing or diminishing the risk of PTSD among trauma victims. An important class of risk factors that modify the probability of PTSD consists of trauma characteristics, and chief among them is trauma severity. An implicit assumption in *DSM* is that the risk of PTSD is uniformly high across the distinct set of stressors in Criterion A. *DSM-III* introduced another idea when it noted that "[s]ome stressors frequently produce the disorder (e.g., torture) and others produce it only occasionally (e.g., car accident)" (p. 236). Certain types of traumatic stressors are more pathogenic than others. Trauma severity has gained a central role in the PTSD literature. Surprisingly, there is limited empirical evidence supporting the importance of trauma severity in producing PTSD.

Brewin, Andrews, and Valentine (2000) conducted a meta-analysis of 14 risk factors for PTSD, including trauma severity, and reported pervasive heterogeneity in effect size (ES) for each risk factor. They examined severity separately in military and civilian studies. In civilian studies, they examined severity within trauma types, using any objective or subjective measure that could reasonably be regarded as a proxy for trauma severity. For example, in burn victims ES might have included the association between burn area and PTSD symptoms; in motor vehicle accident survivors, it might have involved the association between physical injury and PTSD symptoms (C.R. Brewin, personal communication, July 4, 2010). The average ES in civilian studies was 0.18; in military studies, it was 0.26. The implications of coefficients this low for scientific or policy purposes is ambiguous.

Trauma Severity between and within Event Types: The 1996 Detroit Area Survey of Trauma

To examine severity within event types, I take advantage of unique data available in the 1996 Detroit Area Survey of trauma (Breslau et al., 1998) and compare the PTSD risk associated with the "worst events," as selected by the respondents from their lifetime traumatic events, to the PTSD risk associated with randomly selected events of the same type.

The "Worst Event" and "Random Event" Methods

The "worst event" method solved a practical problem. The vast majority of community residents report multiple qualifying events, and a complete assessment of PTSD for each event would impose too heavy a respondent's burden. The standard shortcut has been to assess PTSD in relation to an event singled out by the respondent as the "worst" of all the traumatic events he or she has experienced. This method gives a close estimate of the prevalence of PTSD. However, it was suspected that with this approach there would be potential for an overestimation of the PTSD effects of traumas (Kessler, Sonnega, Bromet, Hughes, & Nelson, 1995). An overestimation bias can occur in two ways. First, highly severe event types (primarily those involving assaultive violence) might be more likely to be selected as the worst relative to the distribution of traumatic events in the population. Second, within event types, the most severe instances would be more likely to be selected as the worst than typical instances of that type (e.g., the worst disasters among all disasters). Across event types and within event types, the worst events represent the extreme end of the severity distributions in terms of objective features or psychological distress in the aftermath.

The "random event" method was proposed in order to address this problem. It assesses PTSD in relation to an event randomly selected from each respondent's complete account of traumatic events (Kessler et al., 1995). Both methods (the "worst event" and the "random event") generate samples of events from the entire pool of PTSD-level events in the population. The extreme end of the severity distribution of the events in the pool comprises the sample of events generated by the "worst event" method, whereas the "random event" method (with proper weights) is a representative sample of the entire pool of PTSD-level events.

The 1996 Detroit Area Survey gathered PTSD information related to both the worst and random events. The survey is a representative sample of 2,181 persons 18 to 45 years of age in the Detroit primary metropolitan statistical area. (Detailed descriptions of the survey appeared in previous publications [Breslau et al., 1998].) A random-digit dialing method was used to select the sample. The computer-assisted telephone interview begins with a complete enumeration of traumatic events, using a list of 19 event types, which operationalizes the *DSM-IV* stressor definition as explicated in its text. An endorsement of an event type was followed by questions about the number of times an event of that type had occurred and the respondent's age at the time of each event. A computer-assembled list of all events reported by the respondent was read by the interviewer, and the respondent was asked to identify the one event that was the most upsetting—the "worst event." PTSD was evaluated in connection with this event.

Next, a computer-selected random event from the complete list of events reported by each respondent is evaluated with respect to PTSD. After a weighting algorithm is applied, the randomly selected events are representative of the total pool of PTSD-qualifying events reported by the respondents.

Trauma Severity: Variability in the PTSD Risk between Event Types

Events were grouped into four composite categories: assaultive violence (seven events), other directly experienced trauma (seven events), learning about trauma to a close relative/friend (four events), and the sudden unexpected death of a close relative/friend (a single item) (Table 1.1). Based on the randomly selected events, the highest PTSD risk (20.9%) was associated with the category of assaultive violence. The probability of PTSD associated with the second category, which covers other directly experienced events (e.g., accidents, disaster), was 6.6%. The lowest risk (2.2%) was associated with learning about trauma to a close relative/friend. The sudden unexpected death of a close friend/relative had an intermediate risk (14.2%).

Individual event types subsumed under the assaultive violence category varied with respect to their PTSD effects: the two highest were associated with being "shot or stabbed" (53.3%) and rape (49.0%). The lowest risk was associated with being "mugged/threatened with a weapon" (8.0%) (Table 1.1).

Table 1.1 Conditional Probability of PTSD across Specific Event Types

Type of trauma	N	% PTSD (SE)
Assaultive violence	286	**20.9 (3.4)**
Rape	32	49.0 (12.2)
Shot/stabbed	21	15.4 (13.7)
Sexual assault other than rape	27	23.7 (10.8)
Mugged/threatened with weapon	138	8.0 (3.7)
Badly beaten up	53	31.9 (8.6)
Other injury or shock	633	**6.1 (1.4)**
Learning about others' events	564	**2.2 (1.7)**
Sudden unexpected death	474	**14.3 (2.6)**

"Assaultive violence" combines the seven individual events listed under it. Two event types with <10 cases are excluded. "Other injury or shock" combines seven individual events (not listed). "Learning about others' events" combines four individual events occurring to a close friend/relative (not listed). N = number of randomly selected events (one per respondent) on which the probability of PTSD is based.

These data show variability in PTSD risk across event types. They confirm the general understanding that events involving assaultive (interpersonal) violence, such as rape and physical assault, are extremely severe trauma, more so than events that do not involve assaultive violence (e.g., severe accidents, disaster, learning about trauma to others). A similar ranking of event types in relation to PTSD risk was reported in another epidemiological study that used the same comprehensive list of *DSM-IV* events (Breslau, Wilcox, Storr, Lucia, & Anthony, 2004).

Trauma Severity: Variability in PTSD Risk within Event Types

To address variability within event types, we compared the PTSD risk based on the worst events versus randomly selected events of the same type. We assumed that events selected as the worst are more severe than the randomly selected events of the same type.

The results show that the PTSD risk of assaultive violence as a composite category is slightly higher when estimated based on the worst events than on the randomly selected events (28.8% versus 20.9%) (Table 1.2). Within individual event types in the assaultive violence category, PTSD risk varies between the worst event and random event databases, but the difference is rarely more than small. For example, for sexual assault, the figures are 26.0% versus 23.7%, respectively, and for having been badly beaten up they are 27.4% versus 31.9% (a reversal). For rape, the risk based on the worst events was 62.0%, versus 49.0% for the random events.

For the sudden unexpected death of a close relative/friend,[1] which is the single most frequently reported event in the population and an event type considered to include vastly heterogeneous experiences, the PTSD risk based on the worst event is virtually the same as the PTSD risk based on the random events (14.2% versus 14.3%). For learning about trauma to others, the PTSD risk is 2.7% for the worst event and 2.2% for the random event (Table 1.2).

These data fail to show material differences in PTSD risk due to severity within event types. Trauma severity levels, which distinguish the worst (or most distressing) instances from typical instances of the same event type, play a minor role in the probability of PTSD. If we are correct in assuming that the worst events are more severe than the average event of the same type, we must conclude that severity within event types is not as important for predicting PTSD as we have thought.[2]

---

1 A set of findings worth mentioning concerns learning about the sudden unexpected death of a close relative/friend, an event type included in the expanded *DSM-IV* stressor criterion. It was found to have an intermediate risk of PTSD, higher than directly experienced events that do not involve assaultive violence—such as severe accidents or disaster—and learning about events experienced by a close relative/friend. Further, in two independent samples, we found that learning about a sudden unexpected death was selected as the worst event considerably more often than would be expected if all qualifying event types had equal selection probabilities. The importance of these findings stems from the fact that the sudden unexpected death of relative/friend is highly prevalent and, because of its intermediate PTSD risk, is responsible for a considerable proportion of all PTSD cases in the population (31% of all PTSD cases in the Detroit Area Survey) (Breslau et al., 1998).

2 The comparison of the PTSD risk between the worst events and the random events performed in Table 1.2 in order to address the severity question touches on the issue of the potential overestimation bias in the worst event method. That potential bias has two sources. The first is the selection as the worst of an event with higher than average conditional PTSD risk within event types, a possibility tested in the comparison of the worst versus random events within types (Table 1.2). That suspected bias mechanism was not substantiated: by and large, the worst events did not result in a higher PTSD risk than the randomly selected events of the same type. However, this finding in itself does not provide a full answer to the suspicion that the worst event method overestimates the PTSD risk among trauma victims. To do that, it is also necessary to examine the possibility of a selection bias from the second source, that is, across event types. Are more severe event types—those associated with a higher PTSD risk—"over selected" as the worst (compared to their expected probabilities of selection)? That test revealed a substantial bias: the sudden unexpected death of a close friend or relative, which carries an intermediate PTSD risk (14.3%), was selected more frequently than would be expected if all qualifying event types had equal selection probability. This "over selection" bias came at the expense of learning about traumas experienced by a loved one, which carries a very low PTSD risk (2.2%). The overall higher conditional probability of PTSD based on the worst versus random events that we reported (13.6% versus 9.2%) is due to this bias. Direct adjustment (i.e., setting the distribution equal to expected values and applying the observed probabilities of PTSD associated with individual event types) brought the estimate close to the unbiased estimate based on the randomly selected traumas (10.9% versus 9.2%) (Breslau, Peterson, Poisson, Schultz, & Lucia, 2004).

Table 1.2 Conditional Probability of PTSD: Random versus Worst Event

Type of trauma	Worst trauma % PTSD (SE)	Random trauma % PTSD (SE)
Assaultive violence	**28.8 (3.1)**	**20.9 (3.4)**
Rape	62.0 (7.3)	49.0 (12.2)
Held captive/tortured/kidnapped	54.5 (26.8)	53.8 (23.4)
Shot/stabbed	24.4 (10.6)	15.4 (13.7)
Sexual assault other than rape	26.0 (7.4)	23.7 (10.8)
Mugged/threatened with weapon	9.2 (3.4)	8.0 (3.7)
Badly beaten up	27.4 (7.2)	31.9 (8.6)
Other injury or shock	**11.7 (1.7)**	**6.1 (1.4)**
Serious car accident	6.5 (2.3)	2.3 (1.3)
Other serious accident	21.6 (6.6)	16.8 (6.2)
Natural disaster	4.1 (2.5)	3.8 (3.0)
Life-threatening illness	31.2 (8.7)	1.1 (0.9)
Child's life-threatening illness	13.1 (6.9)	10.4 (9.8)
Witnessed killing/serious injury	11.4 (3.1)	7.3 (2.5)
Discovering dead body	8.9 (4.4)	0.2 (0.2)
Learning about others' events	**2.7 (0.8)**	**2.2 (1.7)**
Sudden unexpected death	**14.2 (1.5)**	**14.3 (2.6)**

We are left with the finding that PTSD risk varies across event types. Estimates based on both the "random even" and the "worst event" methods show that events involving assaultive violence are associated with a higher PTSD risk than other categories of events. However, even this observation might have to be qualified. With the possible exception of rape, the higher PTSD associated with assaultive violence might apply primarily to females.

Sex Differences in PTSD Risk by Trauma Severity Revisited

In the 1996 Detroit Area Survey of trauma and in our collaborative study of young adults with Johns Hopkins University (Breslau et al., 2004), we found that the excess PTSD risk of assaultive violence is specific to females (Table 1.3). Among males, the PTSD risk of assaultive violence is not higher than the PTSD risk of other categories and is lower than the PTSD risk associated with the sudden unexpected death of a close relative/friend. The possibility that this sex difference might be largely related to assaultive violence is not unique to our two samples. Results from the National Comorbidity Survey (Kessler et al., 1995) show considerably higher rates of PTSD in females than in males chiefly for events involving nonsexual assaultive violence: "physical attack" (26.5% versus 4.4%) and "threatened with a weapon" (32.6% versus 1.9%). In contrast, both sexes had a similar PTSD risk in relation to "accidents" (8.8% versus 6.3%), "witnessing violence" (7.5% versus 6.4%), and "disaster" (5.4% versus 3.7%). A comprehensive review by Tolin and Foa (2006) found that the female versus male odds ratio (OR) of PTSD for nonsexual assault was considerably higher than for other trauma types (4.7 versus the next highest OR of 2.1 for disaster or fire; for sexual assault, the female versus male PTSD OR = 1.1).

Military Studies and Trauma Severity

An exception to the scarcity of evidence on the role of trauma severity for predicting PTSD has been the studies of military samples. But even regarding this finding, two important points should be considered. The first is the low ES of 0.26 estimated in the meta-analysis of Brewin et al. [2000]). Second, leading PTSD researchers have voiced skepticism regarding the interpretation of reported correlations (King et al., 2000; Roemer, Litz, Orsillo, Ehlich, & Friedman, 1998; Southwick, Morgan, Nicolaou, & Charney, 1997; Wessely et al., 2003). Evidence of pervasive inconsistencies in the memory of war-zone traumas, increases over time of reported events, and a correlation of these changes with PTSD symptoms or with poorer perceived health at follow-up have motivated these researchers to question the place of combat severity in the etiology of PTSD and the notion of a "unidirectional" causal relationship between trauma and PTSD.

Table 1.3 Conditional Probability of PTSD: Sex-Specific Comparisons

	Detroit area[a]		Baltimore	
	Male % (SE)	*Female % (SE)*	*Male %*	*Female %*
Assaultive violence	6.0 (3.3)	35.7 (5.6)	7.1	23.5
Excluding rape/sexual assault	6.0 (3.3)	32.3 (6.4)	4.7	12.7
Other injury or shock	6.6 (1.9)	5.4 (2.0)	7.9	5.2
Learning about others	1.4 (0.8)	3.2 (1.3)	2.8	3.1
Sudden unexpected death	12.6 (3.6)	16.2 (3.6)	9.2	8.8

[a] Breslau, Chilcoat, Kessler, Peterson, & Lucia, 1999.
[b] Breslau et al., 2004.

Trauma Severity and the Role of Predispositions

PTSD's distinctive feature in *DSM* is that traumatic stress is the dominant cause of the disorder, and predispositions are secondary. In 1980 this idea was neither new nor specific to PTSD, as illustrated in the following statement on how stress causes disease, published while *DSM-III* was under construction: "The more rigorous and severe the external situation, the less significant are social and individual characteristics in determining the likelihood and nature of response" (Rabkin & Struening, 1976, p. 1018). In the past 30 years, the range of qualifying events has been expanded, in both clinical psychiatric practice and litigations. The expansion is reflected in the revisions of the stressor criterion in *DSM-IV*. McNally (2003, 2009) observed that the broadening of the stressor criterion to include events of low magnitude—the "conceptual bracket creep"—made it less plausible to assign causal significance to the stressor and more plausible to emphasize personal predispositions. The limited empirical data relevant to this point do not support this expectation.

A revisit of a 2003 meta-analysis on risk factors for PTSD by Ozer, Best, Lipsey, and Weiss revealed information relevant to the question of whether the role of predispositions varies as a function of trauma severity. Ozer et al. (2003)[3] estimated the ES of risk factors for PTSD according to three types of events: (1) combat exposure, (2) interpersonal violence (i.e., human-perpetrated violence that occurred in a civilian context), and (3) accidents. They examined three antecedent risk factors: prior trauma, prior psychological adjustment, and family history of psychopathology. This organization of the meta-analysis (i.e., event type as modifier of risk factors) allows us to see whether preexisting vulnerability factors are less important in explaining the PTSD effect of severe trauma (e.g., interpersonal violence) than accidents, a less severe trauma. Data on prior trauma as a risk factor came from 23 studies (n = 5308), on prior psychological adjustment from 23 studies (n = 6797), and on family history of psychopathology from 9 studies (n = 667). (The meta-analysis also included four "proximate" ["peritraumatic"] predictors that are not relevant to this question.)

---

3 Ozer et al. (2003) reported results from a meta-analysis of seven risk factors for PTSD, among them four factors classified as proximal, occurring at the time of the event or in the aftermath: perceived life threat, peritraumatic emotionality, peritraumatic dissociation, and social support. With the exception of social support, these factors have been viewed by psychologists as trauma characteristics predictive of PTSD. It is this group of predictors, as distinct from antecedent factors, that had an ES above 0.20 (but < 0.30) and thus was recommended by Ozer et al. (2003) for attention in future research. I wish to note a conceptual problem in viewing these peritraumatic variables as predictors of PTSD. Peritraumatic dissociations and emotionality might be manifestations of the same pathological processes as PTSD, the outcome we wish to explain. The predictive capacity of these variables might be an artifact of how researchers divide the phenomenon, spuriously distinguishing early from later pathologic responses, as if they were distinct phenomena.

Ozer et al. (2003) found no evidence that predispositions were less important for interpersonal violence (e.g., assault, rape, domestic violence) than for accidents (mostly motor vehicle accidents). To the extent that there were differences in risk factor–PTSD relationships between event types, they were in the reverse direction. The authors summarize their findings as follows: "The manner in which the type of event affected prediction was nearly uniform—average ESs were stronger for prior trauma, prior adjustment, family history of psychopathology [and life threat]—if the index trauma was interpersonal violence" (p. 67). The ES associated with prior trauma were 0.27 for interpersonal violence and 0.12 for accidents; for prior psychological adjustment, they were 0.31 and 0.28, respectively, and for psychopathology in family of origin they were 0.31 and 0.08, respectively (Table 1.4). (For combat exposure, the ES was lower than that for accidents for each of the three predictors; p < 0.01.)

Ozer et al. (2003, p. 67) decline to offer explanations for these results ("all explanations would be *ad hoc* and not supported by ancillary data"), and it is unclear whether the observed differences in ES between interpersonal violence and accidents make a material difference in understanding the ways in which vulnerability factors work. The important conclusion is that there is no support for the idea that preexisting vulnerability plays a lesser role in the relationship of PTSD to severe (versus low-magnitude) events. Established vulnerability factors for PTSD, such as prior disorders and a family history of psychopathology, were not less important when trauma was more severe.

Findings that presage the observation from Ozer et al. (2003) were reported by Helzer in 1981, although the outcome in that study was depression, not PTSD. Helzer reported results from a follow-up study of Vietnam veterans conducted in the early 1970s. He examined the effects of antecedent factors

Table 1.4 Effect Size of Predispositions for PTSD

	Interpersonal violence	Accidents
Prior trauma (23 studies; n = 5,308)	0.27[a]	0.12
Prior adjustment (23 studies; n = 6,797)	0.31	0.28
Family psychopathology (9 studies; n = 667)	0.31[b]	0.08

[a] p = 0.05.
[b] p = 0.01.
From Ozer et al. (2003).

(failure to graduate from high school, early drug use) on depression across different levels of combat stress, measured by number of combat events. The influence of these antecedents was greater (and statistically significant) at high levels of combat stress. It was also greater among wounded than nonwounded veterans. Helzer concluded that there was no decrease in the impact of predispositions with an increase in the level of combat exposure—in fact, the opposite pattern was observed.

That vulnerability factors might be more, not less, important for interpersonal violence (or high-level combat) than for accidents (or lower level combat) runs directly counter to the core assumption of an inverse relationship between stressor severity and the importance of predisposition. That assumption seems so obvious—it flows logically from the idea of a "dose–response" relationship between stressors and PTSD—that there has been little empirical testing.

Heterogeneity in Chronic PTSD: Multiple Kinds of Memory for Trauma

"Heterogeneity" in the PTSD literature has a distinct meaning. In the general psychiatric literature, "heterogeneity" refers to clinical presentation; that is, not all members of a diagnostic category are homogeneous with regard to their clinical features. *DSM-IV* explains,

> [I]ndividuals sharing a diagnosis are likely to be heterogeneous even in regard to the defining features of the diagnosis . . . . In recognition of the heterogeneity of clinical presentations, DSM-IV often includes polythetic criteria sets, in which the individual needs only present with a subset of items from a longer list . . . . (p. xxii)

In contrast, in PTSD, "heterogeneity" most often refers to variability in the potency of events to cause PTSD. North et al. (2009) call attention to uncertainty concerning events that are not life threatening. Specifically, they question the potential of these less severe events to cause the specific PTSD syndrome and suggest the possibility that less severe events cause milder syndromes or non-specific distress. McNally (2003) warns that the enlarged stressor criterion in *DSM-IV* lumps together true cases (i.e., those caused by severe traumas) with questionable cases (i.e., those caused by milder events added in *DSM-IV*) in which preexisting vulnerability is the responsible factor in the victim's PTSD response. McNally doubts that the biology of cases of severe traumas, such as rape or combat, is the same as that of cases of mild trauma, such as indirect exposure to September 11. The solution for North et al. and McNally is the same: tighten up the stressor criterion.

We wish to call attention to a different kind of heterogeneity in PTSD: hetero-geneity in the underlying etiology of the disorder (i.e., the way stressor and syn-drome are connected). Unlike most psychiatric categories, PTSD has a specified etiology: the event (A) causes recurrent painful memories (B), and the memo-ries cause the symptoms in C and D. It is this structure that transforms PTSD to a distinct disorder. However, the *DSM* memory logic is not the only way in which event and PTSD syndrome can be connected. Other causal pathways are created by memory sequences that do not follow the *DSM* model.

Several kinds of memory sequences that differ from the underlying *DSM* model can be discovered in the psychiatric literature (Young, 2004). One type is attributed memory, in which an individual with current symptoms acquires a connection with a past event. When initially experienced, the event was not markedly distressful; only in retrospect is the experience reassessed and remem-bered as traumatic. Clancy describes a process of this kind in her study of adult victims of child sexual abuse. In most of the cases, the sexual abuse was not a traumatic, overwhelming, or terrifying experience for the victim when it hap-pened. It became traumatic later on "only at this point—when victims under-stood the abuse as such, once they had re-conceptualized these formerly ambiguous and confusing events—did the experience become psychologically traumatic and began to exert its negative effects" (Clancy, 2009, p. 122). As an adult, when the person understands the "real" meaning of the event, the memory of the event acquires an emotional potency that it did not originally possess. It becomes a traumatic (pathogenic) memory, but only belatedly.

Examples related to combat PTSD have been reported in several studies. Southwick and colleagues (1997) published a study on changes in traumatic memories among American veterans of the first Gulf War. A sample of 59 veter-ans were interviewed one month after their return from the war and then reinter-viewed two years later. In each interview, veterans completed a 19-item questionnaire about their combat experiences. At the two-year reinterview, 70% reported at least one combat event that they had not reported at one month. (There were also changes from "yes" to "no"; 46% did not report one or more events they had reported one month after returning home.) The events most commonly reported at two years, but not at one month, after return were "bizarre disfigura-tion of bodies as a result of wounds," "seeing others killed or wounded," and "extreme threat to your personal safety." The two former events, as well as other events that were recalled at two years but not at one month, were objectively described events rather than subjectively evaluated experiences, the authors note.

Increases in recalled events over time can be explained in several ways. Memories might have been influenced by media accounts and by conversations with other veterans about their war experiences. The authors also suggest another possibility: "individuals who became increasingly symptomatic over time unknowingly exaggerated their memory for trauma events as a way to understand or explain their emerging psychopathology" (Southwick et al., 1997, p. 176). This explanation is supported by the study's finding that the level of PTSD symptoms at follow-up was positively correlated with the number of responses that were changed from "no" to "yes." The authors describe the implications as follows: Numerous investigations (including their own) have repeatedly shown that the level of combat exposure is correlated with PTSD risk. It is this consistent correlation that has been taken as evidence for a causal role of trauma in PTSD. Based on the new findings, the authors reconsider the meaning of the evidence: "if memories are inconsistent, then statistical analyses, such as correlations, involving accounts of trauma are highly suspect" (p. 174).

Similar findings have been reported in a larger study of U.S. soldiers who served in the peacekeeping mission in Somalia (Roemer et al., 1998) and in a second sample of veterans of the first Gulf War (King et al., 2000). Instability in recalled events was reported from an epidemiological study of civilians (Hepp et al., 2006). Three findings—(1) pervasive inconsistencies in memory of war-zone traumas, (2) increases over time of reported events, and (3) a correlation of these changes with PTSD symptoms at follow-up—motivated these researchers to question the role of combat severity in the etiology of PTSD and the notion of a "unidirectional" causal relationship between trauma and PTSD.

One might disagree with these conclusions. An alternative view might be that combat experiences did cause PTSD in some veterans, and their memory of details has been unstable for other reasons. Unfortunately, there is no obvious way to find out. What is clear is that Southwick and the other PTSD researchers who reported these findings and drew these conclusions identified a fundamental problem in diagnosing PTSD, a disorder based on remembered trauma. The malleability of memory undermines that essential link between trauma and PTSD syndrome.

Attributed memories are distinguished from factitious memories, in which people unknowingly appropriate for themselves memories that originated in the experience of others. In some of the veterans studied by Southwick et al. (1997), the newly recollected combat events might have been factitious, adopted from compelling accounts of combat experiences told by other veterans, as Southwick et al. note.

An illustration of one type of factitious memory was published in 2001 by Sheen, Kemp, and Rubin in an article entitled "Twins Dispute Memory Ownership: A New False Memory Phenomenon." The results of several experiments confirmed anecdotal evidence that disputed memories existed among twins. Disputed memory ownership differs from other memory discrepancies in that the memory detail that is in dispute is who the protagonist in the event is (p. 779). Here is one example from this article: One pair of 52-year-old twins disagreed about which of them had made a dramatic attempt at running away from home at the age of 6. Both recalled sitting in the back of the car while the mother frantically searched the streets for the missing twin.

A subsequent article by these authors reported that parties in the disputes tend to be self-serving, claiming for themselves memories of achievement and misfortunes and giving away (assigning to others) memories of personal wrong-doing (Sheen, Kemp, & Rubin, 2006). The authors comment that "some of the memories in which we play a leading role might in fact have been the experiences of others" (p. 9).

Based on neuroscience research on motor simulation and mirror neuron activity (interpersonal mirroring), Lindner, Echterhoff, Davidson, and Brand (2010) tested a novel type of false memory. A series of experiments documented that merely observing another person's activity induced substantial rates of the observers' falsely reporting that they themselves performed the activity. Observation of another person's action might trigger a simulation of the action and thus activate motor representations similar to those produced during self-performance:

> Evidence suggests that mirrored motor representations can shape observers' self-related motor memory (Stefan et al., 2005) and neural correlates of conscious memory for these representations are similar to those of memory for self-performed actions . . . they could—erroneously—remember having performed the action. (Lindner et al., 2010, p. 1297)

In conclusion, the term "PTSD" is equivalent to (1) the *DSM* definition and (2) the population of individuals who have been given the diagnosis. Only a subgroup of the PTSD-diagnosed population conforms to the *DSM* conception of "A causes B, and B causes C and D." The problem is that these authentic cases account for only a subgroup of the population with the diagnosis. This larger population is heterogeneous regarding etiology. There are no tools for differentiating "valid" cases from cases in which the causal order progresses from current unexplained symptoms to the acquisition of a past traumatic memory. Consequently, heterogeneity remains an intractable problem.

The memory critique, like the other critiques of PTSD heterogeneity (e.g., McNally, 2009; North et al., 2009), accepts the validity of the *DSM* diagnosis (i.e., that psychological trauma can cause chronic psychopathology of a distinct type). However, these other critiques identify problems and solutions; the memory problem, in contrast, has no obvious solution.

Disclosure Statement

This chapter is based on the Paul Hoch Award Address presented at the 2011 meeting of the American Psychopathological Association. The research reported in this chapter was supported in part by Grants MH4586 and MH71395 from the National Institutes of Health, Bethesda, Maryland.

References

American Psychiatric Association. (1980). *Diagnostic and statistical manual of mental disorders* (3rd ed.). Washington, DC: Author.

American Psychiatric Association. (1994). *Diagnostic and statistical manual of mental disorders* (4th ed.). Washington, DC: Author.

American Psychiatric Association (2010). DSM-5 development. Retrieved from: http://www.dsm5.org/Pages/Default.aspx

Breslau, N., Chilcoat, H. D., Kessler, R. C., Peterson, E. L., & Lucia, V. C. (1999). Vulnerability to assaultive violence: Further specification of the sex difference in post-traumatic stress disorder. *Psychological Medicine, 29,* 813–821.

Breslau, N., Kessler, R. C., Chilcoat, H. D., Schultz, L. R., Davis, G. C., & Andreski, P. (1998). Trauma and posttraumatic stress disorder in the community: The 1996 Detroit Area Survey. *Archives of General Psychiatry, 55,* 626–632.

Breslau, N., Peterson, E. L., Poisson, L. M., Schultz, L. R., & Lucia, V. C. (2004). Estimating post-traumatic stress disorder in the community: Lifetime perspective and the impact of typical traumatic events. *Psychological Medicine, 34*(4), 889–898.

Breslau, N., Wilcox, H. C., Storr, C. L., Lucia, V. C., & Anthony, J. C. (2004). Trauma exposure and posttraumatic stress disorder: A study of youths in urban America. *Journal of Urban Health, 81*(4), 530–544.

Brewin, C. R., Andrews, B., & Valentine, J. D. (2000). Meta-analysis of risk factors for posttraumatic stress disorder in trauma-exposed adults. *Journal of Consulting and Clinical Psychology, 68*(5), 748–766.

Brewin, C. R., Lanius, R. A., Novac, A., Schnyder, U., & Galea, S. (2009). Reformulating PTSD for *DSM-V:* Life after Criterion A. *Journal of Traumatic Stress, 22*(5), 366–373.

Clancy, S. A. (2009). *The trauma myth: The truth about the sexual abuse of children—and its aftermath.* New York: Basic Books.

Goodwin, D., & Guze, S. B. (Eds.). (1984). *Psychiatric diagnosis.* Oxford, UK: Oxford University Press.

Helzer, J. E. (1981). Methodological issues in the interpretations of the consequences of extreme situations. In B. S. Dohrenwend & B. P. Dohrenwend (Eds.), *Stressful life events and their contexts: Monographs in psychosocial epidemiology 2* (pp. 108–129). New York: Prodist.

Hepp, U., Gamma, A., Milos, G., Eich, D., Ajdacic-Gross, V., Rossler, W., et al. (2006). Inconsistency in reporting potentially traumatic events. *British Journal of Psychiatry, 188,* 278–283.

Kessler, R. C., Sonnega, A., Bromet, E., Hughes, M., & Nelson, C. B. (1995). Posttraumatic stress disorder in the National Comorbidity Survey. *Archives of General Psychiatry, 52*(12), 1048–1060.

King, D. W., King, L. A., Erickson, D. J., Huang, M. T., Sharkansky, E. J., & Wolfe, J. (2000). Posttraumatic stress disorder and retrospectively reported stressor exposure: A longitudinal prediction model. *Journal of Abnormal Psychology, 109*(4), 624–633.

Lindner, I., Echterhoff, G., Davidson, P. S. R., & Brand, M. (2010). Observation inflation: Your actions become mine. *Psychological Science, 21*(9), 1291–1299.

McNally, R. J. (2003). Progress and controversy in the study of posttraumatic stress disorder. *Annual Review of Psychology, 54,* 229–252.

McNally, R. J. (2009). Can we fix PTSD in DSM-V? *Depression and Anxiety, 26*(7), 597–600.

North, C. S., Suris, A. M., Davis, M., & Smith, R. P. (2009). Toward validation of the diagnosis of posttraumatic stress disorder. *American Journal of Psychiatry, 166*(1), 34–41.

Ozer, E. J., Best, S. R., Lipsey, T. L., & Weiss, D. S. (2003). Predictors of posttraumatic stress disorder and symptoms in adults: A meta-analysis. *Psychological Bulletin, 129*(1), 52–73.

Rabkin, J. G., & Struening, E. L. (1976). Live events, stress, and illness. *Science, 194*(4269), 1013–1020.

Roemer, L., Litz, B. T., Orsillo, S. M., Ehlich, P. J., & Friedman, M. J. (1998). Increases in retrospective accounts of war-zone exposure over time: The role of PTSD symptom severity. *Journal of Traumatic Stress, 11*(3), 597–605.

Sheen, M., Kemp, S., & Rubin, D. C. (2001). Twins dispute memory ownership: A new false memory phenomenon. *Memory and Cognition, 29*(6), 779–788.

Sheen, M., Kemp, S., & Rubin, D. C. (2006). Disputes over memory ownership: What memories are disputed? *Genes, Brain and Behavior, 5*(Suppl. 1), 9–13.

Southwick, S. M., Morgan, C. A., Nicolaou, A. L., & Charney, D. S. (1997). Consistency of memory for combat-related traumatic events in veterans of Operation Desert Storm. *American Journal of Psychiatry, 154*(2), 173–177.

Spitzer, R. L., First, M. B., & Wakefield, J. C. (2007). Saving PTSD from itself in DSM-V. *Journal of Anxiety Disorders, 21*(2), 233–241.

Stefan, K., Cohen, L. G., Duque, J., Mazzocchio, R., Celnik, P., Sawaki, L., et al. (2005). Formation of a motor memory by action observation. *Journal of Neuroscience, 19,* 67–74.

Strahl, M. O., & Lewis, N. D. C. (Eds.). (1972). *Differential diagnosis in clinical psychiatry: The lectures of Paul H. Hoch, M.D.* New York: Science House.

Tolin, D. F., & Foa, E. B. (2006). Sex differences in trauma and posttraumatic stress disorder: A quantitative review of 25 years of research. *Psychological Bulletin, 132*(6), 959–992.

Wessely, S., Unwin, C., Hotopf, M., Hull, L., Ismail, K., Nicolaou, V., et al. (2003). Stability of recall of military hazards over time. Evidence from the Persian Gulf War of 1991. *British Journal of Psychiatry, 183,* 314–322.

Young, A. (1997). *The harmony of illusions: Inventing post-traumatic stress disorder.* Princeton, NJ: Princeton University Press.

Young, A. (2004). When traumatic memory was a problem: On the historical antecedents of PTSD. In G. M. Rosen (Ed.), *Posttraumatic stress disorder: Issues and controversies* (pp. 127–146). Chichester, UK: Wiley.

PART II

Biological and Genetic Factors in Understanding Trauma, Psychopathology, and Violence

2

Epigenetic Pathways and the Consequences of Adversity and Trauma

TANIA L. ROTH AND FRANCES A. CHAMPAGNE

The experience of adversity can have a lasting impact on physiology, neurobiology, and behavior, with consequences for health and well-being. Though these effects are evident when the exposure occurs in adulthood, it is clear that sensitivity to these experiences is heightened in the early stages of development. The devastating and enduring effect of traumatic and adverse experiences has led to increasing exploration of the mediating and moderating biological pathways. This investigation has led to the development of animal models in which the timing and duration of exposure to trauma/stress and adversity can be carefully controlled and the subsequent neurobiological outcomes assessed. Consistent with human physiological and neuroimaging studies, experimental manipulation of the environment of laboratory rodents and nonhuman primates illustrates that long-term programming of stress physiology and modifications in the structure and sensitivity of multiple brain regions are consequences of exposure to stress and trauma. However, analysis of brains derived from animal studies suggests that these effects can be observed even at the cellular and molecular levels, with these early and later-life exposures being associated with persistent changes in the activity of genes. Thus, there appears to be interplay between environments and our genes that might play a critical role in explaining the mechanistic link between our experiences and our biological and psychological functioning.

In the past decade, there have been advances in molecular biology that have provided new insights into those factors that alter the activity of genes without modifying the underlying sequence of DNA. These "epigenetic" factors play a critical role in development, allowing for the emergence of different cell types and mediating both plasticity and stability in gene expression. More recently, data derived from animal studies have identified variation in these same mechanisms in response to a variety of developmental and later-life experiences. The possibility that specific experiences of an individual can become "encoded" within the epigenetic factors that control gene activity has contributed a novel perspective to discussions of the biological pathways through which trauma, adversity, and stress exert their effects. The relevance of these findings for humans is the focus of increasing philosophical and empirical exploration, with emerging data suggesting that epigenetic mechanisms might contribute to our understanding of the pathways through which adversity becomes part of our biology.

In this chapter, we discuss the evolving field of epigenetics in the context of studies on the impact of early-life neglect, abuse, and stress, as well as later-life exposure to trauma. Though the data here are primarily drawn from animal models of these experiences, we also highlight studies in which the translation of these findings to humans has been explored. The impact of adversity, though certainly evident in exposed individuals, might also have implications for the neurobiology and behavior of subsequent generations. The transgenerational impacts of stress and trauma, which have been documented across species and in human populations, might also involve epigenetic pathways and suggest a molecular mechanism through which environmental experiences can become "heritable". Here, we discuss the impact of adversity across generations and the implications of an epigenetic perspective for the future directions of research on the consequences of traumatic life experiences.

Adversity and Psychopathology: Epidemiological Studies of Neglect, Abuse, and Trauma

Though there are certainly individual differences in the susceptibility to the effects of adverse experiences (Caspi et al., 2003; Ellis, Boyce, Belsky, Bakermans-Kranenburg, & van Ijzendoorn, 2011), the significant impact of neglect, abuse, and trauma on physical and psychological health has been well documented.

Childhood Maltreatment

In humans, childhood neglect and abuse have been demonstrated to reduce cognitive performance and impair social development (Trickett & McBride-Chang, 1995) and are associated with a four-fold increase in personality disorders (Johnson, Cohen, Brown, Smailes, & Bernstein, 1999). The severe neglect experienced by institutionalized infants, most recently explored amongst Romanian orphans, provides further examples of the persistent effects of these experiences. Delays in growth and in social and cognitive development observed in Romanian orphans are associated with later life impairments in attachment, heightened inattention, and increased autistic-like behaviors (Beckett et al., 2006; MacLean, 2003; O'Connor & Rutter, 2000; O'Connor, Rutter, Beckett,

Keaveney, & Kreppner, 2000; Rutter & O'Connor, 2004). Though it is difficult to identify the particular aspect of the neglectful or abusive childhood experience that contributes to this outcome, disruption to the mother–infant relationship is thought to be critical. Variations in the attachment relationship between mother and infant have been associated with either resilience to psychological distress (e.g., secure attachment) or increased incidence of psychopathology (e.g., disorganized attachment) (Sroufe, 2005; Sroufe, Carlson, Levy, & Egeland, 1999). Disorganized attachment patterns, which are observed to occur in 48% to 80% of maltreated/abused infants (versus 17% in comparison samples), predict increased rates of borderline personality disorder, dissociation, and self-harm in adulthood (Carlson, 1998; Carlson, Egeland, & Sroufe, 2009; van Ijzendoorn, Schuengel, & Bakermans-Kranenburg, 1999). Thus, the experience of childhood maltreatment, likely in combination with the disruption to the attachment relationship associated with this form of environmental adversity, can lead to a heightened risk of psychopathology in later life.

Stress and Trauma

Adverse life experiences occurring across the life span can contribute to the onset and severity of psychopathology. This phenomenon is typically conceptualized within the vulnerability-stress model of psychiatric disorder, in which stressful life events combined with an underlying biological vulnerability contribute to risk. A classic, though controversial, example of the role of stressful life events in the emergence of disease risk comes from the study of gene–environment interactions and the risk of depression (Caspi et al., 2003). Amongst individuals with a specific genetic variant (e.g., the short form [s/s] of the serotonin transporter [5-HTT] gene), increasing numbers of stressful life events in adulthood were associated with increasing risk of depression and suicidal ideation/attempts. The stressors assessed in this case included financial, employment, family/marital, and health problems occurring in individuals between the ages of 21 and 26. In addition to genetic vulnerability, childhood adversity (neglect and abuse) can also "sensitize" individuals to the effects of later life stressors. For example, amongst adults with a history of childhood adversity, the experience of increasing numbers of stressful life events is associated with a higher prevalence of depression, anxiety, and post-traumatic stress disorder (PTSD) (McLaughlin, Conron, Koenen, & Gilman, 2010). Thus, vulnerability to psychopathology following the experience of stressors can be considered from both a genetic (e.g., 5-HTT allele) and an environmental (e.g., childhood maltreatment) perspective.

The experience of traumatic life events is one of the defining features of the diagnosis of PTSD and demonstrates the profound effect of stressors on psychological functioning. Both early life (e.g., childhood abuse) and later life (e.g., war, violence) trauma have been found to induce symptoms of PTSD, which include psychologically reexperiencing the traumatic event (leading to distress), hypervigilance, and avoidance of cues associated with the experience. Epidemiological studies of PTSD suggest a lifetime prevalence of 7.8%, with females twice as likely as males to develop PTSD (Kessler, Sonnega, Bromet, Hughes, & Nelson, 1995). Importantly, amongst trauma-exposed individuals, approximately 10% will develop PTSD, suggesting vulnerability to trauma in PTSD patients and resilience to trauma amongst the majority of the population. Currently, the biological mechanisms of vulnerability and resilience have yet to be identified.

Exposure to Adversity: Physiological and Neural Correlates

A critical question within the study of the long-term effects of exposure to adversity regards the biological pathways that are activated and persistently altered by the experience of maltreatment, stress, and trauma. Evidence from human studies suggests an impact of adverse experiences on stress physiology and neurobiological functioning, and these findings are supported by animal studies of early life stress/neglect.

Stress Physiology

Stress responses are mediated by the sympathetic-adrenomedullary and hypothalamic-pituitary-adrenocortical (HPA) systems (Gunnar & Quevedo, 2007; Pruessner et al., 2010). In response to a stressor, the adrenal medulla releases catecholamines (epinephrine and norepinephrine [NE]), and the HPA system produces glucocorticoids (GCs) (cortisol in humans and primates, corticosterone in rodents). Catecholamines bind to receptors on various target organs, producing physiological responses that include increased heart rate and blood supply to muscles and the brain. In parallel within the brain, NE is also produced in the locus coeruleus, which increases arousal and attention. Corticotrophin-releasing factor (CRF) (also known as corticotrophin-releasing hormone [CRH]) and arginine vasopressin (AVP) are released by cells in the paraventricular nucleus (PVN) of the hypothalamus, with CRH and AVP subsequently stimulating the release of adrenocorticotropic hormone (ACTH) from the anterior pituitary. ACTH stimulates the release of GCs from the cortex of the adrenal gland, and GCs bind to glucocorticoid receptors (GRs) and ultimately regulate the transcription of genes that contain glucocorticoid-responsive regions. GCs exert negative feedback inhibition in the pituitary, hypothalamus, and hippocampus, mediated by the density of GRs in these brain regions.

Although the physiological role of the HPA axis described here promotes survival in a threatening situation, prolonged activation of the HPA axis through chronic stress is considered maladaptive and is typically associated with pathological outcomes.

Clinical studies demonstrate that the HPA axis is strongly affected by stressful experiences during development and that the quality of mother–infant interactions is an important factor in determining cortisol reactivity, not only during development but also in later life. For example, children with disorganized attachment show increased cortisol reactivity in response to a stressful situation in the laboratory, whereas children who are characterized as having organized attachment do not show increases in cortisol to the same stress challenge (Bernard & Dozier, 2010). Women who have reported childhood physical abuse have a blunted cortisol response following the Trier Social Stress Test (Carpenter, Shattuck, Tyrka, Geracioti, & Price, 2011), and changes in diurnal cortisol patterns have been associated with early life adversity (Gonzalez, Jenkins, Steiner, & Fleming, 2009; Tarullo & Gunnar, 2006). Furthermore, many studies on HPA axis function in children and adults with a history of abuse and neglect support the idea that dysregulation of the HPA axis is an important etiological link between childhood maltreatment and the later onset of stress-related psychiatric disorders (Bremner, Elzinga, Schmahl, & Vermetten, 2008; Heim, Shugart, Craighead, & Nemeroff, 2010; Teicher, 2010).

Brain Imaging Studies

Alterations in brain structures central to cognitive and emotional processes are common outcomes in brain imaging studies of children reared in stressful environments. Smaller orbitofrontal cortex volumes have been found in children who have suffered physical abuse, and these structural alterations are correlated with disruptions in parent–child relationships and difficulties in academic performance within the classroom (Hanson et al., 2010). Children who have been institutionalized have heightened amygdala activity that corresponds to aberrant social behavior (Tottenham et al., 2010). Furthermore, children and teens with a history of caregiver deprivation and emotional neglect have been shown to have heightened activity in both the amygdala and the hippocampus when processing threatening information in a face-viewing paradigm (Maheu et al., 2010). The enduring and negative effects of early adversity on the brain and emotional functioning are also evident from imaging studies performed on adults who report experiences of childhood maltreatment. Childhood emotional maltreatment has been associated with a smaller medial prefrontal cortex (van Harmelen et al., 2010), and alterations in volume and activation in response to threat cues have been found in regions including the amygdala, the hippocampus, the locus coeruleus, and the cerebellum (Bremner et al., 2008; De Bellis, 2005; McCrory, De Brito, & Viding, 2010; Teicher et al., 2003).

Animal Model Neuroendocrine Studies

Consistent with the human clinical data, animal models of deprivation and variations of maternal care demonstrate lasting changes in stress physiology/neurobiology. Maternal stimulation in infant rats is responsible for what is referred to as a stress hyporesponsive period during the first two weeks of life, and indeed, the separation of infant rats from their mothers during this period significantly elevates GCs and heightens responsiveness to subsequent stressors (Gunnar & Quevedo, 2007; Levine, 2000). Adult offspring that experienced low levels of maternal care (licking and grooming [LG]) during the postnatal period were found to have increases in ACTH and corticosterone following a stressor, reduced levels of hippocampal GRs, and increased CRH receptors in the locus coeruleus (Caldji et al., 1998; Liu et al., 1997). These environmentally induced changes in stress neurobiology are not unique to rodents, and there is evidence of similar changes in nonhuman primates. For example, maternal separation in macaques has been shown to both increase cortisol reactivity to a stress challenge and significantly blunt the diurnal rhythmic secretion of cortisol, and increased brain levels of CRH have been associated with neglectful caregiving (Sanchez, Ladd, & Plotsky, 2001; Sánchez et al., 2005). These studies provide support for the validity of using animal models to explore the biological implications of adversity that are relevant to humans.

Epigenetics: Linking Experience to Long-Term Neurobiological Changes

The parallels established in animal and human studies of the neurobiological impact of early life adversity provide a critical tool for further examining the underlying molecular basis of the effects on the brain. In studies of laboratory rodents, in which brain tissue can be analyzed at a cellular and molecular level, it is evident that early life experiences can induce long-term changes in the activity of genes. For example, low levels of maternal care experienced during infancy are associated with decreased transcription of GRs in the adult hippocampus, leading to reduced levels of GRs and an impaired capacity to down-regulate the HPA response to stressors. The stable modification of gene expression appears to be a common feature of many developmental exposures and is also observed in humans associated with childhood experiences (Champagne, 2010; McGowan et al., 2009). Thus, in order to understand the origins of the stress physiology/ neurobiological outcomes associated with adversity, it might be necessary to better understand the mechanisms through which genes can be dynamically yet stably altered in their expression.

Histone Modifications and DNA Methylation

Gene expression is dependent on the accessibility of the DNA and its regulatory regions to transcription factors and RNA polymerase. There are multiple mechanisms through which this accessibility can be altered, including posttranslational modifications to histone proteins and DNA methylation (Fig. 2.1) (Peterson & Laniel, 2004; Razin, 1998). Within the cell nucleus, DNA is wrapped around a cluster of histone proteins (H2A, H2B, H3, and H4). Within the structure of the histones are N-terminal "histone tails," which can be modified through chemical processes such as acetylation, ubiquitination, and methylation. These modifications change the nature of the interaction between the histones and DNA, with implications for the accessibility of the DNA. For example, the acetylation (the addition of an acetyl group) of histone tails is typically associated with increased accessibility of DNA and elevated gene expression (Fig. 2.1[b]), whereas removal of the acetyl group through histone deacetylation (involving histone deacetylases [HDACs]) is typically associated with decreased accessibility of DNA and reduced gene expression (Fig. 2.1[c]). DNA methylation is a covalent modification to the DNA molecule whereby a methyl group is added to cytosine nucleotides within the gene sequence, typically at cytosine-guanine sites. DNA methyltransferases (DNMT1 and DNMT3a/b) mediate this chemical modification, which also attracts protein complexes, including methyl binding proteins that cluster around the DNA and can modify the structure of the histone proteins (Fan & Hutnick, 2005; Feng, Fouse, & Fan, 2007; Turner, 2001). DNA methylation is typically associated with decreased transcriptional activity and has the capacity to induce the long-term silencing of gene expression (Fig. 2.1[c]).

Epigenetics and Development

Molecular processes such as histone modifications and DNA methylation are considered "epigenetic" mechanisms of gene regulation. "Epigenetics" refers to those mechanisms that alter the expression of DNA without altering the underlying DNA sequence. The temporal control of gene expression/silencing is an important feature of development, and epigenetic mechanisms play an essential role in this process. In particular, DNA methylation has a critical role in stably maintaining cell-specific gene expression patterns during cellular differentiation, and these epigenetic marks are transmitted to daughter cells during the process of mitosis (Fukuda & Taga, 2005; Jones & Taylor, 1980). Without this epigenetic modification, development would not proceed beyond the early

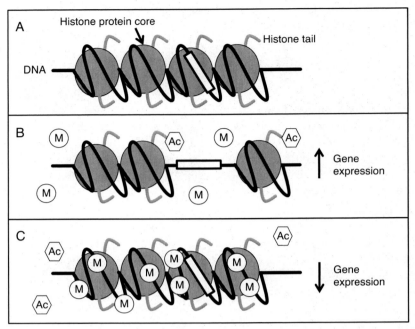

Figure 2.1 Schematic illustrating the epigenetic regulation of gene expression. (A) Within the cell nucleus, DNA (black line) is coiled around a core of histone proteins (grey circles). Part of the structure of these proteins includes a histone tail that dynamically interacts with DNA. Within the sequence of DNA, there are regions that are critical for the regulation of gene activity, such as gene promoter regions (white rectangle). Access to the DNA and, in particular, the promoter is a critical step in initiating transcription (expression) of the gene. (B) When DNA is unmethylated and histone tails are acetylated (Ac), there is increased accessibility to the DNA and the gene promoter region, typically leading to increased gene expression. (C) When DNA is methylated (M) and histones are deacetylated, gene expression is typically reduced.

fetal/postnatal stages. The divergence in cellular phenotype that can be achieved through epigenetic pathways has lead to increasing speculation that divergence in the phenotype of an individual (e.g., neurodevelopment, disease risk, behavior) can likewise be achieved though mechanisms such as DNA methylation. In monozygotic twins, there is emerging evidence for discordance in DNA methylation patterns, and it would appear that this discordance increases over time (Fraga et al., 2005; Mill et al., 2006; Wong et al., 2010). The critical questions raised by these findings are whether epigenetic modifications can be shaped by particular environmental experiences and whether these effects can contribute to our understanding of the long-term impact of these experiences.

Epigenetic Consequences of Prenatal Adversity

The prenatal period of development is a time of heightened susceptibility to environmental adversity. Thus, fetal exposure to undernutrition and stress (in addition to a variety of toxins) has been demonstrated to alter neurodevelopment, with consequences for later life psychopathology. Moreover, there is increasing evidence that epigenetic variation is induced by these developmental exposures.

Maternal Nutrition during Gestation

The quality of the maternal nutritional environment during pregnancy can have a significant impact on the growth and development of the fetus, with long-term consequences for brain development and metabolism (Godfrey & Barker, 2001; Symonds, Stephenson, Gardner, & Budge, 2007; Zeisel, 2009). Laboratory studies in rodents indicate that prenatal protein restriction or folic acid/choline deficiency experienced throughout gestation leads to elevated hepatic GR and peroxisomal proliferator-activated receptor gene expression associated with decreased DNA methylation of these genes (Lillycrop, Phillips, Jackson, Hanson, & Burdge, 2005; Lillycrop et al., 2008). Moreover, these epigenetic effects are not observed when gestational protein restriction is accompanied by folic acid supplementation (Lillycrop et al., 2005). Folic acid supplementation during pregnancy has long been established as a strategy for reducing the risk of neural tube defects, and within epigenetic pathways folic acid serves as a "methyl donor," contributing to the production of methyl groups needed to promote DNA methylation. Dietary effects on levels of the DNA methyltransferase DNMT1 might also account for modifications in global and gene-specific methylation, as DNMT1 expression is increased in hepatic (Lillycrop et al., 2007) and brain tissue (Kovacheva et al., 2007) as a function of protein/choline restriction. These epigenetic effects have likewise been observed in epidemiological studies of human cohorts exposed prenatally to dietary restriction. Analysis of blood samples from famine-exposed versus nonexposed siblings indicates that there is decreased DNA methylation of the insulin-like growth factor II gene as a consequence of maternal periconceptual exposure to famine (Heijmans et al., 2008).

Maternal Stress

The long-term consequences of prenatal stress for brain and behavior have been explored in many species. Recent evidence derived from studies of laboratory mice suggests that altered gene expression and DNA methylation within the placenta and hypothalamus might be possible mediators of these maternal effects. In mice, chronic variable stress during the first trimester is associated with decreased DNA methylation of the CRH gene promoter and increased methylation of the GR exon 17 promoter region in the hypothalamic tissue of adult male offspring (Mueller & Bale, 2008). Gestational stress within these experiments was found to exert sex-specific effects on the expression of DNMT1 in the placenta, which might induce disruption of the epigenetic status of genes within this critical interface between mother and fetus. Maternal antenatal depression in humans, which is associated with an increased risk of psychopathology in offspring, has also been linked to variation in DNA methylation. Analysis of cord blood samples from newborn infants indicates elevated GR promoter DNA methylation levels associated with maternal depressed mood (Oberlander et al., 2008). Moreover, the level of methylation within the neonatal GR promoter predicts increased salivary cortisol levels of infants at three months of age. These data suggest that vulnerability to stress might have its origins in the epigenetic effects of prenatal adversity.

Maternal Influence on the Developing Brain

Though it is perhaps not surprising that extreme forms of adversity during the prenatal and postnatal periods would induce significant changes in offspring development, studies in humans, primates, and laboratory rodents suggest that variations in parental care within the normal range can likewise shift developmental trajectories. Studies of natural variations in postnatal maternal care in laboratory rats have provided a valuable model for exploring the long-term impact of early life experiences and the role of epigenetic modifications in the mediation of these effects (Champagne, 2010; Champagne, Francis, Mar, & Meaney, 2003; Meaney, 2001). The frequency of maternal LG experienced during the postnatal period by rat pups is associated with changes in numerous receptor pathways, with effects on hippocampal GRs being implicated in the high levels of HPA reactivity observed amongst offspring of low LG dams (Liu et al., 1997). Analysis of the GR promoter region suggests that low levels of LG are associated with increased methylation within the GR 17 promoter, decreased GR expression, and an increased HPA response to stress (Weaver et al., 2004). Time course analysis has indicated that these maternally induced epigenetic profiles emerge during the early postnatal period and are sustained into adulthood. Maternal LG also affects gamma-aminobutyric acid (GABA) circuits and receptor subunit composition (Caldji, Diorio, & Meaney, 2003; Caldji, Francis, Sharma, Plotsky, & Meaney, 2000), and in a recent study, reduced hippocampal levels of glutamic acid decarboxylase (GAD1), the rate-limiting enzyme in GABA synthesis, were found in the male offspring of low LG dams associated with increased DNA methylation within the GAD1 promoter (Zhang et al., 2010).

Amongst female offspring, the experience of low levels of LG during the postnatal period is associated with decreased transcription of estrogen receptor alpha (ERα) in the medial preoptic area of the hypothalamus (MPOA) and elevated DNA methylation within the promoter region of this gene (Champagne et al., 2006). Importantly, cross-fostering studies suggest that these epigenetic effects on gene expression are associated with the quality of the care received in infancy rather than prenatal or genetic factors. Though these studies incorporate a candidate gene approach, taken together, it is evident that maternal epigenetic effects can lead to changes in the transcriptional activity of multiple genes within a broad range of brain regions that are established in development and produce long-term variation in gene expression and behavior.

Epigenetic Effects of Early Life Neglect and Abuse

The development of animal models of maternal neglect/separation and abuse has contributed to our understanding of the neurodevelopmental impact of adversity and the long-term biobehavioral outcomes associated with these experiences. More recently, these models have provided an essential tool for studying the epigenetic mechanisms that contribute to these outcomes.

Maternal Separation Studies

Infant separation from the primary caregiver produces long-lasting changes in neuroendocrine regulation, stress responsivity, and behavior. It has been suggested that phenotypic changes resulting from infant separation could reflect epigenetic processes, and there is now evidence in a mouse model of infant separation establishing a link between behavioral outcomes and alterations in the DNA methylation of a key gene involved in the stress regulatory pathway (Murgatroyd et al., 2009). Consistent with previous studies, mouse pups that had been separated from the mother during infancy were found to have increased corticosterone secretion during basal conditions and in response to stress, involution of the thymus, hypertrophy of the adrenals, and an attenuated memory capacity. Biochemical assessment in these mice revealed lower levels of DNA methylation within the AVP gene in the PVN relative to mice that had not been separated as infants. It was also found that hypomethylation of AVP DNA inversely correlated with AVP gene expression, and there were reduced levels of binding of MeCP2 (a methyl binding protein) at the AVP locus containing the unmethylated cytosines. Furthermore, in an additional series of experiments it was shown that the abnormal stress responses in these mice could be partially reversed by pharmacological antagonism of the AVP V1b receptor. Overall, results from this study indicate that infant separation activates neurons within the PVN involved in stress regulation, subsequently leading to stable changes in MeCP2 function and epigenetic reprogramming of the AVP gene and stress-related behavior.

Separation-induced phenotypic changes might also involve epigenetic alterations within the 5-HTT gene. As noted in preceding sections, genetic polymorphisms in the 5-HTT promoter have been shown to interact with stress: carriers of the short allele (which is predictive of less expression of 5-HTT) show increased stress responsivity and more emotional problems in relation to stressful life events, including childhood maltreatment (Aguilera et al., 2009; Caspi et al., 2003). In studies focusing on this same polymorphic region in rhesus macaques, infants who were carriers of the short allele were found to have increased DNA methylation of 5-HTT in peripheral blood mononuclear cells following maternal (and social) separation (Kinnally et al., 2010). This epigenetic change was found to be associated with a decrease in 5-HTT expression and behavioral hyper-reactivity amongst infants who had experienced this form of early life deprivation. Although there is no clear consensus on whether peripheral measures of DNA methylation accurately reflect central nervous system methylation, these data suggest that DNA methylation plays a role in the gene–environment interactions described between the 5-HTT genotype and life stress in predicting the risk of psychopathology.

Maternal Abuse Studies

In primates, infant abuse has been observed both in the lab and in field studies and is associated with increased stress responses and reduced levels of the serotonin metabolite 5-hydroxyindoleacetic acid in abused infants (Maestripieri, 1998; Maestripieri et al., 2006; Sanchez et al., 2010). In laboratory rats, an abuse model has been developed through reduction of the nesting materials provided to dams during the postnatal period. Chronic restriction of nesting material during the first 10 postnatal days has been shown to decrease the duration of dams' LG of pups; increase the frequency of periods during which mothers are away from their pups; and increase dams' stepping on pups, aggressive grooming, and transporting of pups by a limb (Brunson et al., 2005; Ivy, Brunson, Sandman, & Baram, 2008; Raineki, Moriceau, & Sullivan, 2010). This manipulation induces several biobehavioral changes in mothers indicative of heightened stress responsivity, including enlargement of the adrenals, elevated corticosterone levels, altered CRH mRNA levels in the PVN, and reduced exploration in a novel environment. Pups reared in these environments exhibit increased plasma corticosterone levels at basal and stress-evoked conditions, enlarged adrenals, increased amygdala activity, impaired spatial memory and deficits in long-term potentiation of neurons; indicative of reduced neuronal plasticity (Avishai-Eliner, Gilles, Eghbal-Ahmadi, Bar-El, & Baram, 2001; Brunson et al., 2005; Gilles, Schultz, & Baram, 1996; Raineki et al., 2010).

A variation of the limited nesting paradigm has been used to model caregiver maltreatment and to examine the neurobehavioral and epigenetic outcomes associated with exposure to a stressed and abusive caregiver (Roth, Lubin, Funk, & Sweatt, 2009). In order to assess the consequences of abuse, rat pups were given daily exposure to caregivers (nonbiological mothers) that were either in an unfamiliar environment with limited nesting resources (maltreatment condition) or a familiar environment with copious amounts of nesting material (cross-foster care condition). The combination of an unfamiliar environment and impoverished nesting resources was sufficient to induce caretakers to frequently display behaviors that elicited distress responses from pups and which are deemed abusive and potentially harmful in nonhuman primates and humans (Fig. 2.2[a]). In adulthood, offspring that had experienced an abusive caregiver/ adverse nest environment exhibited significantly less expression of the brain-derived neurotrophic factor (BDNF) gene in the prefrontal cortex, an effect that was consistent with DNA hypermethylation of the BDNF gene. Specifically, within an important regulatory region of the BDNF gene (exon IV, which contributes to activity-dependent gene transcription), it was shown that normal adults (i.e., adults with a history of nonabusive infancy or cross-foster care) had either no or very little cytosine methylation. This was in sharp contrast to the

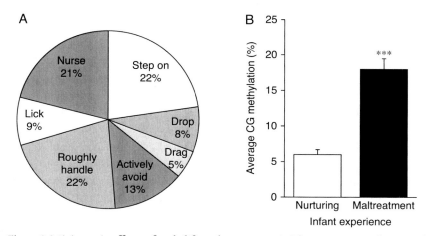

Figure 2.2 Epigenetic effects of early life maltreatment. (A) The assessment of maternal behaviors in a rodent model in which foster dams are placed in a cage with limited bedding material indicates that infants experienced an adverse caregiving environment that was characterized mainly by abusive behaviors. (B) Three months following maltreatment, rats were found to have significant methylation of the BDNF gene (exon IV DNA) in the prefrontal cortex associated with the experience of maltreatment. Figure adapted from Roth et al. (2009). ***p < 0.001.

adults who had experienced maltreatment during infancy, for which sequencing of the BDNF regulatory region revealed that the same cytosine-guanine dinucleotides were all highly methylated (Fig. 2.2[b]). BDNF is known to play a critical modulatory role in the establishment of neuronal connectivity, and the suppression of BDNF expression has been linked to anxiety and depressive-like symptoms. Thus, the adversity-induced effects on BDNF observed in these studies suggest a biological mechanism linking early life stress and later life risk of psychiatric dysfunction.

Stress in Adulthood: Epigenetics and Risk of PTSD

Epidemiological studies suggest that both genetic and environmental factors underlie the development of stress-related psychiatric disorders such as PTSD. Chronic stress paradigms in adult rodents such as predator odor exposure and social defeat are recognized for their ability to produce behavioral and neuroendocrine patterns analogous to symptoms associated with PTSD in humans. The assessment of molecular modifications in these animal models is beginning to highlight the fact that epigenetic changes are a candidate mechanism through which traumatic experiences can moderate the effects of genes and render an individual susceptible to stress-related disorders.

Chronic Stress

Converging evidence from clinical and basic research indicates that neurotrophic factors (such as BDNF) are vulnerable to the effects of traumatic stress. Animal models of chronic stress (such as predator exposure, restraint, and social isolation) have indicated that stress-induced changes in hippocampal function and structure, as well as PTSD-like behavioral stress responses, are typically associated with decreased BDNF activity, including down-regulation of BDNF mRNA and protein levels in the CA1 subregion of the hippocampus (Bazak et al., 2009; Kozlovsky et al., 2007; Lippmann, Bress, Nemeroff, Plotsky, & Monteggia, 2007; Nair et al., 2007; Nibuya, Takahashi, Russell, & Duman, 1999; Rasmusson, Shi, & Duman, 2002; Tsankova et al., 2006). In a recent study, evidence emerged for stress-induced changes in BDNF DNA methylation in a psychosocial stress model of PTSD (Roth, Zoladz, Sweatt, & Diamond, 2011). In order to model PTSD, rats were immobilized (to provide a sense of lack of control) while they were exposed to a cat (a predator stimulus that elicits intense fear and perturbs hippocampal and amygdaloid activity). Rats were also given a second inescapable cat exposure episode 10 days after the first, to provide them with a reminder of their traumatic experience (to model the reexperiencing reported by PTSD patients). Finally, the housing conditions of rats were continually disturbed and randomized over the entire psychosocial stress period (modeling a lack of social support, which has been shown to contribute to PTSD). This stress regimen has been shown to produce physiological and behavioral outcomes in rats that are remarkably similar to those seen in PTSD patients, including increased cardio-vascular and corticosteroid reactivity, increased anxiety, exaggerated startle response, and lasting cognitive impairments (Diamond & Zoladz, 2010; Zoladz, Conrad, Fleshner, & Diamond, 2008). Exposure to trauma/psychosocial stress in this rodent model was found to induce epigenetic effects within the BDNF gene. Several weeks after the second cat exposure, robust hypermethylation of the BDNF gene within the dorsal CA1 region of the hippocampus was detected in stressed rats but not in nonstress controls (Fig. 2.3[a]). Elevated DNA methylation was also detected in the dorsal dentate gyrus of stressed rats, and lower levels were detected in the ventral CA3 subregion. Moreover, within the CA1 hippocampal region, the stress-associated DNA hypermethylation was associated with significantly reduced BDNF gene expression (Fig. 2.3[b]). These data support the notion that increased DNA methylation is one mechanism by which transcriptional suppression of the BDNF gene is induced following exposure to psychosocial stress.

Epigenetic modifications of the glial cell-derived neurotropic factor (GDNF) gene have also been linked to behavioral responses to chronic stress (Uchida et al., 2011). Exposure of mice to six weeks of chronic ultramild stress (random-ized stressors included confinement to a small cage, odor exposure, constant

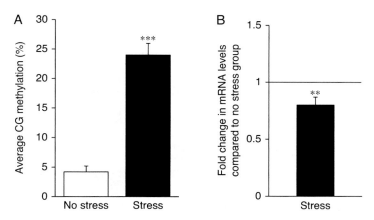

Figure 2.3 Epigenetic effects in a rodent model of PTSD. (A) Rats experiencing a psycho-social stress regimen showed significant increases in BDNF DNA methylation (exon IV) in the dorsal CA1 region of the hippocampus. (B) Consistent with elevated methylation in dorsal CA1, stressed rats had decreased levels of BDNF mRNA (exon IV transcripts). Figure adapted from Roth et al. (2011). **$p < 0.01$. ***$p < 0.001$.

light, and wet bedding) was found to produce significant behavioral effects that were dependent on genotype and the type of epigenetic marks present at the GDNF gene promoter. Specifically, inbred BALB/c mice were found to be more susceptible to the chronic stress regimen and exhibited a depressive-like phenotype in response to stress. In contrast, C57BL/6 (B6) mice exhibited a more adaptive response to the stress regimen. Amongst BALB/c mice, mRNA levels of GDNF in the nucleus accumbens were significantly decreased, whereas GDNF mRNA levels in B6 mice were increased. Histone modifications were found to be associated with these stress-induced effects on gene expression. For example, in stressed BALB/c mice there were reduced levels of histone acetylation and increased expression of the histone deacetylase enzyme HDAC2. Moreover, chronic stress was found to induce hypermethylation of the GDNF promoter and increase MeCP2-HDAC2 binding at the GDNF promoter in stressed BALB/c mice. Histone modifications and DNA methylation of the GDNF promoter thus appear to have crucial roles in behavioral responses to chronic stress.

Social Defeat Stress

Chronic social defeat in mice is commonly used to study the genetic and epigenetic precursors of stress-related psychiatric disorders, particularly depression. In this paradigm, mice are subjected to repeated aggressive encounters with a conspecific, which results in increased avoidance of social contact. This behavioral phenotype can be reversed by chronic treatment with an antidepressant (Tsankova et al., 2006). Amongst defeated mice, there is significant down-regulation in BDNF mRNA levels in the hippocampus, which is correlated with increased levels of the repressive histone mark H3-K9 dimethylation. Chronic imipramine treatment of defeated mice was found to rescue behavior (reducing social avoidance) and increase histone modifications that were consistent with transcriptional activation (acetylation of H3 and dimethylation of H3-K4). Further analysis has indicated that down-regulation of the histone deactylase enzyme HDAC5 in the hippocampus might be a critical mechanism of this antidepressant effect.

Genes regulating the HPA axis are particularly relevant in studies of chronic stress and have been explored within animal models examining the epigenetic consequences of stress and trauma. Using the chronic social defeat paradigm, a recent study has established a link between stress-induced epigenetic marks within the CRF gene in the PVN and subsequent social avoidance behavior (Elliott, Ezra-Nevo, Regev, Neufeld-Cohen, & Chen, 2010). As previously noted, in response to social defeat, some mice are observed to display social avoidance and are thus considered stress susceptible. However, a percentage of mice are unaffected by social defeat (deemed resilient mice). Characterizations of gene expression and DNA methylation patterns of the CRF gene have revealed significant differences between defeated/stress-susceptible and stress-resilient mice. Stress-susceptible mice were found to have increased levels of CRF mRNA in the PVN that corresponded to decreased DNA methylation of the CRF gene. Amongst stressed/defeated mice, there were also decreased levels of DNMT3b and HDAC2. Strikingly, resilient mice did not show changes in mRNA or DNA methylation of the CRF gene. Furthermore, knocking down CRF levels via siRNA attenuated social avoidance in the defeated mice. Overall, these data suggest that differential epigenetic marks, along with genetic factors, might influence either the susceptibility or the resilience of an organism to chronic stressful experiences. These studies are providing important insight into the complex gene-by-environment interactions that are likely responsible for the etiology of stress-related disorders.

Transmission of Adversity: Novel Perspectives on the Inheritance of Risk

The effects of stress are not always confined to the generation experiencing the stress; they can also be observed to alter behavior in subsequent generations. Transgenerational continuity in the effects of stress has traditionally been viewed from a genetic perspective, in which there is an inheritance of genetic polymorphisms that confer susceptibility to stress. However, more recently, the provocative idea of epigenetically determined heritable phenotypes is stimulating much interest and debate. Though our understanding of the mechanisms underlying the transmission of adversity is limited, emerging evidence suggests that epigenetics could provide a biological explanation for the generational persistence of stress-induced phenotypes.

Maternal Behavior and ERα

Natural variations in postnatal maternal LG in rats have a significant impact on the development of infant stress responses (Liu et al., 1997). This form of maternal care is also critical for shaping the maternal brain of female offspring. Females reared by low LG dams have a reduced sensitivity to estrogen-mediated increases in neuronal activation within the MPOA (Champagne, Diorio, Sharma, & Meaney, 2001; Champagne, Weaver, Diorio, Sharma, & Meaney, 2003), and analysis of the levels of ERα in the offspring of high and low LG dams suggests that differences in estrogen sensitivity are mediated by variations in ERα levels. Gene expression of ERα in the MPOA of female offspring of low LG dams is found to be significantly reduced (Champagne, Weaver, et al., 2003). Analysis of levels of DNA methylation within the 1B promoter region of the ERα gene in

MPOA tissue indicates that the experience of high LG is associated with decreased promoter methylation, whereas low LG is associated with increased promoter methylation, leading to reduced gene expression and an attenuated response to hormonally primed behaviors (Champagne et al., 2006). As a consequence of these epigenetic modifications, individual differences in maternal LG are transmitted from mother to offspring (F1 generation) and to grand-offspring (F2 generation) (Champagne, 2008; F.A. Champagne & Meaney, 2007). This transmission of maternal behavior is an experience-dependent inheritance mediated by maternal care itself. The transgenerational continuity in maternal behavior, which is apparent in humans and primates, might be a route through which stress-induced effects are maintained across generations.

Abuse and BDNF

Female rats with a history of maltreatment (using the limited nesting material paradigm described previously) have been found to display increased levels of abusive behaviors toward their own offspring (Roth et al., 2009). Eight-day-old offspring (both males and females) derived from maltreated females are found to have significantly elevated DNA methylation of the BDNF gene in the prefrontal cortex and hippocampus in comparison to offspring derived from normal-treated females (Fig. 2.4[a]). The obvious question raised by these findings is whether the transgenerational epigenetic inheritance was due to the mother's abusive caregiving behaviors. Cross-fostering studies were used to address this issue and revealed that postnatal cross-fostering did not completely reverse the patterns of DNA methylation in second-generation offspring, nor did it induce significant effects on methylation (Fig. 2.4[b]). These data suggest that the perpetuation of maltreatment-induced DNA methylation patterns was not simply a product of the postnatal experience, but likely reflected some prenatal component. These results could reflect a prenatal stress effect (maltreated females in this study were shown to have increased anxiety-like behaviors during the prepartum period), but they could also reflect germ-line epigenetic transmission.

Inheritance of Early Life Stress

A recent study investigated the possibility of germ-line inheritance of stress-induced effects; the DNA methylation profiles of several stress-related and behaviorally relevant genes were examined across multiple generations (Franklin et al., 2010). To create stressful early life conditions for the first generation of infants, dams and litters were subjected to unpredictable separation for three hours daily during the first two postnatal weeks. During separation, mothers were also stressed by a forced swim in cold water and restraint stress, both of which were shown to alter maternal behavior significantly upon reunion.

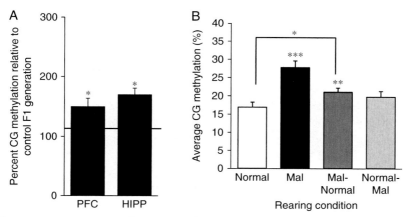

Figure 2.4 Transgenerational epigenetic effects. (A) Offspring of females that had experienced maltreatment had significantly higher levels of methylated BDNF DNA in the prefrontal cortex (PFC) and hippocampus (HIPP) than offspring from females that had a normal infancy. (B) Cross-fostering of these offspring (offspring born to maltreated dams cross-fostered at birth to normal dams [Mal-Normal]) failed to completely rescue central nervous system DNA methylation and did not induce significant changes in DNA methylation in offspring born to normal dams that were fostered to maltreated dams (Normal-Mal). Figure adapted from Roth et al. (2009). *p < 0.05. **p < 0.01. ***p < 0.001.

Offspring were later subjected to behavioral testing. To produce a second generation, first generation (F1) control and stressed males were mated with naïve female mice. To produce a third generation (F3), second-generation (F2) control and stressed males were mated with naïve females. Males were removed from the breeding cage such that they never had any contact with the offspring. The stress regimen was found to produce depressive-like behaviors in the male mice that experienced the early life stress regimen (F1 generation), and these effects persisted in F2 and F3 offspring that were raised normally with nonstressed and nurturing mothers. Strikingly, DNA methylation patterns that were present in the germ-line (sperm) and brains of the male mice that had experienced the early life stress (i.e., the fathers) were also found to be present in the brains of the F2 generation. These patterns included hypermethylation of the MeCP2 gene and hypomethylation of the corticotrophin-releasing factor receptor 2 gene. Methylation changes were consistent with altered expression of these genes. By demonstrating that there were epigenetic changes in the germ-line, this study elegantly demonstrates a mechanism by which stress effects could be passed across generations independent of maternal care or other environmental factors.

Future Directions in the Study of Epigenetics and Adversity

The incorporation of an epigenetic perspective into studies of the long-term effects of adversity has generated novel approaches and methodologies. It is evident that both early life and adult exposure to adversity can shape the activity of genes, with implications for stress physiology, neurobiology, and behavior. These epigenetic effects might also have implications for the stress susceptibility and well-being of subsequent generations, perhaps providing a molecular mechanism with which to explain the transgenerational continuity of the effects of abuse and trauma. Though generally based in laboratory rodent models, there is increasing translation of this research to studies of human exposure to trauma. For example, analysis of postmortem human brain tissue suggests that individuals with a history of childhood abuse have increased DNA methylation within the GR promoter region and decreased hippocampal GR expression compared to nonabused subjects (McGowan et al., 2009). Moreover, there is increasing evidence of epigenetic variation in the brain and in peripheral blood cells that differentiates individuals with various forms of psychopathology, including PTSD (Mill & Petronis, 2007; Uddin et al., 2010). The challenge for these studies will be in the validation of the use of peripheral biomarkers in predicting epigenetic variation that is relevant to both the adverse exposure and the subsequent risk of susceptibility to psychiatric dysfunction. Though our understanding of the dynamics of epigenetic mechanisms is still evolving, continued exploration of epigenetic pathways within the context of these studies will likely continue to be an innovative and informative strategy for understanding the biology of risk and resilience.

Disclosure Statement

This research was supported by Grant No. DP2OD001674 from the Office of the Director, National Institutes of Health (F.A.C.), and by a University of Delaware Research Foundation Award (T.L.R.).

References

Aguilera, M., Arias, B., Wichers, M., Barrantes-Vidal, N., Moya, J., Villa, H., et al. (2009). Early adversity and 5-HTT/BDNF genes: New evidence of gene? Environment interactions on depressive symptoms in a general population. *Psychological Medicine, 39*(9), 1425–1432.

Avishai-Eliner, S., Gilles, E. E., Eghbal-Ahmadi, M., Bar-El, Y., & Baram, T. Z. (2001). Altered regulation of gene and protein expression of hypothalamic-pituitary-adrenal axis components in an immature rat model of chronic stress. *Journal of Neuroendocrinology, 13*(9), 799–807.

Bazak, N., Kozlovsky, N., Kaplan, Z., Matar, M., Golan, H., Zohar, J., et al. (2009). Prepubertal stress exposure affects adult behavioral response in association with changes in circulating corticosterone and brain-derived neurotrophic factor. *Psychoneuroendocrinology, 34*, 844–858.

Beckett, C., Maughan, B., Rutter, M., Castle, J., Colvert, E., Groothues, C., et al. (2006). Do the effects of early severe deprivation on cognition persist into early adolescence? Findings from the English and Romanian adoptees study. *Child Development, 77*(3), 696–711.

Bernard, K., & Dozier, M. (2010). Examining infants' cortisol responses to laboratory tasks among children varying in attachment disorganization: Stress reactivity or return to baseline? *Developmental Psychology, 46*(6), 1771–1778.

Bremner, J. D., Elzinga, B., Schmahl, C., & Vermetten, E. (2008). Structural and functional plasticity of the human brain in posttraumatic stress disorder., *Progress in Brain Research, 167*,171–186.

Brunson, K. L., Kramár, E., Lin, B., Chen, Y., Colgin, L. L., Yanagihara, T. K., et al. (2005). Mechanisms of late-onset cognitive decline after early-life stress. *The Journal of Neuroscience, 25*(41), 9328–9338.

Caldji, C., Diorio, J., & Meaney, M. J. (2003). Variations in maternal care alter GABA(A) receptor subunit expression in brain regions associated with fear. *Neuropsychopharmacology, 28*(11), 1950–1959.

Caldji, C., Francis, D., Sharma, S., Plotsky, P. M., & Meaney, M. J. (2000). The effects of early rearing environment on the development of GABAA and central benzodiazepine receptor levels and novelty-induced fearfulness in the rat. *Neuropsychopharmacology, 22*(3), 219–229.

Caldji, C., Tannenbaum, B., Sharma, S., Francis, D., Plotsky, P. M., & Meaney, M. J. (1998). Maternal care during infancy regulates the development of neural systems mediating the expression of fearfulness in the rat. *Proceedings of the National Academy of Sciences, 95*(9), 5335–5340.

Carlson, E. A. (1998). A prospective longitudinal study of attachment disorganization/disorientation. *Child Development, 69*(4), 1107–1128.

Carlson, E. A., Egeland, B., & Sroufe, L. A. (2009). A prospective investigation of the development of borderline personality symptoms. *Development Psychopathology, 21*(4), 1311–1334.

Carpenter, L., Shattuck, T., Tyrka, A., Geracioti, T., & Price, L. (2011). Effect of childhood physical abuse on cortisol stress response. *Psychopharmacology, 214*(1), 367–375.

Caspi, A., Sugden, K., Moffitt, T. E., Taylor, A., Craig, I. W., Harrington, H., et al. (2003). Influence of life stress on depression: Moderation by a polymorphism in the 5-HT gene. *Science, 301*, 386–400.

Champagne, F., Diorio, J., Sharma, S., & Meaney, M. J. (2001). Naturally occurring variations in maternal behavior in the rat are associated with differences in estrogen-inducible central oxytocin receptors. *Proceedings of the National Academy of Sciences of the United States of America, 98*(22), 12736–12741.

Champagne, F. A. (2008). Epigenetic mechanisms and the transgenerational effects of maternal care. *Frontiers in Neuroendocrinology, 29*(3), 386–397.

Champagne, F. A. (2010). Epigenetic influence of social experiences across the lifespan. *Developmental Psychobiology, 52*(4), 299–311.

Champagne, F. A., Francis, D. D., Mar, A., & Meaney, M. J. (2003). Variations in maternal care in the rat as a mediating influence for the effects of environment on development. *Physiology Behavior, 79*(3), 359–371.

Champagne, F. A., & Meaney, M. J. (2007). Transgenerational effects of social environment on variations in maternal care and behavioral response to novelty. *Behavioral Neuroscience, 121*(6), 1353–1363.

Champagne, F. A., Weaver, I. C., Diorio, J., Dymov, S., Szyf, M., & Meaney, M. J. (2006). Maternal care associated with methylation of the estrogen receptor-alpha1b promoter and estrogen receptor-alpha expression in the medial preoptic area of female offspring. *Endocrinology, 147*(6), 2909–2915.

Champagne, F. A., Weaver, I. C., Diorio, J., Sharma, S., & Meaney, M. J. (2003). Natural variations in maternal care are associated with estrogen receptor alpha expression and estrogen sensitivity in the medial preoptic area. *Endocrinology, 144*(11), 4720–4724.

De Bellis, M. D. (2005). The psychobiology of neglect. *Child Maltreatment, 10*(2), 150–172.

Diamond, D. M., & Zoladz, P. R. (2010). An animal model of PTSD which integrates inescapable predator exposure and social instability. *Culture Pschology Neurosciences, 15*, 6–7.

Elliott, E., Ezra-Nevo, G., Regev, L., Neufeld-Cohen, A., & Chen, A. (2010). Resilience to social stress coincides with functional DNA methylation of the Crf gene in adult mice. *Nature Neuroscience, 13*(11), 1351–1353.

Ellis, B. J., Boyce, W. T., Belsky, J., Bakermans-Kranenburg, M. J., & van Ijzendoorn, M. H. (2011). Differential susceptibility to the environment: An evolutionary–neurodevelopmental theory. *Development Psychopathology, 23*(1), 7–28.

Fan, G., & Hutnick, L. (2005). Methyl-CpG binding proteins in the nervous system. *Cell Research, 15*(4), 255–261.

Feng, J., Fouse, S., & Fan, G. (2007). Epigenetic regulation of neural gene expression and neuronal function. *Pediatric Research, 61*(5 Pt 2), 58R–63R.

Fraga, M. F., Ballestar, E., Paz, M. F., Ropero, S., Setien, F., Ballestar, M. L., et al. (2005). Epigenetic differences arise during the lifetime of monozygotic twins. *Proceedings of the National Academy of Sciences of the United States of America, 102*(30), 10604–10609.

Franklin, T. B., Russig, H., Weiss, I. C., Gräff, J., Linder, N., Michalon, A., et al. (2010). Epigenetic transmission of the impact of early stress across generations. *Biological Psychiatry, 68*(5), 408–415.

Fukuda, S., & Taga, T. (2005). Cell fate determination regulated by a transcriptional signal network in the developing mouse brain. *Anatomical Science International, 80*(1), 12–18.

Gilles, E. E., Schultz, L., & Baram, T. Z. (1996). Abnormal corticosterone regulation in an immature rat model of continuous chronic stress. *Pediatric Neurology, 15*, 114–119.

Godfrey, K. M., & Barker, D. J. (2001). Fetal programming and adult health. *Public Health Nutrition, 4*(2B), 611–624.

Gonzalez, A., Jenkins, J. M., Steiner, M., & Fleming, A. S. (2009). The relation between early life adversity, cortisol awakening response and diurnal salivary cortisol levels in postpartum women. *Psychoneuroendocrinology, 34*(1), 76–86.

Gunnar, M., & Quevedo, K. (2007). The neurobiology of stress and development. *Annual Review of Psychology, 58*(1), 145–173.

Hanson, J. L., Chung, M. K., Avants, B. B., Shirtcliff, E. A., Gee, J. C., Davidson, R. J., et al. (2010). Early stress is associated with alterations in the orbitofrontal cortex: A tensor-based morphometry investigation of brain structure and behavioral risk. *The Journal of Neuroscience, 30*(22), 7466–7472.

Heijmans, B. T., Tobi, E. W., Stein, A. D., Putter, H., Blauw, G. J., Susser, E. S., et al. (2008). Persistent epigenetic differences associated with prenatal exposure to famine in humans. *Proceedings of the National Academy of Sciences of the United States of America, 105*(44), 17046–17049.

Heim, C., Shugart, M., Craighead, W. E., & Nemeroff, C. B. (2010). Neurobiological and psychiatric consequences of child abuse and neglect. *Developmental Psychobiology, 52*(7), 671–690.

Ivy, A. S., Brunson, K. L., Sandman, C., & Baram, T. Z. (2008). Dysfunctional nurturing behavior in rat dams with limited access to nesting material: A clinically relevant model for early-life stress. *Neuroscience, 154,* 1132–1142.

Johnson, J. G., Cohen, P., Brown, J., Smailes, E. M., & Bernstein, D. P. (1999). Childhood maltreatment increases risk for personality disorders during early adulthood. *Archives of General Psychiatry, 56*(7), 600–606.

Jones, P. A., & Taylor, S. M. (1980). Cellular differentiation, cytidine analogs and DNA methylation. *Cell, 20*(1), 85–93.

Kessler, R. C., Sonnega, A., Bromet, E., Hughes, M., & Nelson, C. B. (1995). Posttraumatic stress disorder in the National Comorbidity Survey. *Archives of General Psychiatry, 52*(12), 1048–1060.

Kinnally, E. L., Capitanio, J. P., Leibel, R., Deng, L., LeDuc, C., Haghighi, F., et al. (2010). Epigenetic regulation of serotonin transporter expression and behavior in infant rhesus macaques. *Genes, Brain and Behavior, 9,* 575–582.

Kovacheva, V. P., Mellott, T. J., Davison, J. M., Wagner, N., Lopez-Coviella, I., Schnitzler, A. C., et al. (2007). Gestational choline deficiency causes global- and Igf2 gene-DNA hypermethylation by upregulation of Dnmt1 expression. *Journal of Biological Chemistry, 282*(43), 31777–31788.

Kozlovsky, N., Matar, M. A., Kaplan, Z., Kotler, M., Zohar, J., & Cohen, H. (2007). Long-term down-regulation of BDNF mRNA in rat hippocampal CA1 subregion correlates with PTSD-like behavioural stress response. *The International Journal of Neuropsychopharmacology, 10,* 741–758.

Levine, S. (2000). Influence of psychological variables on the activity of the hypothalamic-pituitary-adrenal axis. *European Journal of Pharmacology, 405*(1–3), 149–160.

Lillycrop, K. A., Phillips, E. S., Jackson, A. A., Hanson, M. A., & Burdge, G. C. (2005). Dietary protein restriction of pregnant rats induces and folic acid supplementation prevents epigenetic modification of hepatic gene expression in the offspring. *Journal of Nutrition, 135*(6), 1382–1386.

Lillycrop, K. A., Phillips, E. S., Torrens, C., Hanson, M. A., Jackson, A. A., & Burdge, G. C. (2008). Feeding pregnant rats a protein-restricted diet persistently alters the methylation of specific cytosines in the hepatic PPAR alpha promoter of the offspring. *British Journal of Nutrition, 100*(2), 278–282.

Lillycrop, K. A., Slater-Jefferies, J. L., Hanson, M. A., Godfrey, K. M., Jackson, A. A., & Burdge, G. C. (2007). Induction of altered epigenetic regulation of the hepatic glucocorticoid receptor in the offspring of rats fed a protein-restricted diet during pregnancy suggests that reduced DNA methyltransferase-1 expression is involved in impaired DNA methylation and changes in histone modifications. *British Jounal of Nutrition, 97*(6), 1064–1073.

Lippmann, M., Bress, A., Nemeroff, C. B., Plotsky, P. M., & Monteggia, L. M. (2007). Long-term behavioural and molecular alterations associated with maternal separation in rats. *European Journal of Neuroscience, 25,* 3091–3098.

Liu, D., Diorio, J., Tannenbaum, B., Caldji, C., Francis, D., Freedman, A., et al. (1997). Maternal care, hippocampal glucocorticoid receptors, and hypothalamic-pituitary-adrenal responses to stress. *Science, 277*(5332), 1659–1662.

MacLean, K. (2003). The impact of institutionalization on child development. *Development and Psychopathology, 15*(4), 853–884.

Maestripieri, D. (1998). Parenting styles of abusive mothers in group-living rhesus macaques. *Animal Behavior, 55*(1), 1–11.

Maestripieri, D., Higley, J. D., Lindell, S. G., Newman, T. K., McCormack, K. M., & Sanchez, M. M. (2006). Early maternal rejection affects the development of monoaminergic systems and adult abusive parenting in rhesus macaques (Macaca mulatta). *Behavioral Neuroscience, 120*(5), 1017–1024.

Maheu, F., Dozier, M., Guyer, A., Mandell, D., Peloso, E., Poeth, K., et al. (2010). A preliminary study of medial temporal lobe function in youths with a history of caregiver deprivation and emotional neglect. *Cognitive, Affective, and Behavioral Neuroscience, 10,* 34–49.

McCrory, E., De Brito, S. A., & Viding, E. (2010). Research review: The neurobiology and genetics of maltreatment and adversity. *Journal of Child Psychology and Psychiatry, 51*(10), 1079–1095.

McGowan, P. O., Sasaki, A., D'Alessio, A. C., Dymov, S., Labonte, B., Szyf, M., et al. (2009). Epigenetic regulation of the glucocorticoid receptor in human brain associates with childhood abuse. *Nature Neuroscience, 12*(3), 342–348.

McLaughlin, K. A., Conron, K. J., Koenen, K. C., & Gilman, S. E. (2010). Childhood adversity, adult stressful life events, and risk of past-year psychiatric disorder: A test of the stress sensitization hypothesis in a population-based sample of adults. *Psychological Medicine, 40*(10), 1647–1658.

Meaney, M. J. (2001). Maternal care, gene expression, and the transmission of individual differences in stress reactivity across generations. *Annual Review of Neuroscience, 24,* 1161–1192.

Mill, J., Dempster, E., Caspi, A., Williams, B., Moffitt, T., & Craig, I. (2006). Evidence for monozygotic twin (MZ) discordance in methylation level at two CpG sites in the promoter region of the catechol-O-methyltransferase (COMT) gene. *American Journal of Medical Genetics Part B: Neuropsychiatric Genetics, 141B*(4), 421–425.

Mill, J., & Petronis, A. (2007). Molecular studies of major depressive disorder: The epigenetic perspective. *Molecular Psychiatry, 12*(9), 799–814.

Mueller, B. R., & Bale, T. L. (2008). Sex-specific programming of offspring emotionality after stress early in pregnancy. *The Journal of Neuroscience, 28*(36), 9055–9065.

Murgatroyd, C., Patchev, A. V., Wu, Y., Micale, V., Bockmuhl, Y., Fischer, D., et al. (2009). Dynamic DNA methylation programs persistent adverse effects of early-life stress. *Nature Neuroscience, 12*(12), 1559–1566.

Nair, A., Vadodaria, K. C., Banerjee, S. B., Benekareddy, M., Dias, B. G., Duman, R. S., et al. (2007). Stressor-specific regulation of distinct brain-derived neurotrophic factor transcripts and cyclic AMP response element-binding protein expression in the postnatal and adult rat hippocampus. *Neuropsychopharmacology, 32,* 1504–1519.

Nibuya, M., Takahashi, M., Russell, D. S., & Duman, R. S. (1999). Repeated stress increases catalytic TrkB mRNA in rat hippocampus. *Neuroscience Letters, 267,* 81–84.

Oberlander, T. F., Weinberg, J., Papsdorf, M., Grunau, R., Misri, S., & Devlin, A. M. (2008). Prenatal exposure to maternal depression, neonatal methylation of human glucocorticoid receptor gene (NR3C1) and infant cortisol stress responses. *Epigenetics, 3*(2), 97–106.

O'Connor, T. G., & Rutter, M. (2000). Attachment disorder behavior following early severe deprivation: Extension and longitudinal follow-up. English and Romanian Adoptees Study Team. *Journal of the American Academy of Child Adolescent Psychiatry, 39*(6), 703–712.

O'Connor, T. G., Rutter, M., Beckett, C., Keaveney, L., & Kreppner, J. M. (2000). The effects of global severe privation on cognitive competence: Extension and longitudinal follow-up. English and Romanian Adoptees Study Team. *Child Development, 71*(2), 376–390.

Peterson, C. L., & Laniel, M. A. (2004). Histones and histone modifications. *Current Biology, 14*(14), R546–551.

Pruessner, J. C., Dedovic, K., Pruessner, M., Lord, C., Buss, C., Collins, L., et al. (2010). Stress regulation in the central nervous system: Evidence from structural and functional neuroimaging studies in human populations—2008 Curt Richter Award Winner. *Psychoneuroendocrinology, 35*(1), 179–191.

Raineki, C., Moriceau, S., & Sullivan, R. M. (2010). Developing a neurobehavioral animal model of infant attachment to an abusive caregiver. *Biological Psychiatry, 67*(12), 1137–1145.

Rasmusson, A. M., Shi, L., & Duman, R. (2002). Downregulation of BDNF mRNA in the hippocampal dentate gyrus after re-exposure to cues previously associated with footshock. *Neuropsychopharmacology, 27*, 133–142.

Razin, A. (1998). CpG methylation, chromatin structure and gene silencing—a three-way connection. *The EMBO Journal, 17*(17), 4905–4908.

Roth, T. L., Lubin, F. D., Funk, A. J., & Sweatt, J. D. (2009). Lasting epigenetic influence of early-life adversity on the BDNF gene. *Biological Psychiatry, 65*(9), 760–769.

Roth, T. L., Zoladz, P. R., Sweatt, J. D., & Diamond, D. M. (2011). Epigenetic modification of hippocampal Bdnf DNA in adult rats in an animal model of post-traumatic stress disorder. *Journal of Psychiatric Research, 45*, 919–926.

Rutter, M., & O'Connor, T. G. (2004). Are there biological programming effects for psychological development? Findings from a study of Romanian adoptees. *Developmental Psychopathology, 40*(1), 81–94.

Sanchez, M. M., Ladd, C. O., & Plotsky, P. M. (2001). Early adverse experience as a developmental risk factor for later psychopathology: Evidence from rodent and primate models. *Development and Psychopathology, 13*, 419–449.

Sanchez, M. M., McCormack, K., Grand, A. P., Fulks, R., Graff, A., & Maestripieri, D. (2010). Effects of sex and early maternal abuse on adrenocorticotropin hormone and cortisol responses to the corticotropin-releasing hormone challenge during the first 3 years of life in group-living rhesus monkeys. *Development and Psychopathology, 22*(1), 45–53.

Sánchez, M. M., Noble, P. M., Lyon, C. K., Plotsky, P. M., Davis, M., Nemeroff, C. B., et al. (2005). Alterations in diurnal cortisol rhythm and acoustic startle response in nonhuman primates with adverse rearing. *Biological Psychiatry, 57*(4), 373–381.

Sroufe, L. A. (2005). Attachment and development: A prospective, longitudinal study from birth to adulthood. *Attachment and Human Development, 7*(4), 349–367.

Sroufe, L. A., Carlson, E. A., Levy, A. K., & Egeland, B. (1999). Implications of attachment theory for developmental psychopathology. *Development and Psychopathology, 11*(1), 1–13.

Symonds, M. E., Stephenson, T., Gardner, D. S., & Budge, H. (2007). Long-term effects of nutritional programming of the embryo and fetus: Mechanisms and critical windows. *Reproduction, Fertility and Development, 19*(1), 53–63.

Tarullo, A. R., & Gunnar, M. R. (2006). Child maltreatment and the developing HPA axis. *Hormones and Behavior, 50*(4), 632–639.

Teicher, M. H. (2010). Commentary: Childhood abuse: New insights into its association with posttraumatic stress, suicidal ideation, and aggression. *Journal of Pediatric Psychology, 35*(5), 578–580.

Teicher, M. H., Andersen, S. L., Polcari, A., Anderson, C. M., Navalta, C. P., & Kim, D. M. (2003). The neurobiological consequences of early stress and childhood maltreatment. *Neuroscience & Biobehavioral Reviews, 27*(1–2), 33–44.

Tottenham, N., Hare, T. A., Quinn, B. T., McCarry, T. W., Nurse, M., Gilhooly, T., et al. (2010). Prolonged institutional rearing is associated with atypically large amygdala volume and difficulties in emotion regulation. *Developmental Science, 13*(1), 46–61.

Trickett, P., & McBride-Chang, C. (1995). The developmental impact of different forms of child abuse and neglect. *Developmental Reviews, 15*, 11–37.

Tsankova, N., Berton, O., Renthal, W., Kumar, A., Neve, R., & Nestler, E. (2006). Sustained hippocampal chromatin regulation in a mouse model of depression and antidepressant action. *Nature Neuroscience, 9*(4), 519–525.

Turner, B. (2001). *Chromatin and gene regulation.* Oxford, UK: Blackwell Science Ltd.

Uchida, S., Hara, K., Kobayashi, A., Otsuki, K., Yamagata, H., Hobara, T., et al. (2011). Epigenetic status of GDNF in the ventral striatum determines susceptibility and adaptation to daily stressful events. *Neuron, 69*(2), 359–372.

Uddin, M., Aiello, A. E., Wildman, D. E., Koenen, K. C., Pawelec, G., de Los Santos, R., et al. (2010). Epigenetic and immune function profiles associated with posttraumatic stress disorder. *Proceedings of the National Academy of Sciences of the United States of America, 107*(20), 9470–9475.

van Harmelen, A.-L., van Tol, M.-J., van der Wee, N. J. A., Veltman, D. J., Aleman, A., Spinhoven, P., et al. (2010). Reduced medial prefrontal cortex volume in adults reporting childhood emotional maltreatment. *Biological Psychiatry, 68*(9), 832–838.

van Ijzendoorn, M. H., Schuengel, C., & Bakermans-Kranenburg, M. J. (1999). Disorganized attachment in early childhood: Meta-analysis of precursors, concomitants, and sequelae. *Development and Psychopathology, 11*(2), 225–249.

Weaver, I. C., Cervoni, N., Champagne, F. A., D'Alessio, A. C., Sharma, S., Seckl, J. R., et al. (2004). Epigenetic programming by maternal behavior. *Nature Neuroscience, 7*(8), 847–854.

Wong, C. C., Caspi, A., Williams, B., Craig, I. W., Houts, R., Ambler, A., et al. (2010). A longitudinal study of epigenetic variation in twins. *Epigenetics, 5*(6), 516–526.

Zeisel, S. H. (2009). Importance of methyl donors during reproduction. *American Journal of Clinical Nutrition, 89*(2), 673S–677S.

Zhang, T. Y., Hellstrom, I. C., Bagot, R. C., Wen, X., Diorio, J., & Meaney, M. J. (2010). Maternal care and DNA methylation of a glutamic acid decarboxylase 1 promoter in rat hippocampus. *The Journal of Neuroscience, 30*(39), 13130–13137.

Zoladz, P. R., Conrad, C. D., Fleshner, M., & Diamond, D. M. (2008). Acute episodes of predator exposure in conjunction with chronic social instability as an animal model of post-traumatic stress disorder. *Stress: The International Journal on the Biology of Stress, 11*, 259–281.

3

Teasing Out the Role of Genotype in the Development of Psychopathology in Maltreated Children

SARA R. JAFFEE

Maltreated youth exhibit elevated rates of psychiatric problems, including depression, conduct and oppositional defiant disorders, anxiety, post-traumatic stress disorder, and attention deficit/hyperactivity disorder (Cicchetti & Valentino, 2006; Kaplan, Pelcovitz, & Labruna, 1999). Compared with nonmaltreated youth, youth who have been maltreated have also been found to display elevated rates of aggression, delinquency, and violence (Jaffee, Caspi, Moffitt, & Taylor, 2004; Smith & Thornberry, 1995; Widom, 1989) and to engage in more frequent substance use and high-risk sexual activity (Thornberry, Ireland, & Smith, 2001; Widom & Kuhns, 1996; Widom & White, 1997). Maltreated youth are also at higher risk for developing personality disorders such as antisocial personality disorder (Horwitz, Widom, McLaughlin, & White, 2001) and borderline personality disorder (Gunderson & Chu, 1993; Widom, Czaja, & Paris, 2009).

Researchers have considered the role of genotype in the development of psychopathology in maltreated youth from three perspectives. The first is whether genes common to parents and children confound the relationship between maltreatment and youth psychopathology, or whether genetically influenced characteristics of children provoke abusive responses from adults. This perspective is concerned with the possibility that genes and environments are correlated. The second is whether genotype moderates the effect of maltreatment on the risk for psychopathology. This perspective is concerned with the possibility that genes interact with maltreatment to increase risk for psychopathology. The third is whether maltreatment leads to epigenetic change. The first two perspectives are considered here in turn; the third is covered in Chapter 2.

Correlations between Genes and Maltreatment

An assumption inherent to most epidemiological studies of maltreated youth is that maltreatment is a cause of psychopathology. Indeed, the evidence that maltreatment plays a causal role in the development of psychopathology has been bolstered by research designs that compare maltreated youth to sociodemographically matched nonmaltreated controls (Kaufman et al., 2004; Toth, Manly, & Cicchetti, 1992; Widom, 1989) and that identify prospective associations between maltreatment and later psychopathology (Stouthamer-Loeber, Loeber, Homish, & Wei, 2001; Thornberry et al., 2001).

However, as noted by DiLalla and Gottesman (1991), the possibility remains that the relationship between maltreatment and psychopathology is accounted for by genes common to parents and children—what behavioral geneticists refer to as a passive gene–environment correlation (Jaffee & Price, 2007). Passive gene–environment correlations arise because the parental genotype not only influences the child's behavior (via the child's genotype) but also influences the child's rearing environment, thus generating a correlation between genotype and environment and a spurious association between the rearing environment and the child's behavior. As an example, because parents who have histories of antisocial behavior (which is moderately heritable) are at elevated risk of abusing their children (Brown, Cohen, Johnson, & Salzinger, 1998; Dinwiddie & Bucholz, 1993; Walsh, McMillan, & Jamieson, 2002), maltreatment might be a marker for genetic risk that parents transmit to children, rather than a causal risk factor for children's conduct problems.

Evocative gene–environment correlations could also account for observed associations between maltreatment and psychopathology. Evocative gene–environment correlations arise when genetically influenced characteristics of an individual evoke some response from the environment. For example, a temperamentally difficult, hard-to-manage child could provoke physically abusive responses from adults, in which case the child's aggressive, oppositional behavior would be a cause of maltreatment rather than the reverse.

Genetically informative research designs are required in order to test whether the relationship between maltreatment and psychopathology is genetically mediated (i.e., accounted for by genotype) or environmentally mediated. Two types of genetically informative designs have been put to this purpose. First, studies of child twins have been used to test whether there are genetic influences on maltreatment consistent with evocative gene–environment correlations. Second, the twin and parents (TaP) design has been used to test whether passive gene–environment correlation accounts for the relationship between maltreatment and youth psychopathology. These research designs are discussed here in turn.

Studies of Child Twins

Quantitative behavioral genetic studies of child twins treat maltreatment like any other characteristic by which individuals in a population differ, and they use quantitative behavioral genetic methods to decompose the variation in maltreatment into genetic, shared environmental, and nonshared environmental components. Thus, this design addresses the question of why some children are more likely to experience maltreatment than others.

The twin method is premised on the observation that monozygotic (MZ) twins share 100% of their genetic material and dizygotic (DZ) twins share 50% of their segregating genetic material, on average. Thus, genetic influences on maltreatment are inferred if MZ twins are more similar to each other than DZ twins. Shared environmental influences (which make twins in a pair similar to each other) are inferred if the DZ twin correlation is more than half the MZ twin correlation, and nonshared environmental influences (which make twins in a pair different from each other) are inferred if MZ twins are not perfectly correlated for a given characteristic. To the extent that there are genetic influences on maltreatment, it is presumed that genetically influenced characteristics of the child evoke maltreatment.

The twin design makes a number of assumptions that, if violated, would potentially bias estimates of genetic and environmental influences. First, the design assumes that *trait-relevant* environments shared by MZ twins are no more similar than the corresponding environments shared by DZ twins. Although it has been widely demonstrated that the environments shared by MZ twins are, overall, more similar than the environments shared by DZ twins (Kendler & Baker, 2007), these environmental similarities do not account for the increased phenotypic similarity shown by MZ versus DZ pairs (Kendler & Gardner, 1998; Kendler, Neale, Kessler, Heath, & Eaves, 1994). Moreover, other genetically informative designs (e.g., the adoption design or sibling comparisons based on genome-wide scans) that do not make the equal-environments assumption generate genetic and environmental estimates similar to those derived using the twin method (Visscher et al., 2006).

Second, the twin design assumes that there is not assortative mating for the characteristic in question. In studies of psychopathology, this assumption is clearly violated, as there is substantial evidence of assortative mating for psychopathology and antisocial behavior (Galbaud du Fort, Bland, Newman, & Boothroyd, 1998; Krueger, Moffitt, Caspi, Bleske, & Silva, 1998; Maes et al., 1998). Because assortative mating will, on average, increase the genetic similarity of DZ twins (and, thus, their phenotypic similarity), the consequence of assortative mating is an inflated estimate of shared environmental effects (and decreased estimates of genetic effects) on the characteristic in question.

Two studies have used the twin design to test whether maltreatment is likely to be a causal risk factor for children's antisocial behavior or whether the relationship is confounded by genotype. Jaffee et al. (2004) used data from the Environmental Risk (E-Risk) Longitudinal Study, a prospective, longitudinal study of 1,116 twin pairs, to study the relationship between child maltreatment (as reported by mothers) occurring before the age of 5 years and children's antisocial behavior (reported by mothers and teachers) at 5 years. The analyses provided four pieces of evidence that were consistent with a causal relationship between children's experiences of maltreatment and their antisocial behavior: (1) physical maltreatment measured at one point in time predicted increases in children's antisocial behavior over time, (2) there was a dose-response relationship between the severity of physical maltreatment and the severity of children's antisocial behavior problems, (3) genetic factors accounted for a small and statistically nonsignificant portion of the variance in physical maltreatment (7%), suggesting that genetically influenced characteristics of children were not provoking an abusive response from adults, and (4) physical maltreatment was uniquely predictive of children's antisocial behavior after controlling for parents' antisocial behavior, although the magnitude of the association was reduced.

Schulz-Heik et al. (2010) used data from 753 twin pairs and 1,248 full sibling pairs in the National Longitudinal Survey of Adolescent Health to test whether the relationship between maltreatment and adolescent conduct problems was genetically mediated. Maltreatment occurring before age 12 years was assessed retrospectively when the participants were young adults. Physical abuse, sexual abuse, and neglect were each measured with one or two items, and scores were combined to reflect increasingly frequent or diverse maltreatment. Consistent with Jaffee et al. (2004), additive genetic factors accounted for a small and statistically nonsignificant portion of the variance in maltreatment (6%) (Schulz-Heik et al., 2009). Nevertheless, the authors tested whether this small genetic effect was shared with genetic influences on conduct problems in adolescence. They found that genetic factors accounted for 70% of the small but significant correlation between maltreatment and adolescent conduct problems. The authors suggest that their results are consistent with the possibility that evocative gene–environment correlations account for the relationship between maltreatment and children's conduct problems. However, power was limited in univariate and bivariate models to distinguish between genetically and environmentally mediated effects, and the only parameter for which the confidence interval did not consistently include zero was the parameter measuring nonshared environmental influences and measurement error.

Twin and Parents Studies

This design estimates the magnitude of genetic and nongenetic pathways by which a parental phenotype (e.g., parental antisocial behavior) is associated with the corresponding phenotype among offspring. Measured environments (e.g., maltreatment) can be included in the model, and their direct effects on the child phenotype can be estimated. The design also estimates the degree of assortative mating between parents. The TaP design assumes that the (genetic and environmental) sources of variation in the parent phenotype are the same as in the offspring phenotype and that the magnitude of the variation in the phenotype is the same in both generations (Fulker, 1982). This assumption is likely to be violated when the parent and offspring phenotypes reflect behavior at different points in development. For instance, it has been shown that gene variants associated with alcohol dependence in adulthood are associated with symptoms of conduct disorder rather than alcohol dependence in adolescence (Dick et al., 2006), and longitudinal data from Eaves, Prom, and Silberg (2010) showed that genetic influences on juvenile antisocial behavior were largely different from genetic influences on adult antisocial behavior in the same individual.

Eaves et al. (2010) used the longitudinal twin and parents (LTaP) design to test whether the association between childhood adversity (indexed by retrospectively reported parental neglect, exposure to interparental violence, and inconsistent parental discipline) and offspring antisocial behavior (as measured by adolescent conduct problems and adult antisocial behavior) was genetically or environmentally mediated. To say that the association is genetically mediated is to imply that genes common to parents and children account for the relationship between childhood adversity and offspring antisocial behavior. To say that the association is environmentally mediated is to imply that childhood adversity has a direct effect on offspring antisocial behavior (or one mediated by other environmental variables). The model tests whether at least some of the environment that makes twins similar to each other reflects childhood adversity.

The use of longitudinal data in this model circumvents some of the more problematic assumptions of the standard TaP model. First, the LTaP design includes measures of the candidate environment (i.e., childhood adversity) and both parents' antisocial behavior, thus providing information about assortative mating and the size of the association between parent antisocial behavior and childhood adversity. Second, the LTaP design includes information about twins' antisocial behavior in adolescence and adulthood, thus providing information about the magnitude of genetic and environmental influences on these behaviors at two different points in development. Third, a model incorporating information about parent antisocial behavior and *adult* offspring antisocial behavior provides information on the extent to which genetic differences in parental behavior account for the relationship between childhood adversity and adult offspring antisocial behavior. Because antisocial behavior is measured at the same point in development for parents and offspring, this model is unlikely to violate the assumption that the same genes influence parent and offspring phenotypes (assuming there are not sizable cohort effects). This model can then be used to identify a model that measures the influence of parental genotype and childhood adversity on juvenile antisocial behavior, including the measure of passive genotype–environment correlation.

Using the LTaP design, Eaves et al. (2010) found that nongenetic effects of parent antisocial behavior on the shared environment were largely mediated by the parental treatment of children, and that childhood adversity directly accounted for shared environmental effects on offspring antisocial behavior, providing evidence for an environmentally mediated effect of parental treatment. Moreover, effects of the shared environment (including parental treatment) on offspring antisocial behavior persisted from adolescence into adulthood. Very small passive gene–environment correlations were detected.

In summary, the two studies that estimated genetic influences on child maltreatment (Jaffee et al., 2004; Schulz-Heik et al., 2010) showed that additive genetic influences on child maltreatment were small, accounting for only 6% to 7% of the variance. Alone, this finding suggests that genetically influenced characteristics of children (including their antisocial behavior) do not provoke adults to abuse them, although it bears noting that assortative mating for psychiatric disorder (and particularly for antisocial behavior) could have artifactually deflated the observed heritability estimates. In addition, Eaves et al. (2010) showed that the relationship between maltreatment-related childhood adversity and offspring antisocial behavior was not merely accounted for by gene variants common to parents and children; rather, childhood adversity was shown to have direct, environmentally mediated effects on youth antisocial behavior, and passive gene–environment correlations were shown to be small. Together, these findings provide stronger support for the hypothesis that maltreatment is a cause of youth antisocial behavior than for alternative hypotheses involving passive or evocative gene–environment correlation.

A limitation of these studies is that none involved documented cases of maltreatment. This limitation is likely to be inherent to some genetically informative designs. For example, although studies of adoptees neatly eliminate the biological relationship between parents and offspring (and, thus, passive genotype–environment correlation), adoptive families are screened so that they have low rates of maltreatment. Although studies of twins (and children of twins) tend not to have information about substantiated maltreatment, it is possible to obtain that information (as demonstrated by Jonson-Reid et al. [2010]). However, even if the information is available, researchers might be rightly concerned about jeopardizing their relationships with study participants by requesting permission to obtain social service records. In practice, obtaining child welfare service records *and* parent and child reports on family functioning and children's behavior could prove challenging.

Genotype × Maltreatment Interactions

The second perspective from which researchers have considered the role of genotype in the development of psychopathology in maltreated children has been the interaction between genes and environments. Gene × environment interactions (GxE), which refer to genetic differences in the effects of exposures like child maltreatment (Kendler & Eaves, 1986), have traditionally been viewed in a diathesis stress framework (but see more recent work by Belsky et al. for a different conceptualization of GxE; Belsky & Pluess, 2009]). Specifically, the effects of adverse childhood experiences are hypothesized to be greater among individuals who carry genetic risk variants (i.e., who have an underlying diathesis or vulnerability for psychopathology) than among individuals who do not carry those genetic risk variants.

Two approaches have been used to test for genotype × maltreatment interactions. The first has been to use the twin design to test whether genetic risk moderates the effect of maltreatment on risk for psychopathology. This approach assigns genetic risk based on information about the pairs' zygosity and the co-twin's psychiatric diagnostic status. Thus, a child who is an MZ twin and whose co-twin has a diagnosis of conduct disorder would be at relatively high risk for conduct problems, whereas a child who is an MZ twin and whose co-twin does not have a diagnosis of conduct disorder would be at relatively low risk for conduct problems. DZ pairs fall between these groups.

Using data from the E-Risk Study of 1,116 twin pairs, Jaffee et al. (2005) showed that genetic risk moderated the effect of maltreatment on youth antisocial behavior, such that the effect of maltreatment on antisocial behavior at age 5 was greater among those at high genetic risk than among those at low genetic risk. However, this finding was not replicated in a sample of 4,432 twins for whom data on maltreatment was obtained from child welfare service records (Jonson-Reid et al., 2010). In addition, data from E-Risk failed to show that genetic risk for psychosis moderated the effect of maltreatment on the risk for psychotic symptoms at age 12 years, although genetic risk and maltreatment had unique additive effects (Arseneault et al., 2011).

The second approach to testing for genotype × maltreatment interaction has been to identify specific gene variants that moderate maltreatment effects. The first evidence that a specific gene variant moderated the effect of maltreatment appeared in 2002 (Caspi et al., 2002). The study involved a cohort of 442 New Zealand men who had participated from birth in the Dunedin Longitudinal Study. Among men who carried the low-activity variant of the monoamine oxidase A (MAOA) gene, those who experienced childhood adversities—including sexual and physical abuse, maternal rejecting behavior, harsh discipline, and frequent caretaker changes—had significantly higher levels of antisocial behavior in childhood and adulthood than those who had not experienced childhood adversity. Among men who carried the high-activity variant, childhood adversity was not associated with later antisocial behavior. In a subsequent paper focused on a variant in the serotonin transporter linked promoter region (5HTTLPR), Caspi et al. (2003) showed that among men and women who were homozygous for the short form of the serotonin transporter polymorphism, experiencing more adverse childhood events was associated with increased levels of depression in adulthood. This association was not observed among individuals who were homozygous for the long form of the serotonin transporter polymorphism.

There is plausible biological evidence from animals and humans that these genotype × environment interactions capture real biological processes (for a review, see Caspi, Hariri, Holmes, Uher, & Moffitt, 2010). MAOA is involved in the metabolism of monoamines in the brain and other organs (Shih & Thompson, 1999), and 5HTTLPR is involved in the reuptake of serotonin at brain synapses (Heils et al., 1995). The results of studies that either knock out or functionally excise these genes support the involvement of MAOA in aggressive traits (Cases et al., 1995; Shih, 2004) and 5HTTLPR in anxious traits (Murphy & Lesch, 2008). Studies of nonhuman primates provide evidence of GxE that is consistent with the findings in humans (for a review, see Caspi et al., 2010), and 5HTTLPR and MAOA have been associated with brain activity in regions implicated in depression and aggression in response to negative stimuli (Buckholtz & Meyer-Lindenberg, 2008; Munafo, Brown, & Hariri, 2008).

Maltreatment × MAOA: Replications

The original publications on GxE have inspired multiple attempts at replication. A meta-analysis of five GxE studies of MAOA and maltreatment-related adversity (Caspi et al., 2002; Foley et al., 2004; Haberstick et al., 2005; Kim-Cohen et al., 2006; Nilsson et al., 2005) showed that there was a robust but small association between maltreatment and risk for antisocial behavior among individuals carrying the low-activity variant, but not among those carrying the high-activity variant (Kim-Cohen et al., 2006). Since 2006 there have been subsequent replications (Ducci et al., 2008; Edwards et al., 2010), some showing that the interaction between maltreatment and MAOA might be specific to antisocial behavior versus substance use (Derringer, Krueger, Irons, & Iacono, 2010), and others replicating the effect for male (Frazzetto et al., 2007; Widom & Brzustowicz, 2006) and Caucasian participants only (Widom & Brzustowicz, 2006). In contrast, others did identify a significant MAOA × maltreatment interaction among female participants (Beach et al., 2010; Ducci et al., 2008). There have also been nonreplications of the original finding, as listed in Table 3.1.

In summary, as shown in Table 3.1, 21 studies have attempted to replicate the original finding by Caspi et al. (2002). Seven of these can be considered replications because the interaction effect was statistically significant and was in the same direction as in the original report in a male population of predominantly European ancestry. We include in this group one study of Native American women (Ducci et al., 2008). One study was considered a partial replication because the interaction was statistically significant for a composite measure of

Table 3.1 Studies that have Attempted to Replicate the MAOA × Maltreatment Effect Reported in Caspi et al. (2002)

Study	Sample	Age at outcome	Measure of maltreatment	Measure of antisocial behavior	Notes
Caspi et al., 2002	442 males; epidemiological sample; Caucasian	Longitudinal (adolescents and adults)	Composite measure of retrospective report, observer ratings, and parent report	Self-report, police records, parent and teacher reports	Maltreatment was associated with elevated levels of antisocial behavior among individuals who carried the low-activity variant, but not among individuals who carried the high-activity variant
Replications					
Foley et al., 2004	514 males; epidemiological sample; Caucasian	Children and adolescents	Composite measure of retrospective report of parenting and interparental violence	Diagnostic interview for conduct disorder	
Nilsson et al., 2005	81 males; epidemiological sample; Caucasian	Adolescents	Retrospective report	Self-report	
Widom & Brzustowicz, 2006	409 males and females; demographically matched cases and controls; mixed ethnicity	Longitudinal (adolescents and adults)	Substantiated maltreatment	Self-report, police records, and clinical interview	Partial replication in white females; nonreplication in non-whites

(*Continued*)

Table 3.1 Studies that have Attempted to Replicate the MAOA × Maltreatment Effect Reported in Caspi et al. (2002) (*Continued*)

Study	Sample	Age at outcome	Measure of maltreatment	Measure of antisocial behavior	Notes
Frazzetto et al., 2007	235 males and females; psychiatric outpatients and controls; Caucasian	Adults	Retrospective report of early life traumatic events	Aggression questionaire	Yes (among males); nonreplication in females
Ducci et al., 2008	291 females; alcoholics and healthy controls; Native American	Adults	Retrospective report of childhood sexual abuse	Clinical interview	Interaction also predicted alcoholism
Derringer et al., 2010	841 males and females; epidemiological sample; Caucasian	Adolescents and young adults	Retrospective self-report of harsh discipline and sexual assault	Clinical interview	Yes
Partial replications					
Edwards et al., 2010	186 males; epidemiological sample; Caucasian	Children and adolescents	Parent report of physical discipline	Youth, parent, and teacher report	
Kim-Cohen et al., 2006	975 males	Children	Parent report	Parent and teacher report	Significant for total mental health composite and ADHD subscale, but not for antisocial behavior subscale
Nonreplications					
Cicchetti et al., 2007 et al.	339 males and females ; maltreated youth and matched controls ; mixed ethnicity	Adolescents	Substantiated maltreatment	Clinical interview, self-report	

Citation	Sample	Age	Exposure measure	Outcome measure	Findings
Huang et al., 2004	766 males and females ; psychiatric outpatients and controls ; mixed ethnicity	Adults	Retrospective report	Aggression, impulsivity, and hostility questionnaires	Significant interaction for impulsivity in males
Haberstick et al., 2005	774 males	Adolescents	Retrospective report	Self-report, police records	
Huizinga et al., 2006	277 males	Adolescents	Retrospective report	Self-report, police records	
Young et al., 2006	247 males ; in treatment for conduct or substance use problems ; mixed ethnicity	Adolescents	Retrospective report	Clinical interview	
Reif et al., 2007	184 males	Adults	Retrospective report of adverse childhood experiences	Police records	
Sjoberg et al., 2007	119 females ; epidemiological sample ; Caucasian	Adolescents	Retrospective report of childhood sexual abuse	Self-report	Significant interaction in direction opposite that of original report
Prom-Wormley et al., 2009	721 females ; twins ; Caucasian	Children and adolescents	Composite measure of retrospective report of parenting and interparental violence	Diagnostic interview for conduct disorder	
van der Vegt et al., 2009	239 males ; adoptees ; Caucasian	Adolescents	Parent report	Parent report	

(Continued)

Table 3.1 Studies that have Attempted to Replicate the MAOA × Maltreatment Effect Reported in Caspi et al. (2002) (*Continued*)

Study	Sample	Age at outcome	Measure of maltreatment	Measure of antisocial behavior	Notes
Weder et al., 2009	114 males and females ; maltreated youth and matched controls ; mixed ethnicity	Children and adolescents	Trauma exposure reflected in Child Protective Services records, parent report, self-report	Teacher report, clinical interview	Significant interaction showing that the low- versus the high-activity variant is associated with elevated symptoms of inattention/hyperactivity when trauma exposure was low versus high
Beach et al., 2010	538 males and females ; adoptees ; Caucasian	Adults	Retrospective report	Clinical interview	Significant interaction in women (but not men), consistent with original report
Enoch et al., 2010	7,500 males and females ; epidemiological ; Caucasian	Children	Maternal report of child's stressful life events, including violence exposure	Maternal report	Significant interaction for girls showing that the high- versus the low-activity variant increases risk for inattention/hyperactivity under conditions of low (but not high) stress

mental health problems that included antisocial behavior, but not the antisocial behavior subscale specifically (Kim-Cohen et al., 2006). Finally, 12 studies can be considered nonreplications because the interaction was not statistically significant for Caucasian men or because it was in a different direction than in the original report. For example, Sjoberg et al. (2007) reported that the high-activity, rather than the low-activity, MAOA variant increased women's risk for antisocial behavior in the context of high levels of childhood adversity.

Of interest, all three of the studies that included samples of preadolescent children (Enoch, Steer, Newman, Gibson, & Goldman, 2010; Kim-Cohen et al., 2006; Weder et al., 2009) detected significant MAOA × maltreatment effects on inattention/hyperactivity but not on conduct problems, although there was heterogeneity among studies in the direction of this effect. For example, two of the studies found that maltreatment was associated with symptoms of inattention/hyperactivity among carriers of the low-activity variant but not among carriers of the high-activity variant (Enoch et al., 2010; Kim-Cohen et al., 2006). Looked at differently, however, the ordinal interactions identified in these studies took different forms and were identified in different subgroups (girls in the former case, boys in the latter). In the former study (Enoch et al., 2010), girls who were homozygous for the high-activity variant had consistently *high* levels of inattention/hyperactivity regardless of stress, whereas girls who were homozgyous for the low-activity variant had low levels of symptoms under conditions of low stress and higher levels of symptoms under conditions of higher stress. In contrast, the latter study showed that boys who carried the high-activity variant had consistently *low* levels of inattention/hyperactivity regardless of maltreatment status, and boys who carried the low-activity variant had low levels of symptomatology if they had not been maltreated and higher levels of symptomatology if they had been maltreated (Kim-Cohen et al., 2006). The third study (Weder et al., 2009) identified a disordinal interaction, such that carriers of the low-activity variant had more symptoms of inattention/hyperactivity if they were exposed to relatively low levels of trauma than if they were exposed to higher levels of trauma. In contrast, carriers of the high-activity variant had more symptoms of inattention/hyperactivity if they were exposed to higher levels of trauma than if they were exposed to lower levels of trauma. Thus, it is possible that in preadolescent samples, the interaction between MAOA and maltreatment is a stronger predictor of inattention/hyperactivity than antisocial behavior, but more research is needed in order to determine whether a consistent pattern of interaction effects can be identified.

Maltreatment × 5HTTLPR: Replications

The interaction between 5HTTLPR and maltreatment-related childhood adversity has also been replicated in subsequent studies (Aguilera et al., 2009; Kumsta et al., 2010; Taylor et al., 2006), although it bears noting that most of these did not measure maltreatment per se (or even a continuum of suboptimal parenting practices) and relied instead on composite measures of adverse childhood events that encompassed a range of experiences (e.g., prolonged periods of parental unemployment, separation from caregivers). Some studies have extended the original findings. Kaufman et al. (2006) not only found that 5HTTLPR moderated the effects of maltreatment on children's risk for depression, but they also detected a three-way interaction among documented maltreatment, 5HTTLPR, and brain derived neurotrophic factor (BDNF) genotype. This finding has been replicated by one group (Wichers et al., 2008) but not by another group, whose measure of childhood adversity did not include maltreatment (Nederhof, Bouma, Oldehinkel, & Ormel, 2010).

Other papers can be seen as partial replications of the original finding by Caspi et al. (2003). For example, in a sample of maltreated children recruited from Child Protective Services and demographically matched nonmaltreated controls, interactions between maltreatment and either MAOA or 5HTTLPR genotype were nonsignificant (Cicchetti, Rogosch, & Sturge-Apple, 2007). However, post hoc analyses showed that sexual assault specifically moderated the effect of 5HTTLPR on risk for internalizing problems, such that sexually abused children had more internalizing symptoms than nonabused children if they were homozygous for the S allele but not if they carried the L allele. Other studies have published evidence of moderation for girls but not boys (Aslund et al., 2009).

As shown in Table 3.2, still others have failed to replicate the original finding. It bears noting that the majority of nonreplications involved studies in which maltreatment was only one of many adverse childhood experiences included in an index of retrospectively reported environmental risk. Thus, heterogeneity in these findings could be accounted for by differences in the specificity with which maltreatment was measured.

In summary, Table 3.2 shows that out of 12 studies, 3 replicated the original report by Caspi et al. (2003) and 3 were partial replications. The remaining six studies failed to replicate the original finding.

Other Genotype × Maltreatment Interactions

Although the majority of research on GxE in the maltreatment literature has involved MAOA and 5HTTLPR, other variants have been identified that increase the risk for psychopathology in the context of maltreatment and related adverse childhood experiences. Briefly, these involve hypothalamic-pituitary-adrenal axis genes, including glucocorticoid receptor variants (Bet et al., 2009), variants on the corticotropin-releasing hormone receptor 1 gene (Bradley et al., 2008; Grabe et al., 2010; Polanczyk et al., 2009; Schmid et al., 2010), and FK506 binding protein 5 (Bradley et al., 2008; Uddin et al., 2010). Other genes that have been shown to moderate the effect of maltreatment on the risk for psychopathology

Table 3.2 Studies that have Attempted to Replicate the 5HTTLPR × Maltreatment Effect Reported in Caspi et al. (2003)

Study	Sample	Age at outcome	Measure of maltreatment	Measure of depression	Notes
Caspi et al., 2003	442 males; epidemiological sample; Caucasian	Longitudinal (adolescents and adults)	Composite measure of retrospective report, observer ratings, and parent report	Self-report and clinical interview	
Replications					
Kaufman et al., 2004, 2006	196 males and females; maltreated youth and matched controls; mixed ethnicity	Children and adolescents	Substantiated maltreatment	Clinical interview	
Taylor et al., 2006	118 males and females; epidemiological; mixed ethnicity	Young adults	Retrospective report of adverse childhood experiences (including maltreatment)	Self-report	
Kumsta et al., 2010	125 males and females	Adolescents	Institutional rearing in Romanian orphanages between the ages of 6 months and 42 months	Clinical interview and parent report	

(Continued)

Table 3.2 Studies that have Attempted to Replicate the 5HTTLPR × Maltreatment Effect Reported in Caspi et al. (2003) *(Continued)*

Study	Sample	Age at outcome	Measure of maltreatment	Measure of depression	Notes
Partial replications					
Cicchetti et al., 2007	339 males and females; maltreated youth and matched controls; mixed ethnicity	Adolescents	Substantiated maltreatment	Clinical interview, self-report	Sexual abuse, but not any maltreatment moderated effect of 5HTTLPR in the same direction as in the original finding
Aguilera et al., 2009	534 males and females; epidemiological; Caucasian	Young adults	Retrospective report (Childhood Trauma Questionnaire)	Self-report	Sexual abuse only, but other forms of maltreatment showed no moderated effect of 5HTTLPR in the same direction as in the original finding
Aslund et al., 2009	1,482 males and females; epidemiological; Caucasian	Adolescents	Retrospective report	Self-report	Significant interaction detected for girls only
Nonreplications					
Surtees et al., 2006	4,175 males and females; selected for high versus low neuroticism	Adults	Retrospective report of adverse childhood experiences (including maltreatment)	Self-report	

Study	Sample	Age group	Measure of maltreatment	Report	Findings
Chipman et al., 2007	2,095 males and females; epidemiological; Caucasian	Adolescents	Retrospective report of adverse childhood experiences (including maltreatment)	Self-report	
Chorbov et al., 2007	238 females; affected twin pairs selected for depression and unaffected control pairs; Caucasian	Adolescents and young adults	Retrospective report of traumatic life events (including maltreatment)	Clinical interview	Genotyped both forms of L allele (L_A and L_C) and found evidence that risk for depression was elevated in high-activity carriers (homozygous for L_A) relative to low- and medium-activity groups, but only in the presence of a single trauma
Wichers et al., 2008	394 females; epidemiological sample; Caucasian	Adults	Retrospective report (Childhood Trauma Questionnaire)	Self-report	No, but three-way interaction among 5HTTLPR, BDNF, and maltreatment
Araya et al., 2009	4,334 males and females; epidemiological; Caucasian	Children	Maternal report of stressful life events (including possible maltreatment)	Parent report	
Antypa & Van der Does, 2010	250 males and females; epidemiological; Caucasian	Young adults	Retrospective report (Childhood Trauma Questionnaire)	Clinical interview	

include BDNF (Aguilera et al., 2009; Perroud et al., 2008), γ-aminobutyric acid receptor 2 (Enoch et al., 2010), and catechol-o-methyltransferase (Savitz, van der Merwe, Newman, Stein, & Ramesar, 2010). A different approach has been to study the effect of multiple gene variants and sum the number of risk variants an individual carries. Using this approach, Beaver (2008) reported that a genetic risk score comprising three dopamine gene variants moderated the effect of sexual abuse on violent delinquency for males but not females.

Methodological Issues in the Study of GxE

Although there is evidence that the effects of maltreatment are moderated by genotype, results from studies of GxE must be read with caution for several reasons. First, studies have rarely used similar measures of maltreatment or outcome. Although some have included documented cases of abuse and neglect (Cicchetti et al., 2007; Kaufman et al., 2004; Widom & Brzustowicz, 2006), others have relied on parent or self-report of maltreatment, harsh discipline, and inter-parental conflict, and still others have aggregated disparate adverse events— only some of which index maltreatment—into a single measure. Retrospective reports of maltreatment can be particularly problematic because they are likely to result in substantial underreporting of abuse and to increase error in the classification of individuals as maltreated or not (Widom & Morris, 1997; Widom & Shepard, 1996). Measures of outcome are similarly heterogeneous and have included retrospective self-reports, prospective self- and other-reports, clinical diagnoses, and criminal records. This heterogeneity in the measurement of environments and outcomes makes it difficult to interpret the overall pattern of replications and nonreplications. For example, although there does appear to be a relationship between how maltreatment is measured and whether GxE involving 5HTTLPR are detected, the same is not true for GxE involving MAOA.

Second, GxE are highly sensitive to transformations of scale (Uher, 2011). As illustrated by Prom-Wormley et al. (2009), evidence for significant MAOA × adversity effects disappeared when the adversity scale was transformed to reflect the number of individuals at each level of the scale. Eaves (2006) has shown that a substantial amount of GxE could be due to Type I error. There is considerable controversy surrounding the replicability of GxE (Caspi et al., 2010; Munafo, Durrant, Lewis, & Flint, 2009; Risch et al., 2009; Uher & McGuffin, 2008, 2010), and reviewers of the literature must be aware of these issues when interpreting published findings.

Implications for Intervention

Research on the role of genotype in the development of psychopathology among maltreated children has generated information about the causal status of maltreatment as a risk factor for psychopathology and has identified groups that are most vulnerable to maltreatment.

To date, there is substantial evidence that maltreatment has environmentally mediated effects on psychopathology. Notably, the results of quantitative genetic studies confirm findings from prospective epidemiological studies showing that (a) characteristics of parents and families, rather than characteristics of children, better explain why some children are more likely to be maltreated than others, and (b) maltreatment has direct effects on youth psychopathology, even controlling for genes common to parents and children. These findings suggest that interventions to prevent maltreatment from occurring or recurring should also produce reductions in rates of psychopathology. Indeed, some evidence for this exists already, with data from the Nurse Family Partnership showing that youth in the intervention group had significantly lower levels of antisocial behavior in adolescence, partially because the intervention successfully reduced rates of maltreatment (Eckenrode et al., 2001).

Findings of genotype × environment interaction have raised the prospect that interventions can be tailored to individuals with specific profiles of genetic and environmental risk. In order for this promise to be realized, researchers must make progress on at least two fronts and grapple with several ethical and practical issues.

First, genotype × environment interactions must be replicated. As described above, detecting GxE is methodologically challenging, and there is considerable controversy about how best to aggregate findings from studies for the purposes of meta-analysis.

Second, researchers must identify the mechanisms by which genes and environments interact to affect behavior, so as to determine how best to intervene. These efforts will require the linking of genetic epidemiology with neuroscience (Caspi & Moffitt, 2006) in order to better identify the biological substrates that mediate environmental effects on behavior in genetically vulnerable individuals. For example, identifying differences at the level of gene expression and neurotransmitter or hormonal function among genetically identical individuals with different environmental exposures could lead to novel treatments for disorders that target those systems specifically. Efforts to identify the mechanisms of GxE effects will also require more investigation of which aspects of the environment provide the active ingredient (e.g., the fear associated with persistent physical abuse or the modeling of aggressive behavior).

Finally, there are ethical and practical problems associated with using GxE to inform prevention or intervention efforts. In theory, researchers or clinicians could direct scarce resources toward preventing maltreatment in families in which it would be predicted to have its worst effects, that is, families in which at least some children carry genetic variants that confer risk for psychopathology in the context of maltreatment. However, prioritizing certain individuals or families for intervention on the basis of genotype could have at least two consequences: it could potentially stigmatize the genetically "vulnerable" and define others as genetically "invulnerable." The latter possibility is especially problematic if certain genetic variants are protective for some outcomes but not others. However, researchers rarely assess a range of outcomes in studies of gene–environment interplay, leaving it unclear, for example, whether the individual whose genotype confers protection against antisocial behavior in the face of maltreatment is also at low risk for depression and anxiety. Practically speaking, such an effort would require mass genotyping of populations in order to identify genetically at-risk individuals and families. Ultimately, these issues might be rendered moot. For example, the risk variants that increase susceptibility to maltreatment are common, affecting around a third of the population. Assuming that several variants interact with maltreatment exposure to increase risk for a broad range of psychiatric symptoms, most individuals will carry at least one of the risk variants, with the result being that even targeted interventions will be directed at the vast majority of the population.

Nevertheless, there is substantial heterogeneity in children's response to maltreatment (Jaffee & Gallop, 2007), and to ignore the possibility that biological factors account for some of that variability could result in missed opportunities to intervene in order to prevent the emergence of psychopathology (Beauchaine, Neuhaus, Brenner, & Gatzke-Kopp, 2008). As we accrue more information about how stressful experiences like maltreatment "get under the skin" (Danese, Pariante, Caspi, Taylor, & Poulton, 2007; Miller & Chen, 2010), it might become possible to identify profiles of biomarkers, including genotype, that mark especially vulnerable individuals. Although any child who presents to child welfare services with symptoms of psychopathology should be referred for treatment, interventions with children who are at high biological risk but are not yet symptomatic could be especially effective in preventing the emergence of mental health problems. Such efforts might be particularly important for the one-third to one-half of children who are reported for maltreatment on multiple occasions following an initial report (Thompson & Wiley, 2009), given that chronic maltreatment is a risk factor for a range of poor cognitive, behavioral, and emotional outcomes (Jaffee & Maikovich-Fong, 2011).

Conclusions

Although the existence of gene–environment interplay has caused some researchers to question the role of maltreatment in the development of children's psychopathology (DiLalla & Gottesman, 1991), findings from genetically informative designs are consistent with those from prospective, longitudinal epidemiological studies in showing that maltreatment is likely to play a causal role in increasing children's risk for psychopathology. However, genetically informative designs have also demonstrated that the effects of maltreatment on children are heterogeneous and that genotype identifies some children who are more vulnerable than others. Research that identifies the biological and sociocognitive mechanisms that underlie effects of maltreatment on the development of psychopathology (particularly in genetically vulnerable groups) will contribute to our understanding of the causes of psychopathology and might inform treatments for psychopathology.

Disclosure Statement

S.R.J. reports no biomedical financial interests or potential conflicts of interest.

References

Aguilera, M., Arias, B., Wichers, M., Barrantes-Vidal, N., Moya, J., Villa, H., et al. (2009). Early adversity and 5-HTT/BDNF genes: New evidence of gene-environment interactions on depressive symptoms in a general population. *Psychological Medicine, 39,* 1425–1432.

Antypa, N., & Van der Does, A. J. W. (2010). Serotonin transporter gene, childhood emotional abuse and cognitive vulnerability to depression. *Genes Brain and Behavior, 9,* 615–620.

Araya, R., Hu, X. Z., Heron, J., Enoch, M. A., Evans, J., Lewis, G., et al. (2009). Effects of stressful life events, maternal depression and 5-HTTLPR genotype on emotional symptoms in pre-adolescent children. *American Journal of Medical Genetics Part B—Neuropsychiatric Genetics, 150B,* 670–682.

Arseneault, L., Cannon, M., Fisher, H. L., Polanczyk, G., Moffitt, T. E., & Caspi, A. (2011). Childhood trauma and children's emerging psychotic symptoms: A genetically sensitive longitudinal cohort study. *American Journal of Psychiatry, 168,* 65–72.

Aslund, C., Leppert, J., Comasco, E., Nordquist, N., Oreland, L., & Nilsson, K. W. (2009). Impact of the interaction between the 5HTTLPR polymorphism and maltreatment on adolescent depression. A population-based study. *Behavior Genetics, 39,* 524–531.

Beach, S. R. H., Brody, G. H., Gunter, T. D., Packer, H., Wernett, P., & Philibert, R. A. (2010). Child maltreatment moderates the association of MAOA with symptoms of depression and antisocial personality disorder. *Journal of Family Psychology, 24,* 12–20.

Beauchaine, T. P., Neuhaus, E., Brenner, S. L., & Gatzke-Kopp, L. (2008). Ten good reasons to consider biological processes in prevention and intervention research. *Development and Psychopathology, 20,* 745–774.

Beaver, K. M. (2008). The interaction between genetic risk and childhood sexual abuse in the prediction of adolescent violent behavior. *Sexual Abuse—A Journal of Research and Treatment, 20,* 426–443.

Belsky, J., & Pluess, M. (2009). Beyond diathesis stress: Differential susceptibility to environmental influences. *Psychological Bulletin, 135,* 885–908.

Bet, P. M., Penninx, B. W. J. H., Bochdanovits, Z., Uitterlinden, A. G., Beekman, A. T. F., van Schoor, N. M., et al. (2009). Glucocorticoid receptor gene polymorphisms and childhood adversity are associated with depression: New evidence for a gene-environ-ment interaction. *American Journal of Medical Genetics Part B—Neuropsychiatric Genetics, 150B,* 660–669.

Bradley, R. G., Binder, E. B., Epstein, M. P., Tang, Y., Nair, H. P., Liu, W., et al. (2008). Influence of child abuse on adult depression—Moderation by the corticotropin-releas-ing hormone receptor gene. *Archives of General Psychiatry, 65,* 190–200.

Brown, J., Cohen, P., Johnson, J. G., & Salzinger, S. (1998). A longitudinal analysis of risk factors for child maltreatment: Findings of a 17-year prospective study of officially recorded and self-reported child abuse and neglect. *Child Abuse and Neglect, 22,* 1065–1078.

Buckholtz, J. W., & Meyer-Lindenberg, A. (2008). MAOA and the neurogenetic architec-ture of human aggression. *Trends in Neurosciences, 31,* 120–129.

Cases, O., Seif, I., Grimsby, J., Gaspar, P., Chen, K., Pournin, S., et al. (1995). Aggressive behavior and altered amounts of brain serotonin and norepinephrine in mice lacking MAOA. *Science, 268,* 1763–1766.

Caspi, A., Hariri, A. R., Holmes, A., Uher, R., & Moffitt, T. E. (2010). Genetic sensitivity to the environment: The case of the serotonin transporter gene and its implications for studying complex diseases and traits. *American Journal of Psychiatry, 167,* 509–527.

Caspi, A., McClay, J., Moffitt, T. E., Mill, J., Martin, J., Craig, I. W., et al. (2002). Role of genotype in the cycle of violence in maltreated children. *Science, 297,* 851–854.

Caspi, A., & Moffitt, T. E. (2006). Gene-environment interactions in psychiatry: Joining forces with neuroscience. *Nature Review Neuroscience, 7,* 583–590.

Caspi, A., Sugden, K., Moffitt, T. E., Taylor, A., Craig, I. W., Harrington, H., et al. (2003). Influence of life stress on depression: Moderation by a polymorphism in the 5-HTT gene. *Science, 31,* 386–389.

Chipman, P., Jorm, A. F., Prior, M., Sanson, A., Smart, D., Tan, X., et al. (2007). No inter-action between the serotonin transporter polymorphism (5HTTLPR) and childhood adversity or recent stressful life events on symptoms of depression: Results from two community surveys. *American Journal of Medical Genetics Part B: Neuropsychiatric Genetics, 144B,* 561–565.

Chorbov, V. M., Lobos, E. A., Todorov, A. A., Heath, A. C., Botteron, K. N., & Todd, R. D. (2007). Relationship of 5-HTTLPR genotypes and depression risk in the presence of trauma in a female twin sample. *American Journal of Medical Genetics Part B—Neuropsychiatric Genetics, 144B,* 830–833.

Cicchetti, D., Rogosch, F. A., & Sturge-Apple, M. L. (2007). Interactions of child maltreat-ment and serotonin transporter and monoamine oxidase A polymorphisms: Depressive symptomatology among adolescents from low socioeconomic status backgrounds. *Development and Psychopathology, 19,* 1161–1180.

Cicchetti, D., & Valentino, K. (2006). An ecological-transactional perspective on child mal-treatment. In D. Cicchetti & D. J. Cohen (Eds.), *Developmental psychopathology* (2nd ed., Vol. 3, pp. 129–201). Hoboken, NJ: John Wiley & Sons, Inc.

Danese, A., Pariante, C. M., Caspi, A., Taylor, A., & Poulton, R. (2007). Childhood mal-treatment predicts adult inflammation in a life-course study. *Proceedings of the National Academy of Sciences, 104,* 1319–1324.

Derringer, J., Krueger, R. F., Irons, D. E., & Iacono, W. G. (2010). Harsh discipline, childhood sexual assault, and MAOA genotype: An investigation of main and interactive effects on diverse clinical externalizing outcomes. *Behavior Genetics, 40,* 639–648.

Dick, D. M., Bierut, L., Hinrichs, A., Fox, L., Bucholz, K. K., Kramer, J., et al. (2006). The role of GABRA2 in risk for conduct disorder and alcohol and drug dependence across developmental stages. *Behavior Genetics, 36,* 577–590.

DiLalla, L. F., & Gottesman, I. I. (1991). Biological and genetic contributions to violence: Widom's untold tale. *Psychological Bulletin, 109,* 125–129.

Dinwiddie, S. H., & Bucholz, K. K. (1993). Psychiatric diagnoses of self-reported child abusers. *Child Abuse and Neglect, 17,* 465–476.

Ducci, F., Enoch, M. A., Hodgkinson, C., Xu, K., Catena, M., Robin, R. W., et al. (2008). Interaction between a functional MAOA locus and childhood sexual abuse predicts alcoholism and antisocial personality disorder in adult women. *Molecular Psychiatry, 13,* 334–347.

Eaves, L. J. (2006). Genotype x environment interaction in psychopathology: Fact or artifact? *Twin Research and Human Genetics, 9,* 1–8.

Eaves, L. J., Prom, E. C., & Silberg, J. L. (2010). The mediating effect of parental neglect on adolescent and young adult anti-sociality: A longitudinal study of twins and their parents. *Behavior Genetics, 40,* 425–437.

Eckenrode, J., Zielinski, D., Smith, E., Marcynyszyn, L. A., Henderson, C. R., Jr., Kitzman, H., et al. (2001). Child maltreatment and the early onset of problem behaviors: Can a program of nurse home visitation break the link? *Development and Psychopathology, 13,* 873–890.

Edwards, A. C., Dodge, K. A., Latendresse, S. J., Lansford, J. E., Bates, J. E., Pettit, G. S., et al. (2010). MAOA-uVNTR and early physical discipline interact to influence delinquent behavior. *Journal of Child Psychology and Psychiatry, 51,* 679–687.

Enoch, M. A., Steer, C. D., Newman, T. K., Gibson, N., & Goldman, D. (2010). Early life stress, MAOA, and gene-environment interactions predict behavioral disinhibition in children. *Genes Brain and Behavior, 9,* 65–74.

Foley, D. L., Eaves, L. J., Wormley, B., Silberg, J. L., Maes, H. H., & Riley, B. (2004). Childhood adversity, monoamine oxidase A genotype, and risk for conduct disorder. *Archives of General Psychiatry, 61,* 744.

Frazzetto, G., Di Lorenzo, G., Carola, V., Proietti, L., Sokolowska, E., Siracusano, A., et al. (2007). Early trauma and increased risk for physical aggression during adulthood: The moderating role of MAOA genotype. *PLoS One, 2*(5), e486.

Fulker, D. W. (1982). Extensions of the classical twin method. *Progress in Clinical and Biological Research, 103,* 395–406.

Galbaud du Fort, G., Bland, R. C., Newman, S. C., & Boothroyd, L. J. (1998). Spouse similarity for lifetime psychiatric history in the general population. *Psychological Medicine, 28,* 789–803.

Grabe, H. J., Schwahn, C., Appel, K., Mahler, J., Schulz, A., Spitzer, C., et al. (2010). Childhood maltreatment, the corticotropin-releasing hormone receptor gene and adult depression in the general population. *American Journal of Medical Genetics Part B—Neuropsychiatric Genetics, 158B,* 1483–1493.

Gunderson, J. G., & Chu, J. A. (1993). Treatment implications of past trauma in borderline personality disorder. *Harvard Review of Psychiatry, 1,* 75–81.

Haberstick, B. C., Lessem, J. M., Hopfer, C. J., Smolen, A., Ehringer, M. A., Timberlake, D., et al. (2005). Monoamine oxidase A (MAOA) and antisocial behaviors in the presence of childhood and adolescent maltreatment. *American Journal of Medical Genetics Part B—Neuropsychiatric Genetics, 135B,* 59–64.

Heils, A., Teufel, A., Petri, S., Seemann, M., Bengel, D., Balling, U., et al. (1995). Functional promoter and polyadenylation site mapping of the human serotonin (5-HT) transporter gene. *Journal of Neural Transmission, 102,* 247–254.

Horwitz, A. V., Widom, C. S., McLaughlin, J., & White, H. R. (2001). The impact of child-hood abuse and neglect on adult mental health: A prospective study. *Journal of Health and Social Behavior*, 42, 184–201.

Huang, Y.-Y., Cate, S. P., Battistuzzi, C., Oquendo, M. A., Brent, D., & Mann, J. J. (2004). An association between a functional polymorphism in the monoamine oxidase A gene promoter, impulsive traits, and early abuse experiences. *Neuropsychopharmacology*, 29, 1498–1505.

Huizinga, D., Haberstick, B. C., Smolen, A., Menard, S., Young, S. E., Corley, R. P., et al. (2006). Childhood maltreatment, subsequent antisocial behavior, and the role of monoamine oxidase A genotype. *Biological Psychiatry*, 60, 677–683.

Jaffee, S. R., Caspi, A., Moffitt, T. E., Dodge, K. A., Rutter, M., Taylor, A., et al. (2005). Nature x nurture: Genetic vulnerabilities interact with child maltreatment to promote conduct problems. *Development and Psychopathology*, 17, 67–84.

Jaffee, S. R., Caspi, A., Moffitt, T. E., & Taylor, A. (2004). Physical maltreatment victim to antisocial child: Evidence of an environmentally mediated process. *Journal of Abnormal Psychology*, 113, 44–55.

Jaffee, S. R., & Gallop, R. (2007). Social, emotional, and academic competence among children who have had contact with Child Protective Services: Prevalence and stability estimates. *Journal of the American Academy of Child & Adolescent Psychiatry*, 46, 757–765.

Jaffee, S. R., & Maikovich-Fong, A. K. (2011). Effects of chronic maltreatment and mal-treatment timing on children's behavior and cognitive abilities. *Journal of Child Psychology and Psychiatry*, 52, 184–194.

Jaffee, S. R., & Price, T. S. (2007). Gene-environment correlations: A review of the evidence and implications for prevention of mental illness. *Molecular Psychiatry*, 12, 432–442.

Jonson-Reid, M., Presnall, N., Drake, B., Fox, L., Bierut, L., Reich, W., et al. (2010). Effects of child maltreatment and inherited liability on antisocial development: An official records study. *Journal of the American Academy of Child and Adolescent Psychiatry*, 49, 321–332.

Kaplan, S. J., Pelcovitz, D., & Labruna, V. (1999). Child and adolescent abuse and neglect research: A review of the past 10 years. Part I: Physical and emotional abuse and neglect. *Journal of the American Academy of Child and Adolescent Psychiatry*, 38, 1214–1222.

Kaufman, J., Yang, B.-Z., Douglas-Palumberi, H., Grasso, D., Lipschitz, D., Houshyar, S., et al. (2006). Brain-derived neurotrophic factor-5-HTTLPR gene interactions and envi-ronmental modifiers of depression in children. *Biological Psychiatry*, 59, 673–680.

Kaufman, J., Yang, B. Z., Douglas-Palumberi, H., Houshyar, S., Lipschitz, D., Krystal, J. H., et al. (2004). Social supports and serotonin transporter gene moderate depres-sion in maltreated children. *Proceedings of the National Academy of Sciences*, 101, 17316–17321.

Kendler, K. S., & Baker, J. H. (2007). Genetic influences on measures of the environment: A systematic review. *Psychological Medicine*, 37, 615–626.

Kendler, K. S., & Eaves, L. J. (1986). Models for the joint effect of genotype and environ-ment on liability to psychiatric illness. *American Journal of Psychiatry*, 143, 279–289.

Kendler, K. S., & Gardner, C. O. (1998). Twin studies of adult psychiatric and substance dependence disorders: Are they biased by differences in the environmental experi-ences of monozygotic and dizygotic twins in childhood and adolescence? *Psychological Medicine*, 28, 625–633.

Kendler, K. S., Neale, M. C., Kessler, R. C., Heath, A. C., & Eaves, L. J. (1994). Parental treatment and the equal environment assumption in twin studies of psychiatric illness. *Psychological Medicine*, 24, 579–590.

Kim-Cohen, J., Caspi, A., Taylor, A., Williams, B., Newcombe, R., Craig, I. W., et al. (2006). MAOA, maltreatment, and gene-environment interaction predicting children's mental health: New evidence and a meta-analysis. *Molecular Psychiatry*, 11, 903–913.

Krueger, R. F., Moffitt, T. E., Caspi, A., Bleske, A., & Silva, P. A. (1998). Assortative mating for antisocial behavior: Developmental and methodological implications. *Behavior Genetics*, 28, 173–186.

Kumsta, R., Stevens, S., Brookes, K., Schlotz, W., Castle, J., Beckett, C., et al. (2010). 5HTT genotype moderates the influence of early institutional deprivation on emotional problems in adolescence: Evidence from the English and Romanian Adoptee (ERA) study. *Journal of Child Psychology and Psychiatry*, 51, 755–762.

Maes, H. H. M., Neale, M. C., Kendler, K. S., Hewitt, J. K., Silberg, J. L., Foley, D. L., et al. (1998). Assortative mating for major psychiatric diagnoses in two population-based samples. *Psychological Medicine*, 28, 1389–1401.

Miller, G. E., & Chen, E. (2010). Harsh family climate in early life presages the emergence of a proinflammatory phenotype in adolescence. *Psychological Science*, 21, 848–856.

Munafo, M. R., Brown, S. M., & Hariri, A. R. (2008). Serotonin transporter (5-HTTLPR) genotype and amygdala activation: A meta-analysis. *Biological Psychiatry*, 63, 852–857.

Munafo, M. R., Durrant, C., Lewis, G., & Flint, J. (2009). Gene x environment interactions at the serotonin transporter locus. *Biological Psychiatry*, 65, 211–219.

Murphy, D. L., & Lesch, K. P. (2008). Targeting the murine serotonin transporter: Insights into human neurobiology. *Nature Reviews Neuroscience*, 9, 85–96.

Nederhof, E., Bouma, E. M. C., Oldehinkel, A. J., & Ormel, J. (2010). Interaction between childhood adversity, brain-derived neurotrophic factor val/met and serotonin transporter promoter polymorphism on depression: The TRAILS study. *Biological Psychiatry*, 68, 209–212.

Nilsson, K. W., Sjoberg, R. L., Damberg, M., Leppert, J., Ohrvik, J., Alm, P. O., et al. (2005). Role of monoamine oxidase A genotype and psychosocial factors in male adolescent criminal activity. *Biological Psychiatry*, 59, 121–127.

Perroud, N., Courtet, P., Vincze, I., Jaussent, I., Jollant, F., Bellivier, F., et al. (2008). Interaction between BDNF Val66Met and childhood trauma on adult's violent suicide attempt. *Genes Brain and Behavior*, 7, 314–322.

Polanczyk, G., Caspi, A., Williams, B., Price, T. S., Danese, A., Sugden, K., et al. (2009). Protective effect of CRHR1 gene variants on the development of adult depression following childhood maltreatment replication and extension. *Archives of General Psychiatry*, 66, 978–985.

Prom-Wormley, E. C., Eaves, L. J., Foley, D. L., Gardner, C. O., Archer, K. J., Wormley, B. K., et al. (2009). Monoamine oxidase A and childhood adversity as risk factors for conduct disorder in females. *Psychological Medicine*, 39, 579–590.

Reif, A., Rosler, M., Freitag, C. M., Schneider, M., Eujen, A., Kissling, C., et al. (2007). Nature and nurture predispose to violent behavior: Serotonergic genes and adverse childhood environment. *Neuropsychopharmacology*, 32, 2375–2383.

Risch, N., Herrell, R., Lehner, T., Liang, K. Y., Eaves, L., Hoh, J., et al. (2009). Interaction between the serotonin transporter gene (5-HTTLPR), stressful life events, and risk of depression: A meta-analysis. *Journal of the American Medical Association*, 301, 2462–2471.

Savitz, J., van der Merwe, L., Newman, T. K., Stein, D. J., & Ramesar, R. (2010). Catechol-o-methyltransferase genotype and childhood trauma may interact to impact schizo-typal personality traits. *Behavior Genetics,* 40, 415–423.

Schmid, B., Blomeyer, D., Treutlein, J., Zimmermann, U. S., Buchmann, A. F., Schmidt, M. H., et al. (2010). Interacting effects of CRHR1 gene and stressful life events on drinking initiation and progression among 19-year-olds. *International Journal of Neuropsychopharmacology,* 13, 703–714.

Schulz-Heik, R. J., Rhee, S. H., Silver, L. E., Haberstick, B. C., Hopfer, C., Lessem, J. M., et al. (2010). The association between conduct problems and maltreatment: Testing genetic and environmental mediation. *Behavior Genetics,* 40, 338–348.

Schulz-Heik, R. J., Rhee, S. H., Silvern, L., Lessem, J. M., Haberstick, B. C., Hopfer, C., et al. (2009). Investigation of genetically mediated child effects on maltreatment. *Behavior Genetics,* 39, 265–276.

Shih, J., & Thompson, R. (1999). Monoamine oxidase in neuropsychiatry and behavior. *American Journal of Human Genetics,* 65, 593–598.

Shih, J. C. (2004). Cloning, after cloning, knock-out mice, and physiological functions of MAO A and B. *Neurotoxicology,* 25, 21–30.

Sjoberg, R. L., Nilsson, K. W., Wargelius, H. L., Leppert, J., Lindstrom, L., & Oreland, L. (2007). Adolescent girls and criminal activity: Role of MAOA-LPR genotype and psychosocial factors. *American Journal of Medical Genetics Part B—Neuropsychiatric Genetics,* 144B, 159–164.

Smith, C., & Thornberry, T. P. (1995). The relationship between childhood maltreatment and adolescent involvement in delinquency. *Criminology,* 33, 451–481.

Stouthamer-Loeber, M., Loeber, R., Homish, D. L., & Wei, E. (2001). Maltreatment of boys and the development of disruptive and delinquent behavior. *Development and Psychopathology,* 13, 941–955.

Surtees, P., Wainwright, N., Willis-Owen, S., Luben, R., Day, N. E., & Flint, J. (2006). Social adversity, the serotonin transporter (5-HTTLPR) polymorphism and major depressive disorder. *Biological Psychiatry,* 59, 224–229.

Taylor, S. E., Way, B. M., Welch, W. T., Hilmert, C. J., Lehman, B. J., & Eisenberger, N. I. (2006). Early family environment, current adversity, the serotonin transporter promoter polymorphism, and depressive symptomatology. *Biological Psychiatry,* 60, 671–676.

Thompson, R., & Wiley, T. R. (2009). Predictors of re-referral to child protective services: A longitudinal follow-up of an urban cohort maltreated as infants. *Child Maltreatment,* 14, 89–99.

Thornberry, T. P., Ireland, T. O., & Smith, C. A. (2001). The importance of timing: The varying impact of childhood and adolescent maltreatment on multiple problem outcomes. *Development and Psychopathology,* 13, 957–979.

Toth, S. L., Manly, J. T., & Cicchetti, D. (1992). Child maltreatment and vulnerability to depression. *Development and Psychopathology,* 4, 97–112.

Uddin, M., Koenen, K. C., de los Santos, R., Bakshis, E., Aiello, A. E., & Galea, S. (2010). Gender differences in the genetic and environmental determinants of adolescent depression. *Depression and Anxiety,* 27, 658–666.

Uher, R. (2011). Gene-environment interactions. In K. S. Kendler, S. R. Jaffee, & D. Romer (Eds.), *The dynamic genome and mental health: The role of genes and environments in youth development* (pp. 29–58). Oxford, UK: Oxford University Press.

Uher, R., & McGuffin, P. (2008). The moderation by the serotonin transporter gene of environmental adversity in the aetiology of mental illness: Review and methodological analysis. *Molecular Psychiatry,* 13, 131–146.

Uher, R., & McGuffin, P. (2010). The moderation by the serotonin transporter gene of environmental adversity in the etiology of depression: 2009 update. *Molecular Psychiatry*, 15, 18–22.

van der Vegt, E. J. M., Oostra, B. A., Rias-Vasquez, A., van der Ende, J., Verhulst, F. C., & Tiemeier, H. (2009). High activity of monoamine oxidase A is associated with external-izing behaviour in maltreated and nonmaltreated adoptees. *Psychiatric Genetics*, 19, 209–211.

Visscher, P. M., Medland, S. E., Ferreira, M. A. R., Morley, K. I., Zhu, G., Cornes, B. K., et al. (2006). Assumption-free estimation of heritability from genome-wide identity-by-descent sharing between full siblings. *PLoS Genetics*, 2, 316–325.

Walsh, C., McMillan, H., & Jamieson, E. (2002). The relationship between parental psy-chiatric disorder and child physical and sexual abuse: Findings from the Ontario Health Supplement. *Child Abuse and Neglect*, 26, 11–22.

Weder, N., Yang, B. Z., Douglas-Palumberi, H., Massey, J., Krystal, J. H., Gelernter, J., et al. (2009). MAOA genotype, maltreatment, and aggressive behavior: The changing impact of genotype at varying levels of trauma. *Biological Psychiatry*, 65, 417–424.

Wichers, M., Kenis, G., Jacobs, N., Mengelers, R., Derom, C., Vlietinck, R., et al. (2008). The BDNF Val(66)Met x 5-HTTLPR x child adversity interaction and depressive symp-toms: An attempt at replication. *American Journal of Medical Genetics Part B: Neuropsychiatric Genetics*, 147, 120–123.

Widom, C. S. (1989). The cycle of violence. *Science*, 244, 160–166.

Widom, C. S., & Brzustowicz, L. M. (2006). MAOA and the "cycle of violence:" Childhood abuse and neglect, MAOA genotype, and risk for violent and antisocial behavior. *Biological Psychiatry*, 60, 684–689.

Widom, C. S., Czaja, S. J., & Paris, J. (2009). A prospective investigation of borderline personality disorder in abused and neglected children followed up into adulthood. *Journal of Personality Disorders*, 23, 433–446.

Widom, C. S., & Kuhns, J. B. (1996). Childhood victimization and subsequent risk for promiscuity, prostitution, and teenage pregnancy: A prospective study. *American Journal of Public Health*, 86, 1607–1612.

Widom, C. S., & Morris, S. (1997). Accuracy of adult recollections of childhood victimiza-tion: Part 2. Childhood sexual abuse. *Psychological Assessment*, 9, 34–46.

Widom, C. S., & Shepard, R. L. (1996). Accuracy of adult recollections of childhood vic-timization: Part 1. Childhood physical abuse. *Psychological Assessment*, 8, 412–421.

Widom, C. S., & White, H. R. (1997). Problem behaviours in abused and neglected chil-dren grown up: Prevalence and co-occurrence of substance abuse, crime and violence. *Criminal Behaviour and Mental Health*, 7, 287–310.

Young, S. E., Smolen, A., Hewitt, J. K., Haberstick, B. C., Stallings, M. C., Corley, R. P., et al. (2006). Interaction between MAO-A genotype and maltreatment in the risk for conduct disorder: Failure to confirm in adolescent patients. *American Journal of Psychiatry*, 163, 1019–1025.

PART III

Trauma in Childhood and Risk of Psychopathology and Violence

4

The Intergenerational Transmission of Family Violence

The Neurobiology of the Relationships among Child Victimization, Parental Mental Health, and Addiction

MICHAEL D. DE BELLIS

Maltreatment in Childhood and the Intergenerational Cycle of Violence

Child victimization includes child maltreatment, which is defined by law as neglect, physical abuse, sexual abuse, and emotional or psychological abuse. In 2009, 3.3 million children nationally were referred for investigation to Child Protective Services (U.S. Department of Health and Human Services, 2010). Of these cases, about two-thirds were investigated, and only 0.1% were identified as intentionally false. Neglect, defined as a failure to supervise or provide, continues to be the most common form of maltreatment. Although child maltreatment rates have been stable, child death rates due to neglect or physical abuse have been rising since 2005, to 1,770 in 2009 (U.S. Department of Health and Human Services, 2010). Of these deaths, about 80% were of children younger than 4 years of age. It should be noted that investigated cases have behavioral and developmental outcomes just as poor as those deemed to not have enough evidence to be substantiated (Hussey et al., 2005; Leiter, Myers, & Zingraff, 1994). A lack of available government services might contribute to the proportion of cases that are not investigated.

Children who are victims of maltreatment commonly experience chronic and multiple forms of abuse and neglect (Kaufman, Jones, Stieglitz, Vitulano, & Mannarino, 1994; Levy, Markovic, Chaudry, Ahart, & Torres, 1995; McGee, Wolfe, Yuen, Wilson, & Carnochan, 1995; Widom, 1989). In our studies of neglected children, in which detailed interviews regarding a variety of life events were conducted, almost all children reported for neglect identified repeated experiences of witnessing family violence and related post-traumatic stress symptoms (De Bellis, Hooper, Spratt, & Woolley, 2009). Child maltreatment continues to be the single most preventable cause of mental illness.

In order to break the intergenerational cycle of child abuse and neglect, it is important to identify the role parental mental health and parental maltreatment histories play in child victimization and to address these illnesses before an individual becomes a parent. Although there has been little empirical work done on parental mental health and maltreatment, one study suggested that mothers of maltreated children have lifetime histories of the comorbidity of two or more nonpsychotic psychiatric disorders including post-traumatic stress disorder (PTSD), dysthymia, major depression, and substance abuse or dependence (including alcoholism) and histories of suicide attempts compared to a sociodemographically similar comparison group of mothers (De Bellis, Broussard, Wexler, Herring, & Moritz, 2001). In this study, mothers of maltreated children had a lifetime relative risk of 3.01 for any mood disorders, 1.90 for any anxiety disorder, and 1.79 for any substance abuse or dependence, and relative risk of 2.62 and 2.57 for two and for three or more lifetime disorders, respectively, compared to the general female population, whereas male role models had a relative risk of 2.40 for any substance abuse or dependence compared to the general male population (De Bellis, Broussard, et al., 2001). Other studies have also demonstrated increased psychopathology in maltreating parents (Famularo, Fenton, & Kinscherff, 1993; Famularo, Kinscherff, & Fenton, 1992; Kaufman et al., 1998). Almost half of child onset mental disorders and one-third of adult onset mental disorders are preceded by child maltreatment and family dysfunction (Green et al., 2010). Although the mental disorders found in maltreating parents are serious, they are thought to be amenable to prevention and treatment.

Child maltreatment prevention programs such as home visiting (Mikton & Butchart, 2009), particularly during an expectant mother's first pregnancy, address these and other issues of high-risk new mothers. For example, home visiting of an expectant mother by nurses for low-income, at-risk families has been promoted as a promising strategy for preventing child abuse and neglect (Kitzman et al., 1997; Olds et al., 1997). Several studies of this Nurse-Family Partnership Program have demonstrated the following: (1) improved grade-point averages and achievement test scores in math and reading in grades 1 through 3 in children during their age 9 follow-up assessment (Olds et al., 2007); (2) decreased mood and anxiety symptoms and decreased rates of tobacco, alcohol, and marijuana use, along with improved reading and math scores at age 12 follow-up assessment (Kitzman et al., 2010); and (3) decreased antisocial behaviors at age 19 follow-up assessment (Eckenrode et al., 2010). However, when a parent becomes maltreating, even an intensive program of home visitation by nurses in addition to standard treatment is not enough to prevent the recurrence of physical abuse and neglect (MacMillan et al., 2005). Maltreated children in foster care showed higher grades and less self-destructive behavior, substance use, and total risk behavior problem standardized scores than maltreated children who were reunified with their biological families when interviewed during their sixth-year follow-up (Taussig, Clyman, & Landsverk, 2001). These studies indicate that there are two opportunities to break the cycle of maltreatment. The first opportunity is during the expectant parent's first pregnancy, to avoid the neurobiological consequences of childhood maltreatment (De Bellis, 2001b; Heim & Nemeroff, 2001; Kaufman & Charney, 2001). These types of early prevention programs are cost effective (Foster, Prinz, Sanders, & Shapiro, 2008). However, if this cannot be done, the second opportunity is to treat victims of maltreatment after the fact. In order to do this, we need to understand the neurobiological consequences of chronic stress on a child's developing brain and body, so we can treat the adverse medical and mental health outcomes of early life stress (Felitti et al., 1998).

In this critical review, we consider childhood maltreatment as a form of violence that affects the development of the biological stress systems of the body and brain and leads to serious mental illness, particularly depression and addictions. These changes to the biological stress systems increase the risk that an untreated formerly victimized first-time parent will maltreat his or her child by increasing his or her risk for mental illness, particularly depression and addictions, thus perpetuating an intergenerational cycle of maltreatment. In recent years, the effects of genetics (i.e., having a specific polymorphism) and adverse environments have revolutionized the genetic (G) versus environment (E) issue. Studies show that individuals with certain polymorphisms are more likely to have depression (Caspi, Hariri, Holmes, Uher, & Moffitt, 2010) or addiction (Agrawal & Lynskey, 2009; Enoch et al., 2010; Xie et al., 2009) if they grow up in adversity. However, understanding the neurobiological effects of maltreatment (e.g., the "E" in the G×E interaction), and how these effects can increase the risk of parental mental illness, will inform the field on how best to decrease the individual and societal burden of maltreatment, because having a specific genetic polymorphism alone does not cause maltreatment, its consequences (Risch et al., 2009), and/or the intergenerational cycle of violence. This understanding is the mission of the field of developmental traumatology, which is in its infancy.

The Effects of the Chronic Stress of Child Maltreatment during Development

The first major principle of developmental traumatology is that although there are an infinite number of stressors that can cause a subjective sense of overwhelming stress and distress, there are finite ways in which the brain and the body (i.e., biological stress systems) can respond (for a review, see De Bellis [2001b]). The second principle, illustrated in Figure 4.1, involves the nature of the chronic stressors, which are dysfunctional and traumatized interpersonal relationships. Child maltreatment is chronic, and victims usually experience multiple forms of abuse or chronic interpersonal stress long before a first report is made to Child Protective Services. Child maltreatment is associated with high rates of PTSD. The diagnosis of PTSD is made after a person experiences a *Diagnostic and Statistical Manual of Mental Disorders, Fourth Edition* (*DSM-IV*) type A life-threatening traumatic event and reacts with fear or disorganized behavior, followed by three categorical clusters of symptoms that persist for at least one month: Cluster B, intrusive reexperiencing of the trauma(s); Cluster C, persistent avoidance of stimuli associated with the trauma(s) or numbing of responsiveness; and Cluster D, persistent symptoms of increased physiological arousal (American Psychiatric Association, 2000).

PTSD prevalence rates in maltreated children are high (Copeland, Keeler, Angold, & Costello, 2007). Neglect is the most common reason for Child Protective

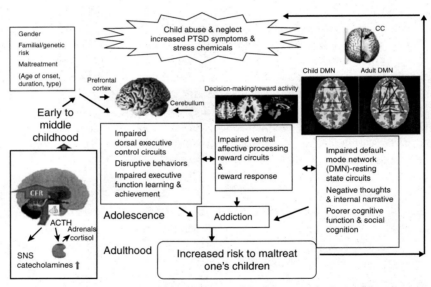

Figure 4.1 The developmental traumatology model of the neurobiology of the intergenerational transmission of child abuse and neglect. In this model, child maltreatment increases baseline levels of stress chemicals (e.g., cortisol from the hypothalamic-pituitary-adrenal [HPA] axis and catecholamines from the locus coeruleus and sympathetic nervous system [SNS]), which in turn adversely affects the development of prefrontal and cerebellar executive brain circuits, leading to immaturity of control and reward inhibitory brain regions, and disrupting the development of the brain default mode network (DMN). The DMN is connected through myelinated circuits in the corpus callosum (CC). These adverse effects lead to psychopathology (e.g., anxiety, depression, PTSD symptoms) and addiction. Parental psychopathology and addiction, in turn, lead to the intergenerational transmission of child maltreatment. (See color insert.)

Services involvement. Preclinical studies strongly suggest that childhood neglect is experienced by a human child, a member of a social species, as traumatic, causing anxiety and dysregulation of biological stress systems and leading to adverse brain development (De Bellis, 2005; Fries, Shirtcliff, & Pollak, 2008). Domestic violence is commonly witnessed by neglected children (Burns et al., 2004; De Bellis et al., 2009). Children who witness intimate partner violence have high rates of PTSD (Pynoos & Eth, 1985). PTSD prevalence rates in abused children are high; 40% to 60% of non–clinically referred sexually abused children have PTSD in the two months following abuse disclosure (Famularo et al., 1993; McLeer et al., 1998). Follow-up studies revealed that many of these children continue to have chronic PTSD (Famularo, Fenton, Augustyn, & Zuckerman, 1996). Physical abuse is associated with rates of PTSD as high as 50% (Dubner & Motta, 1999; Green, 1985). Finally, child maltreatment increases risk for mood disorders, anxiety, and later onset addictions (Clark, Lesnick, & Hegedus, 1997; Clark et al., 1997; De Bellis, 2001a).

Traumatic experiences engender fear. Fearful stimuli and traumatic reminders are processed through the brain's thalamus, activating the amygdala, a brain structure that is part of the fear-detection circuit. Projections from the amygdala then transmit fear signals to connections in the prefrontal cortex, the paraventricular nucleus of the hypothalamus, and the locus coeruleus in the brainstem (for a review, see De Bellis [2003]). Intense fear or anxiety activates the locus coeruleus, an ancient structure that indirectly activates the sympathetic nervous system, leading to the biologic changes of the "fight-or-flight or freeze reaction." Effects of this activation include increases in catecholamine turnover in the brain, the sympathetic nervous system, and the adrenal medulla. The adrenals, endocrine glands located above the kidneys, secrete the stress hormones cortisol and epinephrine. This fight-or-flight or freeze reaction, caused by elevated levels of epinephrine and sympathetic nervous system activity, increases heart rate, blood pressure, metabolic rate, and alertness. These changes prepare the body to fight, run, or in some other way protect itself from ancient enemies (e.g., snakes, lions). This sequence of events results in tachycardia, hypertension, increased metabolic rate, hypervigilance, and increased levels of stress chemicals including catecholamines. Catecholamines contribute to dilation of the pupils, diaphoresis, renal inhibition, and decreases in peripheral blood flow. Activation of the biological stress system results in behaviors consistent with anxiety, hyperarousal, and hypervigilance, which are the core symptoms of PTSD. These stress chemicals impair the brain's prefrontal cortex and executive functions (Arnsten, 1998).

Prolonged exposure to stress leads individuals to display increased stress levels at rest and enhanced stress responsiveness. Maltreated children with and without PTSD show greater levels of catecholamines at baseline than nonmaltreated children (De Bellis, Baum, et al., 1999; De Bellis, Lefter, Trickett, & Putnam, 1994).

Thus chronic activity of the biological stress response is characterized by elevations in catecholamine levels. Higher than expected levels of catecholamines not only cause PTSD and anxiety, but also can lead to medical problems such as hypertension, cardiovascular disease (Dong et al., 2004), and immune dysregulation (De Bellis, Burke, Trickett, & Putnam, 1996; Dube et al., 2009; Shirtcliff, Coe, & Pollak, 2009).

Stress is associated with elevated levels of corticotrophin-releasing hormone (CRH) or factor (CRF) from the paraventricular nucleus of the hypothalamus (Chrousos & Gold, 1992). CRH and CRF are two terms for a single hypothalamic peptide that is a major regulator of mammalian stress response systems. During prolonged stressful events, CRF levels are raised. CRF forms the central component of the limbic hypothalamic-pituitary-adrenal axis, a major neuroendocrine stress response system. CRF is released into the hypothalamic hypophysial portal circulation and to the anterior pituitary, where it binds to CRF receptors, stimulating the production/release of adrenocorticotropin (ACTH). ACTH stimulates the secretion of cortisol from the adrenal cortex. Cortisol triggers a wide range of metabolic and immune-modulating effects in the fight, flight, or freeze reaction and is counter-regulated by negative feedback at the pituitary and hypothalamus (for reviews see De Bellis, 2001b; Heim & Nemeroff, 2001; Kaufman & Charney, 2001). CRF cell bodies and receptors are located in the amygdala and throughout the brain and are also responsible for increasing arousal.

Maltreated children with mood and anxiety symptoms show evidence of hypothalamic-pituitary-adrenal axis dysregulation (De Bellis, Baum, et al., 1999; De Bellis, Chrousos, et al., 1994; De Bellis, Lefter, et al., 1994; Hart, Gunnar, & Cicchetti, 1996; Kaufman, 1991; Kaufman et al., 1997). Baseline cortisol measures taken at home well after maltreatment disclosure and interventions show that maltreated children with PTSD had greater baseline 24-hour urinary cortisol levels than controls (De Bellis, Baum, et al., 1999), suggesting elevations of the body's major stress systems in childhood PTSD. Measures of 24-hour urinary cortisol levels are positively correlated with abuse duration and PTSD symptoms. Diurnal salivary cortisol levels are higher in maltreated children with PTSD and subclinical PTSD (Carrion, Weems, Ray, Glaser, et al., 2002). Elevated salivary cortisol levels were seen in 6- to 12-year-old children raised in Romanian orphanages for more than the first 8 months of their lives as compared to children who were adopted at an earlier age (Gunnar, Morison, Chisholm, & Schuder, 2001). It should be noted that both children who meet the criteria for *DSM-IV* PTSD and those who are not eligible for the diagnosis because they have fewer PTSD symptoms are equally impaired and distressed (Carrion, Weems, Ray, & Reiss, 2002). This work and the work of Scheeringa and colleagues suggests that the *DSM-IV* diagnosis for children might not be developmentally sensitive (Scheeringa, Zeanah, Myers, & Putnam, 2005).

Studies of hypothalamic-pituitary-adrenal axis challenge in maltreated children with depression or in adults with histories of maltreatment have not been consistent, with some studies showing greater cortisol or ACTH reactivity (Heim et al., 2000; Heim et al., 2002; Kaufman et al., 1997) and some showing no differences in cortisol but lower ACTH responses (De Bellis, Chrousos, et al., 1994; MacMillan et al., 2009). However, these studies are consistent with an interpretation of elevated baseline CRF in children and adults as a result of the chronic early life stress of child maltreatment. Lower ACTH levels than in controls likely result from a biological adaptation to chronically higher CRF (i.e., enhanced negative feedback inhibition of ACTH and thus cortisol) (De Bellis, Chrousos, et al., 1994). Adults with PTSD (Baker et al., 1999; Bremner et al., 1997) and adults with histories of abuse and current depression (Heim et al., 2002; Stein, Yehuda, Koverola, & Hanna, 1997) show evidence of higher brain concentrations of CRF. Indeed, in a unique longitudinal study, sexually abused girls demonstrated higher cortisol levels during childhood but lower levels as adults than their nonabused controls (Trickett, Noll, Susman, Shenk, & Putnam, 2010), suggesting developmental alterations to the ACTH response resulting from permanently high baseline levels of CRF in childhood due to chronic sexual abuse. Even though these women with a history of sexual abuse had mood and anxiety symptoms but not PTSD, their lower cortisol levels were similar to those reported in other studies of male and female adult patients with PTSD (Yehuda, 2009).

In summary, maltreatment and maltreatment-related PTSD might cause elevated central CRF levels, which lead to an increased risk for adolescent and later adult depressive and anxiety disorders. Chronic or excessive exposure to stress such as child abuse can lead to dysregulation of stress response systems (De Bellis, Baum, et al., 1999), increased risk for depression (Kaufman & Charney, 2001), and adverse brain development (De Bellis & Keshavan, 2003; De Bellis, Keshavan, et al., 1999; De Bellis, Keshavan, & Frustaci, 2002; De Bellis & Kuchibhatla, 2006). Adverse brain development likely leads to addictions and psychopathologies that are commonly seen in maltreating parents.

Child Maltreatment: Effects on the Developing Brain

Human brain development is marked by the acquisition of progressive skills in physical, behavioral, cognitive, and emotional domains. Myelination of newly formed neuronal networks parallels these changes. Myelin, a fatty white substance produced by supportive glial cells, is a vital component of the brain. Myelin encases the axons of neurons, forming an insulator, the myelin sheath, which is responsible for the color of white matter. Brain development occurs with an overproduction of neurons in utero and increases in synaptic neuropil (neuron size and synapses or neural connections) during childhood and during adolescence; the selective elimination of some neurons (apoptosis), with corresponding decreases in some connections and strengthening of others and corresponding increases in myelination, hastens these connections. Synapses, dendrites, cell bodies, and unmyelinated axons, which form the brain's gray matter, decrease during development (for a review, see Paus [2005]).

The advent of magnetic resonance imaging (MRI) has provided a revolutionary and safe approach for measuring brain maturation. Cross-sectional and longitudinal MRI studies of high-functioning healthy children and adolescents have greatly advanced our knowledge of human brain development and allowed investigators to examine these maturational changes (for a review, see Durston et al. [2001]). Cortical myelination, the growth of white matter, can be easily examined through MRI-based morphometry of cerebral white matter volume and the midsagittal area of the corpus callosum, a white matter structure comprising axons that connects major subdivisions of the left and right cerebral hemispheres. There are regionally specific nonlinear preadolescent increases, followed by postadolescent decreases, in cortical gray matter (Giedd, Blumenthal, Jeffries, Castellanos, et al., 1999; Thompson et al., 2000). The most dramatic increase in myelination takes place in the corpus callosum and peaks in early childhood but continues linearly into young adulthood (Giedd, Blumenthal, Jeffries, Rajapakse, et al., 1999). The prefrontal gyri, which subserve executive and inhibitory cognitive and resting state functions and regulate the stress response, continue their development into young adulthood (Shaw et al., 2008).

During brain maturation, stress and elevated levels of stress hormones and neurotransmitters can lead to adverse brain development through the mechanisms of accelerated loss (metabolism or apoptosis) of neurons (Edwards, Harkins, Wright, & Menn, 1990; Sapolsky, Uno, Rebert, & Finch, 1990; Simantov et al., 1996), delays in myelination (Dunlop, Archer, Quinlivan, Beazley, & Newnham, 1997), abnormalities in developmentally appropriate pruning (Lauder, 1988; Todd, 1992), the inhibition of neurogenesis (Gould, McEwen, Tanapat, Galea, & Fuchs, 1997; Gould, Tanapat, & Cameron, 1997; Gould, Tanapat, McEwen, Flugge, & Fuchs, 1998), or a stress-induced decrease in brain growth factors (e.g. brain-derived neurotrophic factor) (Pizarro et al., 2004). In fact, maternal deprivation increases the death of infant rat brain cells (Zhang et al., 2002). Consequently, dysregulation of a maltreated child's major stress systems likely contributes to adverse brain development and leads to psychopathology (De Bellis, Keshavan, et al., 1999).

Sex hormones influence neurodevelopment throughout the life span (for a review, see McEwen, DeKloet, and Rostene [1986]). In one pediatric neuroimaging study, boys showed a significantly greater loss of gray matter volume and an increase in both white matter volume and corpus callosum area as compared to girls over a similar age range, suggesting sex differences in the maturational processes of both cerebral gray and white matter in childhood (De Bellis, Keshavan et al. 2001). Maltreated males might be more vulnerable to the adverse psychosocial (McGloin & Widom, 2001) and neurobiological (De Bellis & Keshavan, 2003) consequences of maltreatment.

In adults, executive control functions, reward circuits, and default network (or resting state) activity are dysregulated in PTSD and in substance abuse and dependence. In animal models, trauma during development decreases the number of dopamine D2 receptors in the nucleus accumbens and ventral medial prefrontal cortex, brain regions that process reward (Morgan et al., 2002; Papp, Klimek, & Willner, 1994). Adults with child abuse histories had reduced activation in reward regions during a reward task (Dillon et al., 2009). Resting state dysregulation is seen in adult PTSD related to past child abuse (Bluhm et al., 2009; Daniels, Frewen, McKinnon, & Lanius, 2011; Lanius et al., 2010) and substance abuse and dependence (Roberts & Garavan, 2010).

It is not known, but it is highly likely, that preexisting vulnerability to addiction involves dysregulation of control, reward, and resting state circuits related to child trauma, because these systems actively mature during childhood and adolescence (Bjork et al., 2004; Ernst et al., 2005; Fair et al., 2008). Understanding these neurobiological mechanisms might lead to primary prevention of mental disorders and addiction in those maltreated children at risk for continuing the cycle of violence, and this is an important area for future investigations. We now address the association between maltreatment and addiction, the neurobiology of addiction, and the default node network, with emphasis on the brain regions affected by chronic stress.

Child Maltreatment History and Addiction in Adolescence

Studies of adolescents suffering from cannabis and alcohol abuse and dependence show that these individuals have high rates of childhood trauma and PTSD symptoms prior to their alcohol and substance problems (Clark, Lesnick, et al., 1997; Clark, Pollock, et al., 1997; De Bellis, 2001a; Dube et al., 2006; Moran, Vuchinich, & Hall, 2004). In a large cross-sectional survey, Kilpatrick et al. (2000) reported that physical abuse increased the odds ratio (OR) for alcohol and marijuana abuse/dependence to 3.93 and 4.84, respectively; witnessing violence resulted in an OR = 4.87 for alcohol and 8.42 for marijuana, and sexual abuse yielded an OR = 4.55 for alcohol and 8.42 for marijuana. Having adolescent PTSD increases the risk for adolescent substance abuse and dependence (OR = 3.98 for alcohol and 6.17 for marijuana) (Kilpatrick et al., 2000).

In a unique longitudinal study, court-identified abused and neglected children (onset: 0 to 11 years of age) were closely matched with non–court identified nonmaltreated children and followed prospectively in order to assess drug abuse in young adulthood (Widom, Weiler, & Cottler, 1999). In this study, more maltreated children had a current drug abuse diagnosis at young adult follow-up, but the relationship was not significant after Bonferroni correction. However, there was causal evidence for the development of alcohol abuse in maltreated females in this young adult sample (Schuck & Widom, 2001). In another study that followed this sample to middle adulthood, significant gender differences demonstrated that maltreated females had a higher risk of illicit drug abuse through other maltreatment-related behavioral problems (prostitution, homelessness, antisocial behavior, and history of school problems) (Wilson & Widom, 2009).

Adolescents with substance abuse or dependence are at increased risk of having teenage pregnancies and risky health behaviors (Dong et al., 2005). Their offspring are at risk of prenatal substance exposure and its adverse neurobiological consequences (Albrecht et al., 1999; De Genna, Cornelius, & Donovan, 2009; Liu et al., 2009). Cross-sectional studies have repeatedly demonstrated increased histories of child abuse and neglect in adults with a variety of substance abuse or dependence disorders. In community adult samples, sexual abuse histories are associated with increased alcohol consumption (Widom, Ireland, & Glynn, 1995; Wilsnack, Vogeltanz, Klassen, & Harris, 1997). Childhood maltreatment was found to moderate the relationship between parental alcoholism and young adult alcoholism in offspring (Sher, Gershuny, Peterson, & Raskin, 1997). A large health maintenance organization sample found that adults with a history of adverse childhood experiences had an increased incidence of alcohol and substance use disorders (Felitti et al., 1998). In female twin pairs discordant for sexual abuse, the twin exposed to sexual abuse was found to have a substantially increased risk of developing alcohol and other drug dependence (Kendler et al., 2000). These results led the authors to state that childhood sexual abuse is causally related to an increased risk for adult psychiatric and alcohol and substance abuse disorders.

However, there are no published neurobiological studies to date that directly assess maltreatment in childhood and follow these children into adolescence in order to prospectively determine their neurobiological risk for substance abuse or dependence. This is an area in need of future research studies that might shed some light on the differences between the prospective and retrospective findings in the field.

The Neurobiology of Reward Circuits and Addiction

Volkow et al. proposed a model of the addicted brain based on primate and human imaging research (Volkow, Fowler, & Wang, 2003). This model proposes a network of four circuits: (1) the reward circuit, located in the nucleus accumbens and the ventral pallidum; (2) the motivation circuit, located in the orbitofrontal cortex, the amygdala, and the subcallosal cortex; (3) the memory and learning circuit, located in the amygdala and the hippocampus; and (4) the executive or control circuit, located in the prefrontal cortex. These four circuits receive direct innervations from dopaminergic neurons but also are connected with one another through direct or indirect projections (e.g., glutamatergic and serotonergic neurons) (Volkow et al., 2003). Control brain regions can be inhibitory in that their activation inhibits the more primitive brain subcortical regions that are responsible for arousal and impulsive behaviors (e.g., amygdala). It is important to note that in the complex human brain, other brain regions are involved in each of these circuits, and one brain region might participate in more than one circuit.

Each circuit is currently being studied extensively. The human reward circuit, originating in the midbrain, provides dopaminergic inputs to the ventral striatum (which includes the nucleus accumbens) and the ventromedial prefrontal cortex (Schott et al., 2008). In imaging studies of primates and humans, the experience of reward versus no reward elicits activations in brain regions typically implicated in decision and reward processing (i.e., the anterior cingulate, inferior frontal gyrus, middle frontal gyrus, insular, putamen, and ventral striatum) (Apicella, Ljungberg, Scarnati, & Schultz, 1991; Delgado, Locke, Stenger, & Fiez, 2003; Elliott, Newman, Longe, & Deakin, 2003; O'Doherty, Kringelbach, Rolls, Hornak, & Andrews, 2001; Roesch & Olson, 2004; Schultz, Tremblay, & Hollerman, 2000). The orbitofrontal cortex is involved in processing the individual need of the stimulus for the specific reward (Rolls, 2000; Schultz et al., 2000).

The second circuit, the motivation circuit, is located in the orbitofrontal cortex, the amygdala, and the subcallosal cortex. Volkow et al. (2003) hypothesize that the perceived value of a drug as a reinforcer is so much greater than that of any natural reinforcer (e.g., bonding with one's child) that natural reinforcers can no longer compete as viable alternative choices. The orbitofrontal cortex evaluates the value of the need for a specific reward (e.g., a social need for reassurance versus an alcoholic drink during stressful social situations). The orbitofrontal cortex is hypoactive in individuals with addictions during withdrawal and sobriety (Adinoff et al., 2001; Volkow et al., 1992). In these individuals, the decreased activity in the orbitofrontal cortex is associated with reductions in the numbers of DA D2 receptors in striatum (Volkow et al., 1993, 2001). Furthermore, the orbitofrontal cortex and amygdala are active during exposure to drug-related cues and cravings (Bechara, 2005; Volkow & Fowler, 2000). The orbitofrontal cortex is not only involved in reward value. It is less active when individuals, particularly adolescents, are motivated to take greater risks for higher reward values (Eshel, Nelson, Blair, Pine, & Ernst, 2007). It is involved in decision making, response inhibition of impulsive behaviors, and cognitive flexibility (Schoenbaum & Roesch, 2005; Walton, Devlin, & Rushworth, 2004). The orbitofrontal cortex is smaller in individuals with nicotine dependence

(Kühn, Schubert, & Gallinat, 2010), cocaine dependence (Franklin et al., 2002), alcoholism, and polysubstance abuse (Tanabe et al., 2009).

The third circuit, the memory and learning circuit, is located in the amygdala and the hippocampus. The hippocampus places a memory in its context, and the amygdala attaches the emotion of "getting high" or temporarily feeling better to the memory. Multiple memory systems have been proposed in drug addiction (see White [1996] for a review). These include conditioned-incentive learning (mediated in part by the nucleus accumbens and the amygdala), in which a neutral stimulus, coupled with the drug of abuse, acquires reinforcing properties and motivational importance even in the absence of the drug; habit learning (mediated in part by the striatum [also called the caudate and the putamen]), in which well-learned sequences of behaviors are elicited automatically by a stimulus such as stress; and declarative memory (mediated in part by the hippocampus), in which one learns to improve affective states by abusing the drug of addiction. These complex memory circuits are intimately involved in decision and reward circuits and in the brain default mode network. Memory circuits are active during drug intoxication (Volkow, Fowler, & Wang, 2002) and drug craving (Bechara, 2005; Kilts et al., 2001; Wang et al., 1999). One brain area that has been intensely studied in trauma is the hippocampus, because it is sensitive to stress-related glucocorticoid damage (Sapolsky et al., 1990). We discuss how stress affects the brain regions involved in depressed mood and addictions later.

Last, and most important to drug addiction and many psychiatric disorders, is dysfunction of the executive or control circuits located in the prefrontal cortex, including the anterior cingulate gyrus (Volkow et al., 2003) and dorsolateral prefrontal cortex. These brain regions of interest are involved in decision making and in inhibitory executive control, and dysregulation can result in disruptions in self-monitoring and decision-making behaviors, which are executive functions (Bechara, 2005). Impaired executive control might lead an addicted individual (e.g., a parent) to take a drug even when he or she expresses the desire to refrain from taking the drug (Goldstein & Volkow, 2002). Executive functions are impaired in addicted individuals (Crews, He, & Hodge, 2007). These functions develop during childhood and adolescence (Blakemore & Choudhury, 2006) and are also impaired in maltreated children who do not suffer from addictions (Beers & De Bellis, 2002; De Bellis et al., 2009; Pollak et al., 2010).

The Neurobiology of the Brain Default Mode Network or Resting State

The brain default mode network or resting state includes dorsal and ventral structures and exhibits correlated low-frequency activity at rest when individuals generate internal thoughts but decreased activity during social cognition

(Gobbini, Koralek, Bryan, Montgomery, & Haxby, 2007; Mitchell, 2006) or engagement in an active task (Eichele et al., 2008; Fox et al., 2005; Fransson, 2005, 2006; Raichle et al., 2001). The default mode network has also been called the network of self-narrative or of the social brain; it is the circuit that is responsible for perspective-taking of the desires, beliefs, and intentions of others and for remembering the past, as well as planning for the future (Buckner, Andrews-Hanna, & Schacter, 2008; Raichle & Snyder, 2007). The default mode network includes the executive systems: the dorsal lateral prefrontal cortex, dorsal anterior cingulate, intraparietal sulcus, supramarginal and temporal gyrus, and related subcortical structures (e.g., basal ganglia, amygdala, hippocampus, and thalamus). Its ventral structures include the emotional circuits that process emotional stimuli and mediate stress and reward responses. They are complexly connected systems with the dorsal structures and include ventral structures such as the amygdala, orbitofrontal cortex, ventral medial prefrontal cortex, hypothalamus, and other subcortical regions.

During infancy and early childhood, the default mode network is connected laterally to anatomically homologous areas (Fair et al., 2008; Fransson et al., 2007), and it further integrates during optimal developmental periods of myelination in frontal to posterior brain regions both within and between hemispheres from age 9 to 16 years (Fair et al., 2008). During adolescence, white matter is increasing and the corpus callosum, the major area of hemispheric integration, is maturing. This is a neurodevelopmentally sensitive time for the effects of child maltreatment (see Fig. 4.1). Abnormal brain default mode network connectivity is associated with self-directed negative thoughts and impaired executive function. Abnormal default mode network functional connectivity is associated with depression (Greicius et al., 2007; Grimm et al., 2009; Sheline et al., 2009; Sheline, Price, Yan, & Mintun, 2010; Yao, Wang, Lu, Liu, & Teng, 2009), anxiety (Gentili et al., 2009; Liao et al., 2010; Zhao et al., 2007), and trauma history and PTSD (Bluhm et al., 2009; Broyd et al., 2009; Lanius et al., 2010). Abnormal functional connectivity is seen in decision-making and reward and resting state circuits in nicotine dependence (Hahn et al., 2007) and in abstinent individuals with histories of substance use disorders such as alcoholism (Park et al., 2010) and cannabis (Cornelius, Aizenstein, & Hariri, 2010; Hester, Nestor, & Garavan, 2009; Roberts & Garavan, 2010), heroin (Ma et al., 2010), stimulant (Tomasi et al., 2009), and cocaine (Kelly et al., 2011) dependence. Most important, resting state connectivity develops over the first 16 years of life (Fair et al., 2008), and the severe and chronic stress of maltreatment likely impairs the brain default mode network functional connectivity in vulnerable individuals, leading to mental illness, including comorbid disorders such as depression and anxiety, which the individual then self-medicates with addiction.

Based on the description of the neurobiology of the reward system above, there is important overlap between the developing reward system and the development of the default mode network. We now review the evidence suggesting that reward and default mode network brain regions are damaged in maltreated children who do not yet suffer from addictions.

The Neurobiological Consequences of Maltreatment in the Brain's Executive and Reward Circuits and Brain Default Mode Network or Resting State: Implications for Addiction and the Cycle of Violence

Pediatric research studies from different laboratories show that both cerebral and cerebellar volumes are smaller in abused and neglected children than in nonmaltreated children (Bauer, Hanson, Pierson, Davidson, & Pollak, 2009; Carrion et al., 2001; De Bellis & Kuchibhatla, 2006; De Bellis, Keshavan, et al., 1999; De Bellis, Keshavan, Shifflett, et al., 2002). In one study, 43 maltreated children and adolescents with maltreatment-related PTSD and 61 nonmaltreated controls underwent comprehensive clinical assessments and an anatomical MRI brain scan (De Bellis, Keshavan, et al., 1999). Maltreated subjects with PTSD had 7.0% smaller intracranial and 8.0% smaller cerebral volumes than nonmaltreated children. The total midsagittal area of the corpus callosum—the major interconnection between the two hemispheres, which is broadly conceptualized as facilitating intercortical communication and the default mode network—was smaller in maltreated children. Intracranial volume robustly correlated positively with age of onset of PTSD trauma (i.e., smaller cerebral volumes were associated with earlier onset of trauma) and negatively with duration of abuse.

The positive correlation of intracranial volumes with age of onset of PTSD trauma suggests that traumatic stress is associated with disproportionately negative consequences if it occurs during early childhood. The negative correlation of intracranial volumes with abuse duration suggests that childhood maltreatment experiences have global and adverse influences on brain development that might be cumulative. Symptoms of intrusive thoughts, avoidance, hyperarousal, and dissociation correlated negatively with intracranial volume and total corpus callosum measures. In another study from a separate research group, smaller brain and cerebral volumes and attenuation of frontal lobe asymmetry were seen in children with maltreatment-related PTSD or subthreshold PTSD relative to archival nonmaltreated controls (Carrion et al., 2001).

However, these two previously described imaging studies did not control for low socioeconomic status, which can also influence brain maturation through ecological variables. In another study from our group that controlled for socioeconomic status, 28 psychotropic-naïve children and adolescents with maltreatment-related PTSD and 66 sociodemographically similar healthy nonmaltreated children underwent comprehensive clinical assessments and anatomical brain imaging (De Bellis, Keshavan, Shifflett, et al., 2002). Compared with nonmal-treated children, children with maltreatment-related PTSD had smaller intracranial, cerebral, and prefrontal cortex; prefrontal cortical white matter; and right temporal lobe volumes, as well as smaller volumes of areas of the corpus callosum and its subregions and larger frontal lobe cerebral spinal fluid (CSF) volumes than controls. The total midsagittal area of the corpus callosum and middle and posterior regions remained smaller, whereas right, left, and total lateral ventricles and frontal lobe CSF were proportionally larger than in controls, after adjustment for cerebral volume. Brain volumes positively correlated with age of onset of PTSD trauma and negatively correlated with duration of abuse. The larger lateral ventricles were seen only in maltreated males, leading to the conclusion that males are more vulnerable to the neurotoxic effects of childhood maltreatment (De Bellis & Keshavan, 2003).

Our group also found smaller cerebellar volumes in maltreated children with PTSD (De Bellis & Kuchibhatla, 2006). A younger age of onset and longer trauma duration significantly predicted smaller cerebellum volumes. The cerebellum is a complex posterior brain structure that is involved not only with motor functions but also with cognitive functions (Riva & Giorgi, 2000), decision making and reward circuits (Bellebaum & Daum, 2007; Thoma, Bellebaum, Koch, Schwarz, & Daum, 2008), and default mode network or resting state activity (Fransson, 2006). Thus, it is highly likely that abuse and neglect in childhood have detrimental effects on the brain networks that establish an individual's sense of self, integrity, and behaviors.

Child maltreatment is associated with global adverse effects not only on the cerebrum and cerebellum but on individual brain structures that are involved in reward and default network processing. In a study of 61 medically healthy children and adolescents (31 males and 30 females) with chronic PTSD secondary to abuse who had similar trauma and mental health histories and 122 healthy nonmaltreated controls (62 males and 60 females), the midsagittal area of corpus callosum subregion 7 (splenium) was smaller in both boys and girls with maltreatment-related PTSD than in gender-matched comparison subjects (De Bellis & Keshavan, 2003). Children with PTSD did not show the normal age-related increases in the area of the total corpus callosum and its region 7 (splenium) that are seen in nonmaltreated children. This was an important finding for several reasons. The maltreated children were not prenatally exposed to controlled substances, had no pregnancy or birth trauma, were psychotropically naïve, and had no history of substance abuse or dependence. The axons in the splenium of the corpus callosum myelinate during adolescence and are important to the posterior reward circuits and posterior default networks (Fair et al., 2008). Therefore, it was not surprising that we found that clinical symptoms of PTSD (intrusive, avoidant, and hyperarousal symptoms), symptoms of childhood dissociation, and the child behavioral checklist internalizing T score were significantly and negatively correlated with corpus callosum measures (De Bellis & Keshavan, 2003). Children with maltreatment-related PTSD had reduced fractional anisotropy values on diffusion tensor imaging brain scans of white matter in the medial and posterior corpus, a region that contains intrahemispheric projections from brain structures involved in circuits that mediate emotional and memory processing, core disturbances associated with trauma history (Jackowski et al., 2008). Fractional anisotropy values decrease with age as myelination of the corpus callosum matures (Morriss, Zimmerman, Bilaniuk, Hunter, & Haselgrove, 1999; Schmithorst, Wilke, Dardzinski, & Holland, 2005). Lower fractional anisotropy values might reflect fewer posterior default network neurons and less white matter organization. Smaller corpus callosum area measures were seen in neglected children with psychiatric disorders in another anatomical MRI brain study comparing them to nonmaltreated children with psychiatric disorders, indicating that smaller corpus callosum measures might be a consequence of maltreatment (Teicher et al., 2004). Dissociation (defined as disruptions in the usually integrated functions of consciousness, memory, identity, or perception of the environment that interfere with the associative integration of information) is commonly found in traumatized children (Putnam, 1997). Lack of dissociation and an intact corpus callosum are essential to an intact default node network and child mental health.

Furthermore, areas of executive function show evidence of adverse brain development in children with maltreatment-related PTSD. Decreased N-acetylaspartate (NAA) concentrations are associated with increased metabolism and loss of neurons (for a review, see Prichard [1996]). For example, brain NAA levels decrease when someone has neuronal loss, such as from a stroke. A preliminary investigation suggested that maltreated children and adolescents with PTSD demonstrated lower NAA/creatine ratios in the medial prefrontal cortex than sociodemographically matched controls (De Bellis, Keshavan, Spencer, & Hall, 2000). These findings suggest neuronal loss in the anterior cingulate region of the medial prefrontal cortex, an executive brain region, in maltreatment-related PTSD. Another group found decreased left ventral and left inferior prefrontal gray matter volumes in maltreated children with impairing PTSD symptoms that were negatively correlated with bedtime salivary cortisol levels, further suggesting that stress damages executive regions (Carrion, Weems, Richert, Hoffman, & Reiss, 2010). One functional imaging study of maltreated children and adolescents with PTSD symptoms shows significant differences in inhibitory processes relative to nonmaltreated controls (Carrion, Garrett, Menon, Weems, & Reiss, 2008), and another showed impaired cognitive control in adopted children with a history of maltreatment who were formerly raised in foster care (Mueller et al., 2010). These investigations strongly suggest that childhood maltreatment interferes with executive or control circuits, the dys-regulation of which is an important contributor to addiction.

Another important contributor to the reward circuits and the default mode network is the hippocampus. Unlike findings in adult PTSD, in which hippocampal atrophy was reported in several studies (Smith, 2005), maltreated children and adolescents with PTSD or subthreshold PTSD showed no anatomical differences in limbic (hippocampal or amygdala) structures cross-sectionally (Carrion et al., 2001; De Bellis, Keshavan, et al., 1999; De Bellis, Keshavan, Frustaci, et al., 2002) or longitudinally (De Bellis, Hall, Boring, Frustaci, & Moritz, 2001). However, investigators are now finding functional differences in the amygdala and hippocampus of maltreated youth compared to those of non-maltreated children (Carrion, Haas, Garrett, Song, & Reiss, 2010; Maheu et al., 2010). One study suggests that hippocampal atrophy might be a more latent developmental effect of childhood maltreatment (Carrion, Weems, & Reiss, 2007).

Child maltreatment is also associated with adverse development of brain reward regions involved in recognizing emotions and social cognition, such as the superior temporal gyrus (De Bellis, Keshavan, Shifflett, et al., 2002) and the orbital frontal cortex (Hanson et al., 2010). In carefully screened young adult subjects, those with a history of parental verbal abuse and no other form of maltreatment had reduced fractional anisotropy on diffusion tensor imaging brain scans of white matter in the arcuate fasciculus in the left superior temporal gyrus, the cingulum bundle by the posterior tail of the left hippocampus, and the left body of the fornix, indicating decreased integrity of these language neural pathways (Choi, Jeong, Rohan, Polcari, & Teicher, 2009). Furthermore, fractional anisotropy values were negatively correlated with emotional maltreatment experiences. In healthy adult women, a history of sexual abuse was specifically associated with hippocampal, corpus callosum, or frontal cortex reductions if the abuse occurred during specific developmental age periods, indicating vulnerable windows for the brain effects of severe stress (Andersen et al., 2004). In another study, investigators found higher T2 relaxation times (an indirect index of resting blood volume) in the cerebellar vermis of healthy adult women with a history of sexual abuse than in nonmaltreated women, which correlated strongly with Limbic System Checklist ratings of temporal lobe epilepsy and frequency of substance use (Anderson, Teicher, Polcari, & Renshaw, 2002). Corporal punishment, defined as the administration of physical force with the intention to cause pain but not injury to a child for the purpose of correction or behavioral control, is associated with psychopathology, including substance abuse and dependence (MacMillan et al., 1999). In studies of carefully characterized healthy adults who experienced only corporal punishment without other forms of maltreatment, T2 relaxation times were increased in dopamine-rich brain decision-making and reward regions such as the caudate and putamen, dorsolateral prefrontal cortex, substantia nigra, thalamus, and accumbens (Sheu, Polcari, Anderson, & Teicher, 2010). In the latter study, regional T2 relaxation times were significantly associated with the use of drugs and alcohol. These studies provide further evidence that specific types of abuse and neglect contribute to the intergenerational cycle of addiction via their impact on the brain's developing reward circuit and default mode network.

Future Directions

The chronic stress of childhood maltreatment is strongly implicated as the origin of the intergenerational cycle of violence through its effects on the brain's reward and default mode networks. These effects can lead to psychopathology and addiction in maltreating parents who were maltreated as children. These results also provide indirect evidence that PTSD in maltreated children may be regarded as a *complex environmentally induced developmental disorder*. However, understanding the neurobiological effects of maltreatment, and how these effects can increase the risk of parental mental illness, will inform the field on how best to decrease the individual and societal burden of maltreatment. Although new research shows that some individuals are resilient to some of the effects of maltreatment, "resilience" is a relative trait and does not signify invulnerability. Having certain polymorphisms is not deterministic. There is evidence that the presence of strong social supports in genetically vulnerable children with maltreatment (i.e., those with two short 5-HTTLPR alleles) might reduce depression scores to levels only slightly above those of nonmaltreated children with the same genotype (Kaufman et al., 2004). The researchers reporting these findings later extended them to demonstrate that the met allele of the brain-derived neurotrophic factor interacted with the short alleles of 5-HTTLPR to confer the highest vulnerability to depression in maltreated children, but again the availability of social support moderated this risk (Kaufman et al., 2006). Although there is growing evidence that early interventions can decrease the intergenerational transmission of maltreatment-related PTSD and violence, society is still coping with millions of victims. Helping victims of childhood maltreatment through this neurobiological understanding is the mission of the field of developmental traumatology.

Disclosure Statement

This work was supported by a grant from the National Institute of Drug Abuse (Grant No. K24DA028773).

References

Adinoff, B., Devous, M. D., Sr., Best, S. M., George, M. S., Alexander, D., & Payne, K. (2001). Limbic responsiveness to procaine in cocaine addicted subjects. *American Journal of Psychiatry, 158,* 390–398.

Agrawal, A., & Lynskey, M. T. (2009). Candidate genes for cannabis use disorders: Findings, challenges and directions. *Addiction, 104,* 518–532.

Albrecht, S. A., Cornelius, M. D., Braxter, B., Reynolds, M. D., Stone, C., & Cassidy, B. (1999). An assessment of nicotine dependence among pregnant adolescents. *Journal of Substance Abuse Treatment, 16,* 337–344.

American Psychiatric Association. (2000). *Diagnostic and Statistical Manual of Mental Disorders: Fourth Edition, Text Revision.* Washington, DC: Author.

Andersen, S. L., Tomada, A., Vincow, E. S., Valente, E., Polcari, A., & Teicher, M. H. (2004). Preliminary evidence for sensitive periods in the effect of childhood sexual abuse on regional brain development. *Journal of Neuropsychiatry and Clinical Neuroscience, 20*(3), 292–301.

Anderson, C. M., Teicher, M. H., Polcari, A., & Renshaw, P. F. (2002). Abnormal T2 relaxation time in the cerebellar vermis of adults sexually abused in childhood: Potential role of the vermis in stress-enhanced risk for drug abuse. *Psychoneuroendocrinology, 27,* 231–244.

Apicella, P., Ljungberg, T., Scarnati, E., & Schultz, W. (1991). Responses to reward in monkey dorsal and ventral striatum *Experimental Brain Research, 85,* 491–500.

Arnsten, A. F. T. (1998). The biology of being frazzled. *Science, 280,* 1711–1712.

Baker, D. G., West, S. A., Nicholson, W. E., Ekhator, N. N., Kasckow, J. W., Hill, K. K., et al. (1999). Serial CSF corticotropin-releasing hormone levels and adrenocortical activity in combat veterans with posttraumatic stress disorder. *American Journal of Psychiatry, 156,* 585–588.

Bauer, P. M., Hanson, J. L., Pierson, R. K., Davidson, R. J., & Pollak, S. D. (2009). Cerebellar volume and cognitive functioning in children who experienced early deprivation. *Biological Psychiatry, 66,* 1100–1106.

Bechara, A. (2005). Decision making, impulse control and loss of willpower to resist drugs: A neurocognitive perspective. *Nature Neuroscience, 8*(11), 1458–1463.

Beers, S. R., & De Bellis, M. D. (2002). Neuropsychological function in children with maltreatment-related posttraumatic stress disorder. *American Journal of Psychiatry, 159,* 483–486.

Bellebaum, C., & Daum, I. (2007). Cerebellar involvement in executive control. *The Cerebellum, 6,* 184–192.

Bjork, J. M., Knutson, B., Fong, G. W., Caggiano, D. M., Bennett, S. M., & Hommer, D. W. (2004). Incentive-elicited brain activation in adolescents: Similarities and differences from young adults. *Journal of Neuroscience, 24,* 1793–1802.

Blakemore, S. J., & Choudhury, S. (2006). Development of the adolescent brain: Implications for executive function and social cognition. *Journal of Child Psychology and Psychiatry, 47,* 296–312.

Bluhm, R. L., Williamson, P. C., Osuch, E. A., Frewen, P. A., Stevens, T. K., Boksman, K., et al. (2009). Alterations in default network connectivity in posttraumatic stress disorder related to early-life trauma. *Journal of Psychiatry & Neuroscience 34*(3), 187–194.

Bremner, J. D., Licinio, J., Darnell, A., Krystal, J. H., Owens, M. J., Southwick, S. M., et al. (1997). Elevated CSF corticotropin-releasing factor concentrations in posttraumatic stress disorder. *American Journal of Psychiatry, 154,* 624–629.

Broyd, S. J., Demanuele, C., Debener, S., Helps, S. K., James, C. J., & Sonuga-Barke, E. J. S. (2009). Default-mode brain dysfunction in mental disorders: A systematic review. *Neuroscience & Biobehavioral Reviews, 33*(3), 279–296.

Buckner, R., Andrews-Hanna, J., & Schacter, D. (2008). The brain's default network: Anatomy, function, and relevance to disease *Annals of the New York Academy of Science, 1124*, 1–38.

Burns, B. J., Phil, S. D., Wagner, H. R., Barth, R. P., Kolko D. J., Campbell, Y., & Landsverk, J.(2004). Mental health need and access to mental health services by youths involved with child welfare: A national survey. *Journal of the American Academy of Child & Adolescent Psychiatry, 43*, 960–970.

Carrion, V. G., Garrett, A., Menon, V., Weems, C. F., & Reiss, A. L. (2008). Posttraumatic stress symptoms and brain function during a response-inhibition task: An fMRI study in youth. *Depression & Anxiety, 25*(6), 514–526.

Carrion, V. G., Haas, B. W., Garrett, A., Song, S., & Reiss, A. L. (2010). Reduced hippocampal activity in youth with posttraumatic stress symptoms: An FMRI study. *Journal of Pediatric Psychology, 35*(5), 559–569.

Carrion, V. G., Weems, C. F., Eliez, S., Patwardhan, A., Brown, W., Ray, R. D., et al. (2001). Attenuation of frontal asymmetry in pediatric posttraumatic stress disorder. *Biological Psychiatry, 50*, 943–951.

Carrion, V. G., Weems, C. F., Ray, R. D., Glaser, B., Hessl, D., & Reiss, A. L. (2002). Diurnal salivary cortisol in pediatric posttraumatic stress disorder. *Biological Psychiatry, 51*, 575–582.

Carrion, V. G., Weems, C. F., Ray, R., & Reiss, A. L. (2002). Toward an empirical definition of pediatric PTSD: The phenomenology of PTSD symptoms in youth. *Journal of the American Academy of Child & Adolescent Psychiatry, 41*(2), 166–173.

Carrion, V. G., Weems, C. F., & Reiss, A. L. (2007). Stress predicts brain changes in children: A pilot longitudinal study on youth stress, posttraumatic stress disorder, and the hippocampus. *Pediatrics, 119*(3), 509–516.

Carrion, V. G., Weems, C. F., Richert, K., Hoffman, B. C., & Reiss, A. L. (2010). Decreased prefrontal cortical volume associated with increased bedtime cortisol in traumatized youth. *Biological Psychiatry, 68*(5), 491–493.

Caspi, A., Hariri, A. R., Holmes, A., Uher, R., & Moffitt, T. E. (2010). Genetic sensitivity to the environment: The case of the serotonin transporter gene and its implications for studying complex diseases and traits. *American Journal of Psychiatry, 167*, 509–527.

Choi, J., Jeong, B., Rohan, M. L., Polcari, A., & Teicher, M. H. (2009). Preliminary evidence for white matter tract abnormalities in young adults exposed to parental verbal abuse. *Biological Psychiatry, 65*, 227–234.

Chrousos, G. P., & Gold, P. W. (1992). The concepts of stress and stress system disorders: Overview of physical and behavioral homeostasis. *Journal of the American Medical Association, 267*, 1244–1252.

Clark, D. B., Lesnick, L., & Hegedus, A. (1997). Trauma and other stressors in adolescent alcohol dependence and abuse. *Journal of the American Academy of Child and Adolescent Psychiatry, 36*, 1744–1751.

Clark, D. B., Pollock, N., Bukstein, O. G., Mezzich, A. C., Bromberger, J. T., & Donovan, J. E. (1997). Gender and comorbid psychopathology in adolescents with alcohol dependence. *Journal of the American Academy of Child and Adolescent Psychiatry, 36*(9), 1195–1203.

Copeland, W., Keeler, G., Angold, A., & Costello, E. (2007). Traumatic events and posttraumatic stress in childhood. *Archives of General Psychiatry, 64*, 577–584.

Cornelius, J. R., Aizenstein, H. J., & Hariri, A. R. (2010). Amygdala reactivity is inversely related to level of cannabis use in individuals with comorbid cannabis dependence and major depression. *Addictive Behaviors, 35*, 644–646.

Crews, F., He, J., & Hodge, C. (2007). Adolescent cortical development: A critical period of vulnerability for addiction. *Pharmacology, Biochemistry and Behavior, 86*, 189–199.

Daniels, J. K., Frewen, P., McKinnon, M. C., & Lanius, R. A. (2011). Default mode alterations in posttraumatic stress disorder related to early-life trauma: A developmental perspective. *Journal of Psychiatry & Neuroscience, 36*, 56–59.

De Bellis, M., Hooper, S., Spratt, E., & Woolley, D. (2009). Neuropsychological findings in childhood neglect and their relationship to pediatric PTSD. *Journal of International Neuropsychology, 15*, 868–878.

De Bellis, M., & Kuchibhatla, M. (2006). Cerebellar volumes in pediatric maltreatment-related posttraumatic stress disorder. *Biological Psychiatry, 60*(7), 697–703.

De Bellis, M. D. (2001a). Developmental traumatology: A contributory mechanism for alcohol and substance use disorders. *Special Review in Psychoneuroendocrinology, 27*, 155–170.

De Bellis, M. D. (2001b). Developmental traumatology: The psychobiological development of maltreated children and its implications for research, treatment, and policy. *Development and Psychopathology, 13*, 537–561.

De Bellis, M. D. (2003). The neurobiology of posttraumatic stress disorder across the life cycle. In J. C. Soares & S. Gershon (Eds.), *The handbook of medical psychiatry* (pp. 449–466). New York: Marcel Dekker Inc.

De Bellis, M. D. (2005). The psychobiology of neglect. *Child Maltreatment, 10*, 150–172.

De Bellis, M. D., Baum, A., Birmaher, B., Keshavan, M., Eccard, C. H., Boring, A. M., et al. (1999). A. E. Bennett Research Award. Developmental Traumatology Part I: Biological stress systems. *Biological Psychiatry, 45*, 1259–1270.

De Bellis, M. D., Broussard, E., Wexler, S., Herring, D., & Moritz, G. (2001). Psychiatric co-morbidity in caregivers and children involved in maltreatment: A pilot research study with policy implications *Child Abuse and Neglect, 25*, 923–944.

De Bellis, M. D., Burke, L., Trickett, P. K., & Putnam, F. W. (1996). Antinuclear antibodies and thyroid function in sexually abused girls *Journal of Traumatic Stress, 9*, 369–378.

De Bellis, M. D., Chrousos, G. P., Dorn, L. D., Burke, L., Helmers, K., Kling, M. A., et al. (1994). Hypothalamic-pituitary-adrenal axis dysregulation in sexually abused girls. *Journal of Clinical Endocrinology and Metabolism, 78*, 249–255.

De Bellis, M. D., Hall, J., Boring, A. M., Frustaci, K., & Moritz, G. (2001). A pilot longitudinal study of hippocampal volumes in pediatric maltreatment-related posttraumatic stress disorder. *Biological Psychiatry, 50*, 305–309.

De Bellis, M. D., Keshavan, M., Beers, S. R., Hall, J., Frustaci, K., Masalehdan, A., et al. (2001). Sex differences in brain maturation during childhood and adolescence. *Cerebral Cortex, 11*, 552–557.

De Bellis, M. D., Keshavan, M., Clark, D. B., Casey, B. J., Giedd, J., Boring, A. M., et al. (1999). A.E. Bennett Research Award. Developmental Traumatology Part II: Brain development. *Biological Psychiatry, 45*, 1271–1284.

De Bellis, M. D., Keshavan, M., Shifflett, H., Iyengar, S., Beers, S. R., Hall, J., et al. (2002). Brain structures in pediatric maltreatment-related posttraumatic stress disorder: A sociodemographically matched study. *Biological Psychiatry, 52*, 1066–1078.

De Bellis, M. D., & Keshavan, M. S. (2003). Sex differences in brain maturation in maltreatment-related pediatric posttraumatic stress disorder. *Neurosciences and Biobehavioral Reviews, 27*, 103–117.

De Bellis, M. D., Keshavan, M. S., Frustaci, K., Shifflett, H., Iyengar, S., Beers, S. R., et al. (2002). Superior temporal gyrus volumes in maltreated children and adolescents with PTSD. *Biological Psychiatry, 51,* 544–552.

De Bellis, M. D., Keshavan, M. S., Spencer, S., & Hall, J. (2000). N-acetylaspartate concentration in the anterior cingulate in maltreated children and adolescents with PTSD. *American Journal of Psychiatry, 157,* 1175–1177.

De Bellis, M. D., Lefter, L., Trickett, P. K., & Putnam, F. W. (1994). Urinary catecholamine excretion in sexually abused girls. *Journal of the American Academy of Child and Adolescent Psychiatry, 33,* 320–327.

De Genna, N. M., Cornelius, M. D., & Donovan, J. E. (2009). Risk factors for young adult substance use among women who were teenage mothers. *Addictive Behaviors, 34,* 463–470.

Delgado, M. R., Locke, H. M., Stenger, V. A., & Fiez, J. A. (2003). Dorsal striatum responses to reward and punishment: Effects of valence and magnitude manipulations. *Cognitive Affective & Behavioral Neuroscience, 3,* 27–38.

Dillon, D. G., Holmes, A. J., Birk, J. L., Brooks, N., Lyons-Ruth, K., & Pizzagalli, D. A. (2009). Childhood adversity is associated with left basal ganglia dysfunction during reward anticipation in adulthood. *Biological Psychiatry, 66,* 206–213.

Dong, M., Anda, R. F., Felitti, V. J., Williamson, D. F., Dube, S. R., Brown, D. W., et al. (2005). Childhood residential mobility and multiple health risks during adolescence and adulthood: The hidden role of adverse childhood experiences. *Archives of Pediatrics & Adolescent Medicine, 159*(12), 1104–1110.

Dong, M., Giles, W. H., Felitti, V. J., Dube, S. R., Williams, J. E., Chapman, D. P., et al. (2004). Insights into causal pathways for ischemic heart disease: Adverse childhood experiences study. *Circulation, 110*(13), 1761–1766.

Dube, S. R., Fairweather, D., Pearson, W. S., Felitti, V. J., Anda, R. F., & Croft, J. B. (2009). Cumulative childhood stress and autoimmune diseases in adults. *Psychosomatic Medicine, 71*(2), 243–250.

Dube, S. R., Miller, J. W., Brown, D. W., Giles, W. H., Felitti, V. J., Dong, M., et al. (2006). Adverse childhood experiences and the association with ever using alcohol and initiating alcohol use during adolescence. *Journal of Adolescent Health, 38*(4), 444e441–410.

Dubner, A. E., & Motta, R. W. (1999). Sexually and physically abused foster care children and posttraumatic stress disorder. *Journal of Consulting & Clinical Psychology, 67,* 367–373.

Dunlop, S. A., Archer, M. A., Quinlivan, J. A., Beazley, L. D., & Newnham, J. P. (1997). Repeated prenatal corticosteroids delay myelination in the ovine central nervous system. *Journal of Maternal-Fetal Medicine, 6,* 309–313.

Durston, S., Hulshoff Pol, H. E., Casey, B. J., Giedd, J. N., Buitelaar, J. K., & van Engeland, H. (2001). Anatomical MRI of the developing human brain: What have we learned? *Journal of the American Academy of Child & Adolescent Psychiatry, 40,* 1012–1020.

Eckenrode, J., Campa, M., Luckey, D. W., Henderson, C. R., Jr., Cole, R., Kitzman, H., et al. (2010). Long-term effects of prenatal and infancy nurse home visitation on the life course of youths: 19-year follow-up of a randomized trial. *Archives of Pediatric and Adolescent Medicine, 164*(1), 9–15.

Edwards, E., Harkins, K., Wright, G., & Menn, F. (1990). Effects of bilateral adrenalectomy on the induction of learned helplessness. *Behavioral Neuropsychopharmacology, 3,* 109–114.

Eichele, T., Debener, S., Calhoun, V. D., Specht, K., Engel, A. K., Hugdahl, K., et al. (2008). Prediction of human errors by maladaptive changes in event-related brain networks. *Proceedings of the National Academy of Sciences USA, 105,* 6173–6178.

Elliott, R., Newman, J. L., Longe, O. A., & Deakin, J. F. (2003). Differential response patterns in the striatum and orbitofrontal cortex to financial reward in humans: A parametric functional magnetic resonance imaging study. *Journal of Neuroscience, 23,* 303–307.

Enoch, M.-A., Hodgkinson, C. A., Yuan, Q., Shen, P.-H., Goldman, D., & Roy, A. (2010). The influence of GABRA2, childhood trauma, and their interaction on alcohol, heroin, and cocaine dependence. *Biological Psychiatry, 67,* 20–27.

Ernst, M., Nelson, E. E., Jazbec, S., McClure, E. B., Monk, C. S., Leibenluft, E., et al. (2005). Amygdala and nucleus accumbens in responses to receipt and omission of gains in adults and adolescents. *NeuroImage, 25,* 1279–1291.

Eshel, N., Nelson, E. E., Blair, R. J., Pine, D. S., & Ernst, M. (2007). Neural substrates of choice selection in adults and adolescents: Development of the ventrolateral prefrontal and anterior cingulate cortices. *Neuropsychologia, 45,* 1270–1279.

Fair, D. A., Cohen, A. L., Dosenbach, N. U. F., Church, J. A., Miezin, F. M., Barch, D. M., et al. (2008). The maturing architecture of the brain's default network. *Proceedings of the National Academy of Sciences USA, 105*(10), 4028–4032.

Famularo, R., Fenton, T., Augustyn, M., & Zuckerman, B. (1996). Persistence of pediatric post traumatic stress disorder after 2 years. *Child Abuse & Neglect, 20,* 1245–1248.

Famularo, R., Fenton, T., & Kinscherff, R. (1993). Child maltreatment and the development of post traumatic stress disorder. *American Journal of Diseases of Children, 147,* 755–760.

Famularo, R., Kinscherff, R., & Fenton, T. (1992). Psychiatric diagnoses of abusive mothers. *Journal of Nervous and Mental Disease, 180,* 658–661.

Felitti, V. J., Anda, R. F., Nordenberg, D., Williamson, D. F., Spitz, A. M., Edwards, V., et al. (1998). Relationship of childhood abuse and household dysfunction to many of the leading causes of death in adults. *American Journal of Preventive Medicine, 14,* 245–258.

Foster, M. E., Prinz, R. J., Sanders, M. R., & Shapiro, C. J. (2008). The costs of a public health infrastructure for delivering parenting and family support. *Children and Youth Services Review, 30,* 493–501.

Fox, M. D., Snyder, A. Z., Vincent, J. L., Corbetta, M., Van Essen, D. C., & Raichle, M. E. (2005). From the cover: The human brain is intrinsically organized into dynamic, anticorrelated functional networks. *Proceedings of the National Academy of Sciences USA, 102,* 9673–9678.

Franklin, T. R., Acton, P. D., Maldjian, J. A., Gray, J. D., Croft, J. R., Dackis, C. A., et al. (2002). Decreased gray matter concentration in the insular, orbitofrontal, cingulate, and temporal cortices of cocaine patients. *Biological Psychiatry, 51*(2), 134–142.

Fransson, P. (2005). Spontaneous low-frequency BOLD signal fluctuations: An fMRI investigation of the resting-state default mode of brain function hypothesis. *Human Brain Mapping, 26,* 5–29.

Fransson, P. (2006). How default is the default mode of brain function? Further evidence from intrinsic BOLD signal fluctuations. *Neuropsychologia, 44,* 2836–2845.

Fransson, P., Skiold, B., Horsch, S., Nordell, A., Blennow, M., Lagercrantz, H., et al. (2007). Resting-state networks in the infant brain. *Proceedings of the National Academy of Sciences USA, 104,* 15531–15536.

Fries, A. B., Shirtcliff, E. A., & Pollak, S. D. (2008). Neuroendocrine dysregulation following early social deprivation in children. *Developmental Psychobiology, 50*(6), 588–599.

Gentili, C., Ricciardi, E., Gobbini, M. I., Santarelli, M. F., Haxby, J. V., Pietrini, P., et al. (2009). Beyond amygdala: Default mode network activity differs between patients with social phobia and healthy controls. *Brain Research Bulletin, 79*(6), 409–413.

Giedd, J. N., Blumenthal, J., Jeffries, N. O., Castellanos, X., Liu, H., Zijdenbos, A., et al. (1999). Brain development during childhood and adolescence: A longitudinal MRI study. *Nature Neuroscience, 2*, 861–863.

Giedd, J. N., Blumenthal, J., Jeffries, N. O., Rajapakse, J. C., Vaituzis, A. C., Liu, H., et al. (1999). Development of the human corpus callosum during childhood and adolescence: A longitudinal MRI study. *Progress in Neuropsychopharmacology and Biological Psychiatry, 23*, 571–588.

Gobbini, M. I., Koralek, A. C., Bryan, R. E., Montgomery, K. J., & Haxby, J. V. (2007). Two takes on the social brain: A comparison of theory of mind tasks. *Journal of Cognitive Neuroscience, 19*, 1803–1814.

Goldstein, R. Z., & Volkow, N. D. (2002). Drug addiction and its underlying neurobiological basis: Neuroimaging evidence for the involvement of the frontal cortex. *American Journal of Psychiatry, 159*, 1642–1652.

Gould, E., McEwen, B. S., Tanapat, P., Galea, L. A., & Fuchs, E. (1997). Neurogenesis in the dentate gyrus of the adult tree shrew is regulated by psychosocial stress and NMDA receptor activation. *Journal of Neuroscience, 17*, 2492–2498.

Gould, E., Tanapat, P., & Cameron, H. A. (1997). Adrenal steroids suppress granule cell death in the developing dentate gyrus through an NMDA receptor-dependent mechanism. *Developmental Brain Research, 103*, 91–93.

Gould, E., Tanapat, P., McEwen, B. S., Flugge, G., & Fuchs, E. (1998). Proliferation of granule cell precursors in the dentate gyrus of adult monkeys is diminished by stress. *Proceedings of the National Academy of Sciences of the United States of America, 95*, 3168–3171.

Green, A. (1985). *Children traumatized by physical abuse.* Washington, DC: American Psychiatric Press.

Green, J. G., McLaughlin, K. A., Berglund, P. A., Gruber, M. J., Sampson, N. A., Zaslavsky, A. M., et al. (2010). Childhood adversities and adult psychiatric disorders in the National Comorbidity Survey Replication, I: Associations with first onset of DSM-IV disorders. *Archives of General Psychiatry, 67*, 113–123.

Greicius, M. D., Flores, B. H., Menon, V., Glover, G. H., Solvason, H. B., Kenna, H., et al. (2007). Resting-state functional connectivity in major depression: Abnormally increased contributions from subgenual cingulate cortex and thalamus. *Biological Psychiatry, 62*(5), 429–437.

Grimm, S., Boesiger, P., Beck, J., Schuepbach, D., Bermpohl, F., Walter, M., et al. (2009). Altered negative BOLD responses in the default-mode network during emotion processing in depressed subjects. *Neuropsychopharmacology, 34*, 932–943.

Gunnar, M. R., Morison, S. J., Chisholm, K., & Schuder, M. (2001). Salivary cortisol levels in children adopted from Romanian orphanages. *Development & Psychopathology, 13*, 611–628.

Hahn, B. J., Ross, T. J., Yang, Y., Kim, I., Huestis, M. A., & Stein, E. A. (2007). Nicotine enhances visuospatial attention by deactivating areas of the resting brain default network. *The Journal of Neuroscience, 27*(13), 3477–3489.

Hanson, J. L., Chung, M. K., Avants, B. B., Shirtcliff, E. A., Gee, J. C., Davidson, R. J., et al. (2010). Early stress is associated with alterations in the orbitofrontal cortex: A tensor based morphometry investigation of brain structure and behavioral risk. *Journal of Neuroscience, 30*(22), 7466–7472.

Hart, J., Gunnar, M., & Cicchetti, D. (1996). Altered neuroendocrine activity in maltreated children related to symptoms of depression. *Development and Psychopathology, 8*, 201–214.

Heim, C., & Nemeroff, C. B. (2001). The role of childhood trauma in the neurobiology of mood and anxiety disorders: Preclinical and clinical studies. *Biological Psychiatry, 49,* 1023–1039.

Heim, C., Newport, D. J., Heit, S., Graham, Y. P., Wilcox, M., Bonsall, R., et al. (2000). Pituitary-adrenal and autonomic responses to stress in women after sexual and physical abuse in childhood. *Journal of the American Medical Association, 284,* 592–597.

Heim, C., Newport, D. J., Wagner, D., Wilcox, M. M., Miller, A. H., & Nemeroff, C. B. (2002). The role of early adverse experience and adulthood stress in the prediction of neuroendocrine stress reactivity in women: A multiple regression analysis. *Depression & Anxiety, 15,* 117–125.

Hester, R., Nestor, L., & Garavan, H. (2009). Impaired error awareness and anterior cingulate cortex hypoactivity in chronic cannabis users. *Neuropsychopharmacology, 34*(11), 2450–2458.

Hussey, J. M., Marshall, J. M., English, D. J., Knight, E. D., Laud, A. S., Dubowitz, H., et al. (2005). Defining maltreatment according to substantiation: Distinction without a difference? *Child Abuse & Neglect, 29,* 479–492.

Jackowski, A. P., Douglas-Palumberi, H., Jackowski, M., Win, L., Schultz, R. T., Staib, L. W., et al. (2008). Corpus callosum in maltreated children with posttraumatic stress disorder: A diffusion tensor imaging study. *Psychiatry Research: Neuroimaging, 162,* 256–261.

Kaufman, J. (1991). Depressive disorders in maltreated children. *Journal of the American Academy of Child and Adolescent Psychiatry, 30,* 257–265.

Kaufman, J., Birmaher, B., Brent, D., Dahl, R., Bridge, J., & Ryan, N. (1998). Psychopathology in the relatives of depressed abused children. *Child Abuse and Neglect, 22*(7), 171–181.

Kaufman, J., Birmaher, B., Perel, J., Dahl, R. E., Moreci, P., Nelson, B., et al. (1997). The corticotropin-releasing hormone challenge in depressed abused, depressed nonabused, and normal control children. *Biological Psychiatry, 42,* 669–679.

Kaufman, J., & Charney, D. (2001). Effects of early stress on brain structure and function: Implications for understanding the relationship between child maltreatment and depression. *Development & Psychopathology, 13*(3), 451–471.

Kaufman, J., Jones, B., Stieglitz, E., Vitulano, L., & Mannarino, A. (1994). The use of multiple informants to assess children's maltreatment experiences. *Journal of Family Violence, 9,* 227–248.

Kaufman, J., Yang, B. Z., Douglas-Palumberi, H., Grasso, D., Lipschitz, D., Houshyar, S., et al. (2006). Brain-derived neurotrophic factor-5-HTTLPR gene interactions and environmental modifiers of depression in children. *Biological Psychiatry, 59,* 673–680.

Kaufman, J., Yang, B. Z., Douglas-Palumberi, H., Houshyar, S., Lipschitz, D., Krystal, J. H., et al. (2004). Social supports and serotonin transporter gene moderate depression in maltreated children. *Proceedings of the National Academy of Sciences USA, 101,* 17316–17321.

Kelly, C., Zuo, X.-N., Gotimer, K., Cox, C. L., Lynch, L., Brock, D., et al. (2011). Reduced interhemispheric resting state functional connectivity in cocaine addiction. *Biological Psychiatry, 69,* 684–692.

Kendler, K. S., Bulik, C. M., Silberg, J., Hettema, J. M., Myers, J., & Prescott, C. A. (2000). Childhood sexual abuse and adult psychiatric and substance use disorders in women. *Archives of General Psychiatry, 57,* 953–959.

Kilpatrick, D. G., Acierno, R., Schnurr, P. P., Saunder, B., Resnick, H. S., & Best, C. L. (2000). Risk factors for adolescent substance abuse and dependence: Data from a national sample. *Journal of Consulting and Clinical Psychology, 68*(1), 19–30.

Kilts, C. D., Schweitzer, J. B., Quinn, C. K., Gross, R. E., Faber, T. L., Muhammad, F., et al. (2001). Neural activity related to drug craving in cocaine addiction. *Archives of General Psychiatry, 58*, 334–341.

Kitzman, H., Olds, D. L., Cole, R., Hanks, C. A., Anson, E. A., Arcoleo, K. J., et al. (2010). Enduring effects of prenatal and infancy home visiting by nurses on children. *Archives of Pediatric and Adolescent Medicine, 164*(5), 412–418.

Kitzman, H., Olds, D. L., Henderson, C. R., Jr., Hanks, C., Cole, R., Tatelbaum, R., et al. (1997). Effect of prenatal and infancy home visitation by nurses on pregnancy outcomes, childhood injuries, and repeated childbearing: A randomized controlled trial. *Journal of the American Medical Association, 278*, 644–652.

Kühn, S., Schubert, F., & Gallinat, J. (2010). Reduced thickness of medial orbitofrontal cortex in smokers. *Biological Psychiatry, 68*, 1061–1065.

Lanius, R. A., Bluhm, R. L., Coupland, N. J., Hegadoren, K. M., Rowe, B., Theberge, J., et al. (2010). Default mode network connectivity as a predictor of post-traumatic stress disorder symptom severity in acutely traumatized subjects. *Acta Psychiatrica Scandinavica, 121,* 33–40.

Lauder, J. M. (1988). Neurotransmitters as morphogens. *Progress in Brain Research, 73,* 365–388.

Leiter, J., Myers, K. A., & Zingraff, M. T. (1994). Substantiated and unsubstantiated cases of child maltreatment: Do their consequences differ? *Social Work Research, 18*(2), 67–82.

Levy, H. B., Markovic, J., Chaudry, U., Ahart, S., & Torres, H. (1995). Reabuse rates in a sample of children followed for 5 years after discharge from a child abuse inpatient assessment program. *Child Abuse & Neglect, 11,* 1363–1377.

Liao, W., Chen, H., Feng, Y., Mantini, D., Gentili, C., Pan, Z., et al. (2010). Selective aberrant functional connectivity of resting state networks in social anxiety disorder. *NeuroImage, 52,* 1549–1558.

Liu, J., Bann, C., Lester, B., Tronick, E., Das, A., Lagasse, L., et al. (2009). Neonatal neurobehavior predicts medical and behavioral outcome. *Pediatrics, 125,* e90–e98.

Ma, N., Liu, Y., Li, N., Wang, C.-X., Zhang, H., Jiang, X.-F., et al. (2010). Addiction related alteration in resting-state brain connectivity. *NeuroImage, 49,* 738–744.

MacMillan, H. L., Boyle, M. H., Wong, M. Y., Duku, E. K., Fleming, J. E., & Walsh, C. A. (1999). Slapping and spanking in childhood and its association with lifetime prevalence of psychiatric disorders in a general population sample. *Canadian Medical Association Journal, 161,* 805–809.

MacMillan, H. L., Georgiades, K., Duku, E. K., Shea, A., Steiner, M., Niec, A., et al. (2009). Cortisol response to stress in female adolescents exposed to childhood maltreatment: Results of the Youth Mood Project. *Biological Psychiatry, 66*(1), 62–68.

MacMillan, H. L., Thomas, B. H., Jamieson, E., Walsh, C. A., Boyle, M. H., Shannon, H. S., et al. (2005). Effectiveness of home visitation by public-health nurses in prevention of the recurrence of child physical abuse and neglect: A randomised controlled trial. *Lancet, 365,* 1786–1793.

Maheu, F. S., Dozier, M., Guyer, A. E., Mandell, D., Peloso, E., Poeth, K., et al. (2010). A preliminary study of medial temporal lobe function in youths with a history of caregiver deprivation and emotional neglect. *Cognitive, Affective, & Behavioral Neuroscience, 10*(1), 34–49.

McEwen, B. S., DeKloet, E. R., & Rostene, W. (1986). Adrenal steroid receptors and actions in the nervous system. *Physiological Reviews, 66,* 1121–1188.

McGee, R., Wolfe, D., Yuen, S., Wilson, S., & Carnochan, J. (1995). The measurement of maltreatment: A comparison of approaches. *Child Abuse & Neglect, 19,* 233–249.

McGloin, J. M., & Widom, C. S. (2001). Resilience among abused and neglected children grown up. *Development and Psychopathology, 13,* 1021–1038.

McLeer, S. V., Dixon, J. F., Henry, D., Ruggiero, K., Escovitz, K., Niedda, T., et al. (1998). Psychopathology in non-clinically referred sexually abused children. *Journal of the American Academy of Child & Adolescent Psychiatry, 37,* 1326–1333.

Mikton, C., & Butchart, A. (2009). Child maltreatment prevention: A systematic review of reviews. *Bulletin of the World Health Organization, 87,* 353–361.

Mitchell, J. P. (2006). Mentalizing and Marr: An information processing approach to the study of social cognition. *Brain Research, 1079,* 66–75.

Moran, P. B., Vuchinich, S., & Hall, N. K. (2004). Associations between types of maltreatment and substance use during adolescence. *Child Abuse & Neglect, 28,* 565–574.

Morgan, D., Grant, K. A., Gage, H. D., Mach, R. H., Kaplan, J. R., Prioleau, O., et al. (2002). Social dominance in monkeys: Dopamine D2 receptors and cocaine self-administration. *Natural Neuroscience, 5,* 169–174.

Morriss, M. C., Zimmerman, R. A., Bilaniuk, L. T., Hunter, J. V., & Haselgrove, J. C. (1999). Changes in brain water diffusion during childhood. *Neuroradiology, 41,* 929–934.

Mueller, S. C., Maheu, F. S., Dozier, M., Peloso, E., Mandell, D., Leibenluft, E., et al. (2010). Early-life stress is associated with impairment in cognitive control in adolescence: An fMRI study. *Neuropsychologia, 48,* 3037–3044.

O'Doherty, J., Kringelbach, M. L., Rolls, E. T., Hornak, J., & Andrews, C. (2001). Abstract reward and punishment representations in the human orbitofrontal cortex. *Nature Neuroscience, 4,* 95–102.

Olds, D. L., Eckenrode, J., Henderson, C. R., Jr., Kitzman, H., Powers, J., Cole, R., et al. (1997). Long-term effects of home visitation on maternal life course and child abuse and neglect: Fifteen-year follow-up of a randomized trial. *Journal of the American Medical Association, 278*(8), 637–643.

Olds, D. L., Kitzman, H., Hanks, C., Cole, R., Anson, E., Sidora-Arcoleo, K., et al. (2007). Effects of nurse home visiting on maternal and child functioning: Age-9 follow-up of a randomized trial. *Pediatrics, 120,* e832.

Papp, M., Klimek, V., & Willner, P. (1994). Parallel changes in dopamine D2 receptor binding in limbic forebrain associated with chronic mild stress-induced anhedonia and its reversal by imipramine. *Psychopharmacology, 115,* 441–446.

Park, S. Q., Kahnt, T., Beck, A., Cohen, M. X., Dolan, R. J., Wrase, J., et al. (2010). Prefrontal cortex fails to learn from reward prediction errors in alcohol dependence. *The Journal of Neuroscience, 30,* 7749–7753.

Paus, T. (2005). Mapping brain maturation and cognitive development during adolescence. *TRENDS in Cognitive Sciences, 9*(2), 60–68.

Pizarro, J. M., Lumley, L. A., Medina, W., Robison, C. L., Changa, W. E., Alagappana, A., et al. (2004). Acute social defeat reduces neurotrophin expression in brain cortical and subcortical areas in mice. *Brain Research, 1025,* 10–20.

Pollak, S. D., Nelson, C. A., Schlaak, M. F., Roeber, B. J., Wewerka, S. S., Wiik, K. L., et al. (2010). Neurodevelopmental effects of early deprivation in postinstitutionalized children. *Child Development, 81*(1), 224–236.

Prichard, J. W. (1996). *MRS of the brain-prospects for clinical application.* London: The Livery House.

Putnam, F. W. (1997). *Dissociation in children and adolescents: A developmental perspective.* New York: The Guilford Press.

Pynoos, R. S., & Eth, S. (Eds.). (1985). *Witnessing acts of personal violence.* Washington, DC: American Psychiatric Press.

Raichle, M. E., MacLeod, A. M., Abraham, Z., Snyder, A. Z., Powers, W. J., Gusnard, D. A., et al. (2001). A default mode of brain function. *Proceedings of the National Academy of Sciences USA, 98*, 676–682.

Raichle, M. E., & Snyder, A. Z. (2007). A default mode of brain function: A brief history of an evolving idea *Neuroimage, 37*, 1083–1099.

Risch, N., Herrell, R., Lehner, T., Liang, K.-Y., Eaves, L., Hoh, J., et al. (2009). Interaction between the serotonin transporter gene (5-HTTLPR) stressful life events, and risk for depression. *Journal of the American Medical Association, 301*(23), 2462–2471.

Riva, D., & Giorgi, C. (2000). The cerebellum contributes to higher functions during development. *Brain, 123*, 1051–1061.

Roberts, G. M. P., & Garavan, H. (2010). Evidence of increased activation underlying cognitive control in ecstasy and cannabis users. *NeuroImage, 52*, 429–435.

Roesch, M. R., & Olson, C. R. (2004). Neuronal activity related to reward value and motivation in primate frontal cortex. *Science, 304*, 307–310.

Rolls, E. T. (2000). The orbitofrontal cortex and reward. *Cerebral Cortex, 10*, 284–294.

Sapolsky, R. M., Uno, H., Rebert, C. S., & Finch, C. E. (1990). Hippocampal damage associated with prolonged glucocorticoid exposure in primates. *Journal of Neuroscience, 10*, 2897–2902.

Scheeringa, M. D., Zeanah, C. H., Myers, L., & Putnam, F. W. (2005). Predictive validity in a prospective follow-up of PTSD in preschool children. *Journal of the American Academy of Child and Adolescent Psychiatry, 44*(9), 899–906.

Schmithorst, V. J., Wilke, M., Dardzinski, B. J., & Holland, S. K. (2005). Cognitive functions correlate with white matter architecture in a normal pediatric population: A diffusion tensor MRI study. *Human Brain Mapping, 26*, 139–147.

Schoenbaum, G., & Roesch, M. (2005). Orbitofrontal cortex, associative learning, and expectancies. *Neuron, 47*, 633–636.

Schott, B. H., Minuzzi, L., Krebs, R. M., Elmenhorst, D., Lang, M., Winz, O. H., et al. (2008). Mesolimbic functional magnetic resonance imaging activations during reward anticipation correlate with reward-related ventral striatal dopamine release. *Journal of Neuroscience, 28*(52), 14311–14319.

Schuck, A. M., & Widom, C. S. (2001). Childhood victimization and alcohol symptoms in females: Causal inferences and hypothesized mediators. *Child Abuse & Neglect, 25*, 1069–1092.

Schultz, W., Tremblay, L., & Hollerman, J. R. (2000). Reward processing in primate orbitofrontal cortex and basal ganglia. *Cerebral Cortex, 10*, 272–284.

Shaw, P., Kabani, N. J., Lerch, J. P., Eckstrand, K., Lenroot, R., Gogtay, N., et al. (2008). Neurodevelopmental trajectories of the human cerebral cortex. *The Journal of Neuroscience, 28*(14), 3586–3594.

Sheline, Y. I., Barch, D. M., Price, J. L., Rundle, M. M., Vaishnavi, S. N., Snyder, A. Z., et al. (2009). The default mode network and self-referential processes in depression. *Proceedings of the National Academy of Sciences of the United States of America, 106*(6), 1942–1947.

Sheline, Y. I., Price, J. L., Yan, Z., & Mintun, M. A. (2010). Resting-state functional MRI in depression unmasks increased connectivity between networks via the dorsal nexus. *Proceedings of the National Academy of Sciences of the United States of America, 107*(24), 11020–11025.

Sher, K. J., Gershuny, B. S., Peterson, L., & Raskin, G. (1997). The role of childhood stressors in the intergenerational transmission of alcohol use disorders. *Journal of the Study of Alcohol, 58*, 414–427.

Sheu, Y.-S., Polcari, A., Anderson, C. M., & Teicher, M. H. (2010). Harsh corporal punishment is associated with increased T2 relaxation time in dopamine-rich regions. *NeuroImage, 53*, 412–419.

Shirtcliff, E. A., Coe, C. L., & Pollak, S. D. (2009). Early childhood stress is associated with elevated antibody levels to herpes simplex virus type 1. *Proceedings of the National Academy of Sciences of the United States of America, 106*(8), 2963–2967.

Simantov, R., Blinder, E., Ratovitski, T., Tauber, M., Gabbay, M., & Porat, S. (1996). Dopamine induced apoptosis in human neuronal cells: Inhibition by nucleic acids antisense to the dopamine transporter. *Neuroscience, 74*, 39–50.

Smith, M. E. (2005). Bilateral hippocampal volume reduction in adults with post-traumatic stress disorder: A meta-analysis of structural MRI studies. *Hippocampus, 15*, 798–807.

Stein, M. B., Yehuda, R., Koverola, C., & Hanna, C. (1997). Enhanced dexamethasone suppression of plasma cortisol in adult women traumatized by childhood sexual abuse. *Biological Psychiatry, 42*(8), 680–686.

Tanabe, J., Tregellas, J. R., Dalwani, M., Thompson, L., Owens, E., Crowley, T., et al. (2009). Medial orbitofrontal cortex gray matter is reduced in abstinent substance-dependent individuals. *Biological Psychiatry, 65*, 160–164.

Taussig, H. N., Clyman, R. B., & Landsverk, J. (2001). Children who return home from foster care: A 6-year prospective study of behavioral health outcomes in adolescence. *Pediatrics, 108*(1), 1–7.

Teicher, M. H., Dumont, N. L., Ito, Y., Vaituzis, C., Giedd, J. N., & Andersen, S. L. (2004). Childhood neglect is associated with reduced corpus callosum area. *Biological Psychiatry, 56*, 80–85.

Thoma, P., Bellebaum, C., Koch, B., Schwarz, M., & Daum, I. (2008). The cerebellum is involved in reward-based reversal learning. *Cerebellum, 7*, 433–443.

Thompson, P. M., Giedd, J. N., Woods, R. P., MacDonald, D., Evans, A. C., & Toga, A. W. (2000). Growth patterns in the developing brain detected by using continuum mechanical tensor maps. *Nature, 404*, 190–193.

Todd, R. D. (1992). Neural development is regulated by classical neuro-transmitters: Dopamine D2 receptor stimulation enhances neurite outgrowth. *Biological Psychiatry, 31*, 794–807.

Tomasi, D., Volkow, N. D., Wang, R., Telang, F., Wang, G.-W., Chang, L., et al. (2009). Positive emotionality is associated with baseline metabolism in orbitofrontal cortex and in regions of the default network. *PLoS ONE, 4*(6), e6102–6101–6113.

Trickett, P. K., Noll, J. G., Susman, E. J., Shenk, C. E., & Putnam, F. W. (2010). Attenuation of cortisol across development for victims of sexual abuse. *Development and Psychopathology, 22*, 165–175.

U.S. Department of Health and Human Services. (2010). *Child maltreatment 2009*. Washington, DC: Administration for Children and Families, Administration on Children, Youth, and Families, Children's Bureau.

Volkow, N. D., Chang, L., Wang, G.-J., Fowler, J. S., Ding, Y.-S., Sedler, M., et al. (2001). Low level of brain dopamine D(2) receptors in methamphetamine abusers: Association with metabolism in the orbitofrontal cortex. *American Journal of Psychiatry, 158*, 2015–2021.

Volkow, N. D., & Fowler, J. S. (2000). Addiction, a disease of compulsion and drive: Involvement of the orbitofrontal cortex. *Cerebral Cortex, 10*, 318–325.

Volkow, N. D., Fowler, J. S., & Wang, G. J. (2002). Role of dopamine in drug reinforcement and addiction in humans: Results from imaging studies. *Behavioural Pharmacology, 13*, 355–366.

Volkow, N. D., Fowler, J. S., & Wang, G.-J. (2003). The addicted human brain: Insights from imaging studies. *The Journal of Clinical Investigations, 111*(10), 1444–1451.

Volkow, N. D., Hitzemann, R., Wang, G.-J, Fowler, J. S., Wolf, A. P. Dewey, S. L. et al. (1992). Long-term frontal brain metabolic changes in cocaine abusers. *Synapse, 11,* 184–190.

Volkow, N. D., Fowler, J. S., Wang, G.-J., Hitzemann, R., Logan, J., Schlyer, D. J. et al. (1993). Decreased dopamine D2 receptor availability is associated with reduced frontal metabolism in cocaine abusers. *Synapse, 14,* 169–177.

Walton, M. E., Devlin, J. T., & Rushworth, M. F. (2004). Interactions between decision making and performance monitoring within prefrontal cortex. *Nature Neuroscience, 7,* 1259–1265.

Wang, G.-J., Volkow, N. D., Fowler, J. S., Cervany, P., Hitzemann, R. J., Pappas, N. R., et al. (1999). Regional brain metabolic activation during craving elicited by recall of previous drug experiences. *Life Science, 64,* 775–784.

White, N. M. (1996). Addictive drugs as reinforcers: Multiple partial actions on memory systems. *Addiction, 91,* 921–949.

Widom, C. S. (1989). The cycle of violence. *Science, 244,* 160–166.

Widom, C. S., Ireland, T., & Glynn, P. J. (1995). Alcohol abuse in abused and neglected children followed-up: Are they at increased risk? *Journal of Studies on Alcohol, 56,* 207–217.

Widom, C. S., Weiler, B. L., & Cottler, L. B. (1999). Childhood victimization and drug abuse: A comparison of prospective and retrospective findings. *Journal of Consulting and Clinical Psychology, 67,* 867–880.

Wilsnack, S. C., Vogeltanz, N. D., Klassen, A. D., & Harris, T. R. (1997). Childhood sexual abuse and women's substance abuse: National survey findings. *Journal of the Study of Alcohol, 58,* 264–271.

Wilson, H. W., & Widom, C. S. (2009). A prospective examination of the path from child abuse and neglect to illicit drug use in middle adulthood: The potential mediating role of four risk factors. *Journal of Youth and Adolescence, 38,* 340–354.

Xie, P., Kranzler, H. R., Poling, J., Stein, M. B., Anton, R. F., Brady, K., et al. (2009). Interactive effect of stressful life events and the serotonin transporter 5-HTTLPR genotype on posttraumatic stress disorder diagnosis in 2 independent populations. *Archives of General Psychiatry, 66*(11), 1201–1209.

Yao, Z., Wang, L., Lu, Q., Liu, H., & Teng, G. (2009). Regional homogeneity in depression and its relationship with separate depressive symptom clusters: A resting-state fMRI study. *Journal of Affective Disorders, 115,* 430–438.

Yehuda, R. (2009). Status of glucocorticoid alterations in post-traumatic stress disorder. *New York Academy of Sciences, 1179,* 56–69.

Zhang, L.-X., Levine, S., Dent, G., Zhan, Y., Xing, G., Okimoto, D., et al. (2002). Maternal deprivation increases cell death in the infant rat brain. *Developmental Brain Research, 133,* 1–11.

Zhao, X., Wang, P., Li, C., Hu, Z., Xi, Q., Wu, W., et al. (2007). Altered default mode network activity in patient with anxiety disorders: An fMRI study. *European Journal of Radiology, 63*(3), 373–378.

5

Predictors, Correlates, and Consequences of Trajectories of Antisocial Personality Disorder Symptoms from Early Adolescence to Mid-30s

PATRICIA COHEN, THOMAS CRAWFORD,
HENIAN CHEN, STEPHANIE KASEN,
AND KATHY GORDON

In this chapter we attempt to add usefully to the substantial research over the past 3 decades and longer, on the origins and course of antisocial behaviors in children, adolescents, and adults (Farrington, 1992; Fergusson & Horwood 1998; Larzelere & Patterson 1990; Loeber, Farrington, Stouthamer-Loeber, & VanKammen 1998; McCord, 1991; Patterson, Reid, & Dishion, 1992; Widom 1989). Much of this literature, and particularly the longitudinal follow-up of children, was initiated by Lee Robins (1979; Robins, West, & Herjanic, 1975), a long-term active member of the American Psychopathological Association. We attempt to follow in her footsteps and in the footsteps of others who appreciated the critical importance of prospectively collected longitudinal data (Tonry, Ohlin, & Farrington, 1991).

The most solidly established early environmental risks for antisocial and violent behavior are poverty and childhood maltreatment or neglect (Grant & Compas, 2003). But these also place individuals at risk of a number of other problematic life trajectories, including other personality disorders, psychotic features, alcohol and drug abuse and dependence, and suicidality. Presumably the "choice" of a *particular* negative life trajectory involves more than these risk factors, including the way that the parents and the family as a whole cope with each other and, often, with poverty, the community setting in which the family lives, the origin and kind of maltreatment, and, of course, the genetic "environment" the child presents for these risks (Caspi et al., 2002; Widom & Brzustowicz, 2006).

There is increasing evidence that problematic components of family life and interpersonal interactions might be present and influential at the very beginning of an infant's life. Although much of the empirical work showing problematic mother–infant interactions focuses on offspring of depressed mothers (Field, 2010), there is growing evidence that maternal problems with coping adequately with the demands of a newborn are far from unusual (Beebe et al., 2010; Ritter, Bucci, Beebe, Jaffe, & Maskit, 2007). Other early problematic exposures might be associated with a wide range of personal and situational risks within the family, including behavior problems of one or both parents and interparental conflict.

One of the probable early mechanisms of subsequent trajectories of antisocial behaviors is employed as a diagnostic criterion: namely, problems in understanding and empathizing with others. But this "skill" is one that normatively begins to develop very early in life (Greenspan & Shanker, 2004), and its development process usually occurs via early infancy and subsequent interactions with other people, especially primary caretakers (usually mothers). As individuals move past infancy, their early development is furthered and influenced by the emotional and behavioral models presented to them by parents, siblings, and other persons by whom they are frequently surrounded and with whom they interact. In some circumstances and families, these models teach young children both which persons had better be avoided and what "negative" behaviors are normative.

Of course, a full investigation of the mechanisms of this large risk range with varied manifestations is beyond any single research project. However, here we hope to add some new considerations to our understanding of the origins of antisocial behavior, and we attempt some considerations of the consequences as well.

As a research perspective, it is increasingly appreciated that the optimal empirical evidence promoting understanding of differential health/illness, emotional or interpersonal traits or problems, and adaptive or maladaptive behaviors comes from longitudinal studies. A general focus on current environment and recent events, problems, and behaviors tends to minimize problems of informant memory and recall distortion influenced by more recent phenomena. Longitudinal studies permit the empirical identification of problems with developmental persistence and change over years and decades. Ideally, such studies include a range of subpopulations that vary with regard to likely or potential possession of or exposure to strengths and risks relevant to the study goals. As noted, it is also increasingly appreciated that the individual development of many important negative and positive traits, behaviors, and interactions begins very early in life, making it desirable to begin assessing trajectories of such characteristics during that period.

A fundamental premise underlying the empirical analyses presented here is that *trajectories* over two decades of the diagnostic criteria for this disorder will show substantial empirical statistical strength, despite the modest number of youth who would actually meet the diagnostic criteria. This does not necessarily reflect the reliability of the assessments; rather, the strength is attributable to the fact that trajectories involving multiple assessments over extensive intervals (here over 20 years) tend to strongly reflect the "central" component of a social/emotional/behavioral pattern that is *not* highly vulnerable to "local effects" of temporary positive and/or negative influence. Nevertheless, there might also be points in individual life trajectories at which we see more dramatic changes.

The analyses of trajectories of antisocial personality (ASP) symptoms investigated in these data reflect the following substantive hypotheses:

1. All personality disorders (PDs), including antisocial PD, begin their development early in life with exposure to a range of early environmental risks, including problematic parenting. (Responses and, potentially, exposures to these risks might depend partly on genetic variations among children. However, we do not include in this chapter any analyses of genetic associations on the segment of this cohort on whom such data have been collected.)

2. By mid-childhood, signs of ASP problems will be manifest in traits including poor social skills, misbehavior patterns, and problematic achievement that signal likely future problems.

3. The behavioral and social difficulties that accompany elevated ASP over these developmental trajectories will be reflected in correlated emotional and interpersonal problems.

4. The collective influence of these early risks leads to unrealistic and non-communitarian life goals in adolescence, with effects on ASP lasting to full adulthood.

5. The early and ongoing exposure to failures as many of these young people reach adulthood will lead to more violent expression of the ASP trajectory and consequent arrests, with time spent in jail or prison, independent of the ongoing effects of early risks.

Study Sample

The "Children in the Community" study sample was originally designed and recruited by Leonard Kogan and colleagues in 1975 to reflect, as much as possible, the variation in living conditions of American children. Kogan selected 100 tract/block groups located in rural, small town, suburban, urban, and central city sites in two upstate New York counties. Specific areas were picked to reflect the full range of median family income and to include about 10% African American families. Randomly selected families with one or more children between the ages of 1 and 10 in each site were asked to participate, and one child in this age range per family was randomly selected as the "target" child for maternal interviews covering pregnancy and the birth of the child, health history, child activities and behaviors, parenting, and family environment. Following Dr. Kogan's unanticipated death in the year following the data collection, his colleagues offered the data to Dr. Cohen. The original interview data were so rich that she obtained funding to determine whether the cohort could still be located (because of unrecorded family surnames of recruited families). Although the majority of families were located and almost all agreed to participate, a segment of the cohort could not be located because of the subsequent destruction of an originally sampled central-city area. The W.T. Grant Foundation provided funding for the replacement of this segment of the cohort by newly recruited families. The first follow-up interviews of mothers and study children were initiated and funded by the National Institute of Mental Health (Patricia Cohen, principal investigator) and the National Institute on Drug Abuse (Judith Brook, principal investigator) as a collaborative study.

This cohort of over 800 children has been assessed, via separate maternal and offspring interviews, up to an offspring mean age of 22. Interviews of parents (usually mothers) and cohort members were carried out separately in private locations (usually member homes) for the second, third, and fourth assessments. Interviews in full adulthood were carried out by in-person interviewers and/or via telephone, Internet, and/or mail, as was feasible and preferred by respondents, and the full adult interviews (mean ages 33 and 38) were followed by a clinical interview over the telephone to confirm diagnoses. Questionnaire responses and official records regarding violent experiences, behaviors, arrests, and incarceration were funded by the National Institute of Justice over the cohort's late 20s. Table 5.1 shows the mean birth year, gender, race, and poverty-level income in childhood for participants included in these analyses. In the analyses reported here, we found no race effects to be independent of poverty effects, except incarceration. Race is not included in this chapter. Although there have been virtually no actual response refusals or requests to be removed from the participant list, the sample assessments have declined over the most recent assessments, primarily because of our inability to locate some participants. These difficulties are consistent with the high mobility of this generation (now living in at least 40 states) and the use of cell phones, which deters potential location via telephone books (which had been critical for the first follow-up). The two most recent assessments were limited to 694 of the estimated over 770 surviving respondents. Some interviews of adult participants in New York State prisons have been arranged with the appropriate authorities. Subject loss is not correlated with race or with psychiatric diagnoses, but the lesser

Table 5.1 Characteristics of Study Trajectory Sample, Including Residence at Initial Assessment

Gender		51% male	
Race	Caucasian	90%	
	Black	9%	
		N	% in poverty by location
Early life location	Rural	287	11%
	Small town	38	18%
	Suburban	181	6%
	City	314	18%
Total		820	12.6%

Note: Less than 1% of the sample were of other race/ethnicity, including Asian American, Native American, or a combination of backgrounds.

participation of males in any given adult assessment that generally characterizes longitudinal studies is also found in this study. Participants receive a modest compensation for the time spent on each assessment. All procedures were conducted in accordance with those approved by the New York State Psychiatric Institute Institutional Review Board.

Methods to be Employed in these Analyses

The primary method we will be employing for the analyses of these risks will examine their influence on the trajectory of antisocial PD symptoms as assessed by self-report. This cohort was born over a full decade, and the intervals between the four assessments employed here varied among participants, depending on both funding intervals and participant convenience for scheduling. This variability in intervals between assessments, as well as the substantial birth year variability of this cohort, has led us to adopt the SAS Hierarchical Linear Model (HLM) program for the analyses of these data. The measure of ASP symptoms is taken by means of self-report over four assessments beginning in early adolescence (mean age 13.4, but as young as age 10) and ending when the subjects are as old as age 36. The sum of responses to the items covering the antisocial PD diagnostic criteria permits analyses of the trajectories representing four assessments over 20 years across the entire cohort using this HLM program.

The variables representing this trajectory are not criterion counts but rather responses to scaled items representing *Diagnostic and Statistical Manual of Mental Disorders*, fourth edition (*DSM-IV*) antisocial PD diagnostic criteria, here selected for maximal consistency over the trajectory and strong representation of these criteria by chapter co-author Crawford. The dependent variable in most of these analyses is the *trajectory* of ASP symptoms, rather than any individual assessment. There is no standard way of assessing the reliability of a trajectory centered on a consistent age when the age range of a cohort is so large and the durations between assessments vary substantially both for the sample as a whole and within the sample. The internal consistency reliability of the measure covers the *DSM-IV* ASP criteria in individual assessments at mean age 13.5 (SD = 0.67), mean age 16.5 (SD = 0.73), mean age 21 (SD = 0.75), and mean age 33 (SD = 0.78). Correlations between these assessments averaged 0.54, and those between consecutive assessments averaged 0.61.

In these analyses, the trajectory mean for each participant is estimated at a fixed age of 22, and annual changes in trajectory before and after that age are also an essential component of the "level 1" (or individual) differences being examined. These Bayesian estimates produced by the HLM program also permit tests for nonlinear antisocial trajectories and changes in the magnitude of the effects of risks with age, as well as an examination of the connections of the antisocial trajectory with the trajectories of any other measures also assessed consistently at every interview. Finally, in addition to an analysis of the earlier life risks, these analyses permit examination of the trajectory relationship with adult arrest for violent behavior and any adult incarceration.[1]

Method and Presentation of Findings

As noted, all of the analyses employed here are designed to add to the general understanding of the sources and consequences of ASP symptoms in a general U.S. population sample born in the decade surrounding 1970. In order to maximize understanding and comparison of differential effect size magnitudes associated with the measured risks in addition to standardization of the full ASP trajectory, we standardized each scaled predictor. The exceptions to this rule are dichotomous predictors, such as child abuse, in which the difference between the two levels of the variable are best understood as mean differences between those with a 0 score and those with a score of 1. We graph some associations of predictors with the trajectory of ASP symptoms both to promote understanding of risk-associated differences *over the trajectory*, including gender differences, and, especially, to clarify changes in the magnitude of effects of some predictors over the ages represented by this trajectory.

The sections begin with an identification of the variables representing each of the study hypotheses. Each section includes a tabular display of trajectory findings and a graphic presentation of findings that might otherwise be more difficult to understand. After an analysis of the risk sets, we combine those risks

---

1 Although prison sentence information was available, we used either information from self-reports of incarceration or official records of incarceration to yield a measure of any incarceration.

that showed significant effects when separately considered in order to determine which are sufficiently powerful and/or unique to be viewed as independent predictors of the ASP trajectory.

Study Measures and Analytic Strategy Reflecting the Five Study Hypotheses

Hypothesis 1: Risks for Elevated Trajectories of ASP Symptoms Begin Early in Life with Exposure to a Range of Early Environmental Risks

The first set of analyses estimate (a) which early life environmental exposures and experienced parenting are empirically identified child risks for an elevated subsequent trajectory of ASP symptoms, and (b) which early life risks show independent cumulative influence and which might be better understood as correlates of these independent-effect risks.

Early Childhood Environment Risks

The earliest measured risk in this study was a maternal report (at offspring mean age 5.5) of the mother's feelings and those of the child's father when they first found out she was pregnant with this child. Perhaps surprisingly, although an unwanted pregnancy was a predictor of some other symptom trajectories, it was not a significant predictor of antisocial PD. Family income below the federal poverty level for families of that size (measured dichotomously as "poverty") and parental divorce history are examined as risks. Another mother-reported exposure is whether the child's father has problems with alcohol, substance use, and/or the police, measured dichotomously and labeled as "paternal sociopathy." Parenting practices beginning early in childhood as reported by the mother include "power-assertive punishment"; this is our label for disciplinary methods of the mother and father (if the father was present) including frequent physical punishment, timed isolation in frightening or restricting locations, insulting name-calling, and threats of abandonment. Maternal reports of marital problems including arguments were a significant predictor of ASP trajectory elevation. However, these problems were not assessed until the second maternal interviews, were not available for most divorced fathers, and overlapped substantially with parental divorce; therefore, here we focus on the impact of divorce on the ASP trajectory.

Any well-known set of risks must include childhood or early adolescent severe neglect and/or physical or sexual abuse, here assessed via a combination of official records and youth abuse reports when the children were age 18 or older (consistent with then-constricted investigation via self-report at earlier ages). All risks are examined for differential impact on boys as compared to girls.

Having identified which of these risks are statistically significant when examined separately, we explored them in subsequent analyses as a set of early environmental risks. These analyses estimate whether some of the identified risks might be viewed as mediated by other risks when examined in combination.

In this series we also examine the child's relationship with parents, first measured in the early adolescent assessment. Examined variables include the level of parental involvement with this child and the child's admiration of and wish to be or not be like the parent.

Hypothesis 2: By Mid-childhood, Signs of These Problems Will Be Manifest in Relevant Traits, Misbehavior Patterns, Poor Social Skills, and Poor Achievement

Childhood traits selected as predictors of the ASP symptom trajectory are primarily based on factored trajectories of 78 items covering offspring characteristics and behaviors reported by the mother in the three assessments covering the period from early childhood (wave 1, ages 2 to 10) to late adolescence (ages 12 to 19). In order to "equate" the estimated assessment age across the cohort, each item trajectory mean was estimated for each child at age 9, and the resulting means were factored. We have labeled these "traits" for the high or problematic end as irritable, hyperactive/unsocialized, neurotic, shy introversion, isolated introversion, poor executive function, and aggression. Although not assessed until the children were, on average, age 13, we also include two other theoretically important maternal reports: offspring social competence (covering friendship quality and quantity, bullying, and being bullied) and offspring school performance (average grades). As with the analyses of hypothesis 1, we anticipate overlap in these predictions and examine together those that showed a clear association with the trajectory when considered separately. Gender differences are also examined.

Hypothesis 3: Antisocial Trajectories Partly Reflect Emotional and Interpersonal Problems that Result in the Behavioral and Social Malfunctions of Antisocial Symptoms

Selected variables for this hypothesis are an unusual set of variable trajectories that we believe well represent these problems. These are the trajectories over the same decades of the diverse individual criteria of borderline disorder. We label these diagnostic criteria (presented in the same sequence as described in *DSM-IV*) as (1) fear of abandonment, (2) unstable close relationships, (3) problematic identity, (4) impulsivity, (5) suicidality, (6) unstable affect, (7) severe anger, (8) frequent boredom (our closest measured approximation to the criterion "feelings of emptiness"), and (9) paranoia. These names are, of course, shortcuts to the more detailed descriptions of these problems in *DSM*, and are represented by "miniscales" employed to assess them, typically including two to four Likert scale response items. Our use of these to represent potential emotional promoters (or protectors) of elevated symptoms of antisocial PD is justified by (a) the reasonably strong representation of the major negative emotions, (b) the history of these two disorders as being part of the same "subgroup" of PDs in *DSM*, and (c) our recent examination of these individual borderline PD symptom trajectories in relationship to early life negative experiences (submitted). There are no items that were employed for the assessment of both of these disorders.

Hypothesis 4: The Antisocial Trajectory Will Be Reflected in Unrealistic and Noncommunitarian Life Goals in Adolescence, with Effects Lasting to Full Adulthood

Selected variables come from responses to a "q-sort" task (the Childs Life Priority measure) devised to measure the relative importance to cohort members of 21 major potential life goals (Cohen & Cohen, 1996, pp. 43–53). Respondents grouped these goals into seven piles, with one goal identified as the "most important"; two as the next most important; four ranked as the next most important after those two; seven in the middle category; and then another four, two, and finally one "least important" goal. These goals have been shown in previous analyses to be related to a range of current and young adult Axis I psychiatric disorders and other negative outcomes (Cohen & Cohen, 1996, 2001), but their relationship with ASP symptoms has not been previously examined. This hypothesis is not tested by prediction of the full trajectory of ASP, because at the time of assessment that trajectory was already well underway, particularly for the older members of this cohort. Therefore, these life goals are employed as predictors of ASP symptoms 15 to 20 years later, when the cohort members were in their 30s.

Hypothesis 5: The ASP Trajectory Will Predict Violent and Other Illegal Behavior in Full Adulthood, and Will Do So Independently of the Early Life Risks

For these analyses, we examine the combined effects of the ASP trajectory at a mean age of 22 and the official records of arrest for violent offence and incarceration for the following eight years. We also examine the independence of the ASP trajectory and the early life risks as predictors of adult violence and crime.

Study Findings

The first set of analyses examines the full trajectory of scaled and standardized antisocial criteria from age 10 to age 40 for the sample as a whole and for males and females separately (see Fig. 5.1). For the entire cohort, average antisocial behavior begins its decline in late adolescence, and the mean assessment at age 22 is already about 0.125 standard deviation (SD) lower than its maximum at a mean value of 0.116. Also, the antisocial criteria sum is about 0.5 SD higher for males than for females. This first graph shows the mean antisocial PD symptom trajectories of males and females in this cohort from the first assessment, when the youngest members were ages 9 and 10, to the fourth assessment of these symptoms, when the cohort members were in their mid-30s. This graph, like all the graphs shown here, use symptom sums standardized across the full trajectory in order to provide an understood measure of the size of effects and effect differences, and use age 22 as the trajectory mean age. The vertical scale shows the standardized trajectory mean = 0 and here covers the range from 1 SD unit below the mean to 1 SD above the mean. The horizontal scale shows the ages covered by these data (the ages actually go to the mid-30s, but the trajectories are basically flat after about age 32). Not surprisingly, the male average level of antisocial PD symptoms is consistently higher than the female average (about half the SD of the combined data by age 18). In addition, the overall average symptoms begin to decline at about age 17 for girls and decline later and less for boys, for whom a relative plateau tends to characterize their 30s.

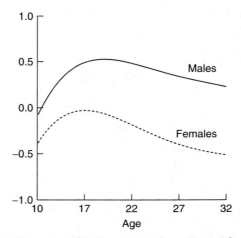

Figure 5.1 Full mean trajectories of ASP symptoms for males and females.

Hypothesis 1. Early Childhood Risks Are Predictors of Elevated Trajectories of Antisocial PD Symptoms

Table 5.2 reports the trajectory mean elevation at age 22 found for each of these early childhood risks for the sample as a whole and separately by gender (if the magnitudes of effects were significantly different). Children in families living below the national poverty level showed a nearly 0.25 SD higher antisocial symptom trajectory (B = 0.228). Offspring of fathers with "sociopathy" (a problem with alcohol, drug use, and/or the police) had a trajectory mean that was 0.29 SD units higher than that of those whose father did not have any of these mother-reported problems. Perhaps surprisingly, this paternal risk showed no significant difference in effects on sons and on daughters.

Parenting via power-assertive punishment was equally predictive of ASP trajectory elevation when assessed in wave 1 (W1) (not shown in the table because 53 children in the cohort were not yet recruited) and in W2, when the cohort was almost eight years older. This effect on ASP symptoms declined on average by 0.004 per year. Because its effect at age 22 is estimated at 0.142, this indicates that at age 12, for example, it was approximately 0.142 + (−10 years × −0.004 = 0.04) = 0.182. Early life parental divorce had a particularly problematic effect on sons, although its effect was not significant on daughters. Divorce prior to offspring adolescence had a strong association with the ASP trajectory for both sons and daughters, with average elevation at the trajectory mean bieng 0.33 SD above the remaining sample mean.

As anticipated, a childhood history of abuse was strongly connected with antisocial behavior. The effects of physical abuse was large and not significantly different for boys and girls: with nearly 1/2 SD elevation of ASP throughout the

Table 5.2 Individual Childhood Risks for Elevated Trajectory of ASP

		Effect (SE)	Change per year (SE)
Poverty		0.228 (0.065)*	
Paternal sociopathy		0.290 (0.065)*	
Power punishment 2		0.142 (0.028)**	−0.004 (0.002)**
Divorce prior to wave 1	Females	0.005 (0.118)	
	Males	0.341 (0.146)	0.063 (0.018)**
Divorce prior to wave 2		0.332 (0.074)*	
Any abuse		0.433 (0.078)*	0.012 (0.005)**
Sex abuse	Females	0.266 (0.084)*	
	Males	0.691 (0.224)*	
Physical abuse		0.439 (0.109)*	

**p < 0.01.
*p < 0.05.

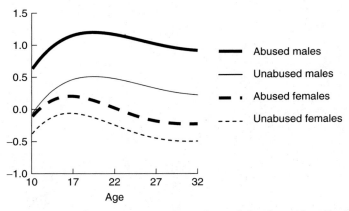

Figure 5.2 Trajectories of ASP symptoms for males and females with and without a history of sexual abuse.

trajectory (0.44) However, the effect of sexual abuse was not the same for girls and boys. As shown in Figure 5.2, a history of sexual abuse of boys was associated with a remarkable elevation of 0.691 SD units of ASP symptoms, with almost no decline over the trajectory. The ASP trajectory history of sexual abuse of girls was 0.266 SD units, not trivial, but certainly much lower. Sexual abuse was associated with trajectory means that were 0.266 SD units higher on average for girls but a remarkable 0.691 SD units higher for the few boys with such a reported or recorded history, and there was almost no subsequent decline throughout the adult years (see Fig. 5.2). This is a controversial finding, although it is supported by many clinicians. The effect of physical abuse was large and not significantly different for males and females, with nearly 0.5 SD elevation throughout the trajectory (0.439).

Of course, these childhood risks are not uncorrelated. Table 5.3 shows the significance of the independent effects of these risks. The overlap in exposure to these risks is reflected in a decline in these estimates, as expected, and the effect

Table 5.3 Early Risks Modeled Together

	Effect (SE)
Poverty	0.070 (0.067)*
Paternal sociopathy	0.138 (0.068)**
Power punishment 2	0.136 (0.027)***
Divorce	0.245 (0.064)***
Any abuse	0.266 (0.078) ***

*NS, not significant.
**p < 0.05.
*** p < 0.01.

of poverty is essentially mediated by the higher likelihood of the other risks in families living in poverty.

*Hypothesis 2. By Mid-childhood, Signs of Early Risk of Later
ASP Will Be Manifest in Relevant Traits, Misbehavior
Patterns, Poor Social Skills, and Poor Achievement that
Will Influence the Subsequent ASP Trajectory*

These risks are mother-reported childhood behavior patterns and traits estimated at age 9 as described earlier. To these we added two measures first reported by mothers at offspring mean age 13.5: social competence (having adequate friendships, not bullying, not being bullied) and academic achievement (summed across academic subjects). As can be seen in Table 5.4, the largest predictor of the subsequent antisocial PD symptom trajectory (+0.41) was what we labeled "hyperactive/unsocialized," which involved a broad range of defiant, rule-breaking behaviors, as well as signs of hyperactivity, a variable that might be viewed as a "prelude" to later measured full ASP symptoms.

Childhood aggression and irritability significantly predicted the subsequent antisocial PD symptom trajectory, with each showing an estimated mean elevation at trajectory age 22 of 0.18 SD units. However, the prediction of elevated ASP by childhood irritability declined somewhat in full adulthood. Neurotic behaviors were more modestly, but significantly, associated with the trajectory (+0.13), as was low executive function (+0.08). Introversion/shyness, considered by itself, did not characterize the children who later showed antisocial symptoms. Social competence as reported by mothers at offspring mean age 13 was modestly but significantly predictive of a lower ASP trajectory. Academic performance was highly predictive of the ASP trajectory, as shown in Figure 5.3. It

Table 5.4 Childhood Traits as Risks for Elevated ASP Trajectory

	Individual effect (SE)	*Change per year (SE)*	*Combined effect*
Hyperactive/unsocialized	0.396 (0.065)**		0.402 (0.034)**
Irritable	0.185 (0.029)**	−0.004 (0.002)*	0.007 (0.032)
Aggressive	0.183 (0.026)**		0.028 (0.029)
Neurotic	0.140 (0.027)**	−0.004 (0.002)*	−0.040 (0.032)
Poor executive function	0.087 (0.027)**	−0.005 (0.002)**	−0.059 (0.027)*
Introverted/shy	−0.015 (0.027)	−0.004 (0.002)*	−0.092 (0.026)**
Introverted/alone	0.036 (0.027)		0.005 (0.027)
School grades	−0.164 (0.028)**	0.007 (0.002)**	−0.073 (0.031)*
Social competency	−0.038 (0.015)*		0.004 (0.015)

*p < 0.05.
**p < 0.01.

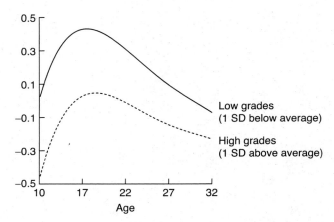

Figure 5.3 Trajectories of ASP symptoms associated with high and low school grades.

can be seen that in the preteen years, low grades were not particularly predictive of elevation in ASP symptoms, but by late adolescence such symptoms were nearly 0.5 SD above the norm for youth with low grades.

As shown in Table 5.4, when we combined these childhood traits for simultaneous prediction the only independent effects were hyperactive/unsocialized (B = 0.402, P < .0001) and introverted/shy (B = −.0.091, P < 0.001), which was somewhat *protective*. An interactive effect (not shown here) indicated that some of those shy children who were not hyperactive/unsocialized at age 9 became subsequently involved in antisocial behaviors, perhaps as a way of becoming part of a group of "peers".

Parent–Child Relationship in Adolescence

Although for the most part we are not reporting findings on parent–youth relationships in mid- to late adolescence, when ASP symptoms might already be established, certain measures reported by youth or mothers at mean age 13.4 were too informative to be ignored. When asked whether they identified with or wanted to be like each parent, unlike most offspring, those with subsequent elevated ASP trajectories tended not to identify with either the father (B = −0.21, P < 0.01) or the mother (B = −0.22, P < 0.01). We also examined the potential interactive effect of identification with the father when the father had early sociopathic symptoms (as reported by the mother). This interaction was statistically significant (p = 0.01) and showed that the ASP trajectory mean associated with the father's sociopathy was lowered from 0.24 to 0.08 (not significant) when the child was one SD unit lower on identification with the father. We interpret this finding as effective resilience on the child's part.

Mothers who reported a low level of involvement with their offspring also had children with higher antisocial trajectories; similarly, youth who reported a significantly low level of paternal involvement also had elevated ASP trajectories (maternal reports on this variable were not asked for because divorces were common).

Hypothesis 3: Antisocial Trajectories Partly Reflect Emotional and Interpersonal Problems that Influence and Reflect the Behavioral and Social Difficulties of Antisocial Symptoms

We employ the trajectories of the nine individual criteria of borderline personality disorder (BDL) as defined earlier in this chapter. Unlike the risks examined earlier, these measures were taken as part of the same sets of interviews as the diagnostic criteria for ASP. Thus we are examining not "predictive" risks but what may be viewed as concurrent emotional correlates. As seen in Table 5.5, the trajectory of only one of these criteria was *not* significantly positively related to the ASP trajectory. This measure, fear of abandonment, was (modestly) related *negatively* to the ASP trajectory, possibly reflecting a constructive response to problematic parenting. For most of the other BDL criteria, excepting suicidality (which had a surprisingly large relationship with ASP symptoms at age 22), the associations of these emotional/social problems were very modest in early adolescence and increased over the full two decades we include in these analyses.

In order to understand the meaning of such trajectories we may compare these effects with the trajectory changes in Figure 5.1, where the norm was shown to be a decline of ASP symptoms in adulthood, and with Table 5.4 where, with the exception of hyperactive and aggression, childhood trait effects on antisocial symptoms declined over time. This table indicates that every emotional and behavioral risk that defines borderline disorder except the fear of abandonment and suicidality showed an <u>increased</u> relationship with ASP over this 20 year period into full adulthood. Paranoid symptoms are associated with 0.089 elevated ASP symptoms at age 22 but this association also increased 0 .015 per year, which would increase paranoid effects to about 0.24, if persistent over the subsequent decade.

As noted earlier, the weakest measure of BDL criteria in this set is "boredom" (used to reflect the criterion "feelings of emptiness"), which was measured by a single (Likert scale) item indicating frequent boredom. Nevertheless, this item had the largest association with the ASP trajectory of this set, and the second largest increase with age. The only significant gender difference in these associations was found with ASP and impulsivity, for which the relationship was greater for males.

Table 5.5 Associations of BDL Emotional Criteria Trajectories with Trajectories of ASP

		Effect on ASP mean (SE)	Change per year (SE)
Fear of abandonment		−0.056 (0.015)*	
Unstable relationships		0.171 (0.018)*	0.009 (0.002)*
Problematic identity		0.157 (0.017)*	0.004 (0.002)**
Impulsivity	Males	0.215 (0.021)*	0.007 (0.002)*
	Females	0.104 (0.021)*	0.007 (0.002)*
Suicidality		0.165 (0.015)*	
Unstable affect		0.202 (0.017)*	0.011 (0.002)*
Anger		0.137 (0.017)*	0.007 (0.002)*
Boredom		0.259 (0.018)*	0.013 (0.002)*
Paranoia		0.089 (0.018)**	0.015 (0.002)*

*$p < 0.05$.
**$p < 0.01$.

Hypothesis 4. Aberrant Rankings of Life Goals in Adolescence Will Predict ASP Symptoms as Assessed in Full Adulthood

In these analyses we did not employ the trajectory of ASP as the dependent variable, because these life goals were assessed until late adolescence. Rather, we identify the adolescent life goals that significantly predicted ASP symptoms at mean age 33. Because there were nontrivial gender differences in the importance of a number of these life goals, and because there were sparse numbers of women who had seriously elevated antisocial symptoms when they were in their 30s, we focus on male importance rankings. Here we note the largest correlations of "rankings" of the life goals in adolescence with ASP symptoms in reporting males some 12 to 14 years later. The strongest predictive goal was "to have a satisfying sex life," which correlated +0.238 with ASP symptoms. The largest negatively predictive goals (indicating rankings much lower than those made by other males) were "to be a really good person" (r = −0.165) and "to really love my work" (−0.147). "To be rich" was ranked somewhat more modestly higher (+0.106) by those adolescent boys who would subsequently have elevated ASP symptoms.

Hypothesis 5. The Trajectory of Antisocial PD Symptoms Will Predict Violence and Incarceration in Adulthood Independent of the Childhood Risks that Led to Such Symptoms

We also examined whether the ASP trajectory can be considered causal of adult crime and violence, as opposed to these being only one more outcome of early life risks and traits. A related question is whether the early life risk effects on adult crime and violence are entirely mediated by ASP symptoms. We employed the following sequence of analyses in order to address this question: First, analyses identified the highest early risks for adult arrest for violence and/or adult incarceration to be family poverty, power-assertive punishment (standardized scale), abuse, paternal sociopathy, and parental divorce. These early risks were then pooled with the (standardized) trajectory mean of ASP symptoms estimated at age 22 as predictors in logistic regression analyses of officially recorded adult violent offenses of females and males, followed by analyses of adult incarceration of men in the sample.

Of the 34 men with a history of adult arrest for assault or violence, despite the significant associations of each of these potential risks when considered separately, when employed as combined predictors the only significant risks were a history of power-assertive punishment (p = 0.01; odds ratio [OR] = 1.80; confidence interval [CI] = 1.53–2.81) and the ASP trajectory mean (p = 0.01; OR = 1.83; CI = 1.15–2.91). Poverty (net of these correlated predictors) was "protective" (OR = 0.33, p = 0.015), as was child abuse history (OR = 0.21, p = 0.001).

For the 11 women with a history of adult arrest for assault or violence, family poverty was also "protective" (net of the correlated early risks) (OR = 0.16, CI = 0.039–0.641) when examined with the significant standardized ASP trajectory mean (p = 0.01; OR = 3.11; CI = 1.29–7.52) per SD elevation.

Findings for the adult incarceration of men were quite different from findings for arrest for violence. As can be seen in Figure 5.4, adult incarceration of men was strongly related to level of ASP symptoms, and also for women in late adolescence. But family poverty history was also an independent risk for adult incarceration (p = 0.022, OR = 3.24), as was power-assertive punishment (p = 0.006, OR = 2.18), when examined in combination with ASP symptoms at age 22 (p = 0.004, OR = 2.12). These variables remained significant when race was added to the predictors. Analysis regarding the adult incarceration of eight women indicated ASP symptoms at age 22 as the only significant independent predictor, with OR = 8.17.

Thus, the answer to the question posed earlier is that the trajectory of ASP symptoms is very predictive of adult violence and incarceration and may be viewed as "carrying the risks" of problematic early life experience to a substantial degree. It is true that for some fraction of these "early vulnerable" youth, early life risks—especially poverty, abuse history, and early semi-abusive "power-assertive" punishment—were associated with reduced risk of arrest for violence. Nevertheless, these early life experiences represent partly independent risks for adult male incarceration.

Overall Findings and Study Limitations

Our goal in this chapter has been to support the existing evidence from a number of other studies that the risks of subsequent antisocial symptoms and behaviors are often present very early in life. A range of early childhood exposures indicate

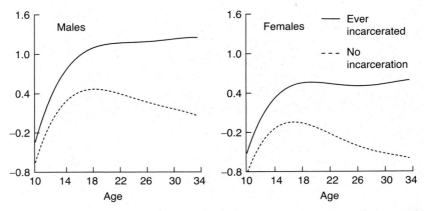

Figure 5.4 ASP symptoms for males and females with and without a history of incarceration.

substantial risk for a subsequent elevated trajectory of antisocial PD symptoms as assessed first in early adolescence and subsequently three times over the next 20 years. These early risks also influence the development of childhood traits that might reflect, lead to, or protect from subsequent unambiguous trajectories of antisocial symptoms. Poor parent–offspring relationship quality might also both reflect and increase these developing symptoms. These trajectories are often accompanied by a range of emotional problems, as we have shown here. Nevertheless, the relationships of ASP symptoms with emotional problems might reflect bidirectional influences.

In addition, many of the variables we explored as predictors of elevated trajectories of ASP symptoms cannot be unambiguously identified as causes rather than intervening mechanisms. Experiences and behaviors are influenced by earlier behaviors and experiences, and identifying the point at which intervention would be most critical is difficult.

Despite the richness of these data, it is quite unlikely that the risks we examined here fully describe the set of influences that result in adolescent or adult antisocial behavior (Kasen, Cohen, Chen, Johnson, & Crawford, 2009). Frequently, certain risks lead to other risks. There will be "local" influences and difficult-to-study combinations of events and settings, more likely to be portrayed in the theatre than readily identified by research. And unlike some—perhaps most—of the PDs we have studied, the clinical "treatments" of antisocial PD (and its early manifestations) might only rarely be carried out in a spirit of helpfulness and concern for the individual, even in adolescence.

One's environment, peers, and activities during adolescence might shape life goals and goal options in a way that enhances or protects from the likelihood of the longer-term persistence in adulthood of elevated antisocial symptoms. Although some of these factors, such as school climate (Kasen et al., 2009), reactions to school, neighborhood qualities, and peer relationships/bullying, were also assessed on this cohort, the inclusion of these required more assessments "during" as well as prior to the assessed trajectory of ASP symptoms. Nevertheless, the comparative analyses reported here strongly support the view that although some additional early risks might have long-term effects on violent and maladaptive behavior, subsequent experiences, achievements, and goals also reflected in and on the ASP trajectory represent a long-term risk for violence and other criminal behavior.

Where might we go from here? There are several interesting findings that bear on controversial issues. One of these is the very substantial negative impact we found of childhood sexual abuse on boys in this study. A meta-analysis of studies of college students (Rind, Tromovitch, & Bauserman, 1998) concluded that the childhood sexual abuse of boys had modest adult effects. That publication elicited a huge outcry, and eventually even a U.S. congressional condemnation of the research and a subsequent American Psychological Association retraction of support for the empirical meta-analysis (McNally, 2003). More recent research (D'Arecca, 2004; Nalavany, 2006) and research reviews, especially Spiegel's 2003 book *Sexual Abuse of Males*, have led to a broader acceptance of the childhood abuse of males as a serious problem, particularly by the clinical world (Campagna, 2005).

Perhaps the most critical issue raised by these and other data is that of early prevention efforts. An empirically based appreciation of the impact of problematic environments in early childhood should bring into focus some of our best chances of minimizing the frequency of antisocial trajectories from childhood to adulthood. There is also a need for an increased understanding of how some fraction of these children manage to develop into emotionally and behaviorally adept adults, and of what might be their biological and environmental "protectors" that allow them to avoid an elevated trajectory of antisocial symptoms.

An essential part of this intervention would seek to correct the maladaptive understanding of other people that encourages, or even produces, antisocial behavior. This will probably require early interventions that would help mothers, and ideally both parents, to provide sufficient and mutually satisfying interactions with their offspring in infancy and continuing throughout the early years. Prevention efforts relevant to these risks are now underway, including early offspring life positive parenting training of mothers, preschool child training, and other efforts (Murray & Farrington, 2010). However, a range of both policy and prevention efforts are likely to be needed before we find solutions that are both accepted and effective (Yirmiya, 2010).

Acknowledgments

This chapter was delivered in conjunction with the presentation of the Joseph Zubin Award at the 2011 meeting of the American Psychopathology Association to Patricia Cohen. We particularly thank our statistical collaborator Jack McArdle, who introduced the SAS Hierarchical Linear Model and trained our group of investigators.

Disclosure Statement

The authors have no conflicts of interest to disclose.

References

Beebe, B., Jaffe, J., Markese, S., Buck, K., Chen, H., Cohen, P., et al. (2010). The origins of 12-month attachment: A microanalysis of 4 month mother-infant interaction. *Attachment & Human Development*, 12(1–2), 6–141.

Campagna, A. F. (2005). Review of sexual abuse of males: The SAM model of theory and practice. *Journal of the American Academy of Child & Adolescent Psychiatry*, 44(10), 1064–1065.

Caspi, A., McClay, J., Moffit, T. E., Mill, J., Martin, J., & Craig, I. A. (2002). Role of genotype in cycle of violence in maltreated children. *Science*, 297, 851–854.

Cohen, P., & Cohen, J. (2001). Life values and adolescent mental health. In P. Schmuck & K. M. Sheldon (Eds.), *Life goals and well-being* (pp. 167–181). Goettingen, Germany: Hogrefe.

Cohen, P., Crawford, T. N., Johnson, J. G., & Kasen, S. (2005). The children in the community study of developmental course of personality disorder. *Journal of Personality Disorders*, 19(5), 466–486.

D'Arecca, T. L. (2004). Childhood sexual abuse: Trauma symptoms, coping responses, and cognitive distortions between adult male offenders and non-offenders. *Dissertation Abstracts International Section B*, 64(8), 4029.

Farrington, D. P. (1992). Explaining the beginning, progress and ending of antisocial behavior in adulthood. In J. McCord (Ed.), *Facts, frameworks and forecasts: Advances in criminology* (pp. 253–286). Brunswick, NJ: Transaction.

Farrington, D. P., & Welsh, B. C. (2007). *Saving children from a life of crime: Early risks and interventions*. Oxford, UK: Oxford University Press.

Fergusson, D. M., & Horwood, L. J. (1998). Exposure to interparental violence in childhood and adjustment in young adulthood. *Child Abuse & Neglect*, 22, 339–357.

Field, T. (2010). Postpartum depression effects on early interactions, parenting, and safety practices: A review. *Infant Behavior & Development*, 33(1), 1–6.

Grant, K. E., & Compas, B. E. (2003). Stressors and child and adolescent psychopathology: Moving from markers to mechanisms of risk. *Psychological Bulletin*, 129(3), 447–466.

Greenspan, S., & Shanker, S. G. (2004). *The first idea: How symbols, language, and intelligence evolved from our primate ancestors to modern humans*. Cambridge, MA: Perseus Books.

Kasen, S., Cohen, P., Chen, H., Johnson, J. G., & Crawford, T. N. (2009). School climate and continuity of adolescent personality disorder symptoms. *Journal of Child Psychology & Psychiatry*, 50(12), 1504–1512.

Larzelere, R. E., & Patterson, G. R. (1990). Parental management: Mediator of the effect of parent status on early delinquency. *Criminology*, 28(2), 301–323.

Loeber, R., Farrington, D. P., Stouthamer-Loeber, M., & VanKammen, W. B. (1998). *Antisocial behavior and mental health problems: Explanatory factors in childhood and adolescence*. Mahwah, NJ: Lawrence Erlbaum Associates.

McCord, J. (1991). Family relationships, juvenile delinquency, and adult criminality. *Criminology*, 29(3), 397–417.

McNally, R. J. (2003). Progress and controversy in the study of post-traumatic stress disorder. *Annual Review of Psychology*, 34, 229–252.

Moffit, T. E. (1993). Adolescence-limited and life-course-persistent antisocial behavior. *Psychological Review*, 100, 674–701.

Murray, J., & Farrington, D. P. (2010). Risk factors for conduct disorder and delinquency: Key findings from longitudinal studies. *Canadian Journal of Psychiatry*, 55(10), 633–642.

Nalavany, B. (2006). The impact of preadoptive childhood sexual abuse on adopted boys. *Dissertation Abstracts International Section A*, 67(4), 1536.

Patterson, G. R., Reid, J. B., & Dishion, T. J. (1992). *Antisocial boys: A social interactional approach* (Vol. 4). Eugene, OR: Castalia.

Rind, B., Tromovitch, P., & Bauserman, R. (1998). A meta-analytic examination of assumed properties of child sexual abuse using college samples. *Psychological Bulletin*, 124(1), 22–53.

Ritter, M., Bucci, W., Beebe, B., Jaffe, J., & Maskit, B. (2007). Do mothers of secure infants speak differently than mothers of avoidant infants in natural conversations? *Journal of the American Psychoanalytic Association*, 55(1), 269–275.

Robins, L. N. (1979). Sturdy childhood predictors of adult outcomes. In J. E. Barrett, R. M. Rose, & G. L. Klerman (Eds.), *Stress and mental disorder*. New York: Raven Press.

Robins, L. N., West, P. A., & Herjanic, B. L. (1975). Arrests in two generations of black urban families and their children. *Journal of Child Psychology and Psychiatry*, 16, 125–140.

Spiegel, J. (2003). *Sexual abuse of males: The SAM model of theory and practice*. New York: Brunner-Routledge.

Tonry, M., Ohlin, L. E., & Farrington, D. P. (1991). *Human development and criminal behavior: New ways of advancing knowledge*. New York: Springer-Verlag.

Widom, C. S. (1989). The cycle of violence. *Science*, 244, 160–166.

Widom, C. S., & Brzustowicz, L. M. (2006). MAOA and the "cycle of violence": Childhood abuse and neglect, MAOA genotype, and risk for violent and antisocial behavior. *Biological Psychiatry*, 60, 684–689.

Yirmiya, N. (2010). Editorial: Early prevention and intervention—The five W (and one H) questions. *Journal of Child Psychology & Psychiatry*, 51(12), 1297–1299.

6

Children and Adolescents in Disaster, War, and Terrorism

Developmental Pathways to Psychopathology and Resilience

ANGELA J. NARAYAN AND ANN S. MASTEN

The decade following the attacks on the twin towers of the World Trade Center has witnessed a devastating sequence of wars, natural disasters, acts of terror, and extreme political violence that has affected the lives of millions of children worldwide. As a result, there is growing concern about the effects of such extreme trauma experiences on child development (American Psychological Association [APA], 2010; Becker-Blease, Turner, & Finkelhor, 2010; Furr, Comer, Edmunds, & Kendall, 2010; Masten & Narayan, 2012). An understanding of the processes of adaptation in disaster holds the promise of revealing how best to prevent or ameliorate risk and promote resilience or recovery. However, theory and data both suggest that it will be challenging to unravel the complex processes involved. Many influences contribute to the exposure of children to extreme adversities, and also to their adaptation during or following exposure. These influences are likely to include qualities of the individual, both strengths and vulnerabilities; qualities of the family, including the quality of parenting and attachment relationships; environmental conditions pre- and postexposure; and the quality and timing of interventions targeting biological, social, or larger ecological processes. Recent advances in multiple-levels-of-analysis research have also underscored the important and complex roles of genes, epigenetic programming, and neuroendocrine systems in informing child development research on the effects of disasters.

The purpose of this review is to highlight recent findings and issues in research on pathways to psychopathology and resilience for children and adolescents in the aftermath of disasters and mass trauma. The chapter is focused on the developmental timing of exposure, individual differences in response, and the interplay of biological and environmental factors that might influence child adaptation or maladaptation. This discussion is informed by a sequence of reviews on disasters and child development published since 2010 (e.g., Betancourt, 2011; Bonanno, Brewin, Kaniasty, & La Greca, 2010; Masten & Narayan, 2012; Masten & Osofsky, 2010; National Commission on Children in Disasters [NCCD], 2010), in addition to recent exemplary empirical studies. It is conceptually grounded in developmental psychopathology, dynamic systems, and resilience frameworks.

In order to limit the scope of the review, we have focused on disasters and trauma with widespread effects on large groups of youth. More localized traumatic exposures are not discussed, such as those from child abuse, family violence, and traumatic accidents, although these adversities are important in child development and likely share similar risk and protective mechanisms with the experiences discussed here. In this review, we aimed for an integrative summary of recent findings and empirical advances so as to delineate and disseminate current knowledge about *what matters* for child competence and resilience in the face of disasters.

Contemporary research on child development in disasters is informed by historical research on adversity and is constrained by ongoing research challenges. For example, over the past century scholars have noted consistent phenomena in children's postdisaster responses, such as the importance of the recovery context and, particularly, the availability of supportive parents and communities, in addition to individual differences in promoting resilience. Such observations have been made in children exposed to the horrors of child soldiering who return to families and communities that are supportive versus stigmatizing (e.g., Betancourt et al., 2010; Klasen et al., 2010) and in the context of political violence and natural disasters that undermine child development because they threaten to split families (Qouta, Punamäki, & El Sarraj, 2008; Wickrama & Kaspar, 2007). These findings echo historical accounts of children who fared poorly in World War II, despite being protected from violence, because they were isolated from their parents (Freud & Dann, 1951). Additional findings replicated across time involve dose effects, with greater or more proximal exposure conferring worse prognosis and increased symptomatology (Comer & Kendall, 2007; MacFarlane & Van Hooff, 2009); individual differences in response to disasters, such as "steeling" or strengthening effects in some children and "scarring" or sensitizing effects in others; and the critical role of time in the recovery process (Garmezy & Rutter, 1985; Korol, Kramer, Grace, & Green, 2002; Masten & Narayan, 2012; Norris, Friedman, & Watson, 2002; Rutter, 1983).

Recent reviews of research and prevention efforts also serve as a reminder of the challenges that investigators of adversity face and the conspicuous gaps in knowledge in the disaster literature (APA, 2010; Bonanno et al., 2010; Masten & Osofsky, 2010). In addition to the challenges of assessing children immediately after exposure and gathering information on their pre- and postdisaster functioning, there are also difficulties in accessing the aftermath context, as well as special ethical considerations related to protecting survivors and avoiding harm to investigators. Moreover, there often might be political complications or a lack of rapid or adequate funding. Many mass conflicts and disasters occur in underdeveloped areas where access to resources, technology, and communication tools are less available (Masten & Narayan, 2012). Further, investigators often need to adapt to and comply with the level of access available; such conditions might not allow for rigorous research designs with predisaster baseline data, comparison data, or longitudinal follow-ups (Betancourt, 2011).

A comprehensive understanding of how disasters affect the lives of children would require knowledge of predisaster development, functioning, and context; the nature of the disaster; its consequences for ongoing interactions among individuals, families, and communities and their experiences both in the immediate aftermath and over a longer-term period of adjustment; and how all of the people and environments change over time. This is a tall order, and understandably there are very limited data on many aspects of this complex set of processes, despite wide recognition that many aspects of pre- and postdisaster function in all of these systems are important. Nonetheless, the evidence base has improved in recent years, and reviews are emerging that summarize key findings in this literature (Becker-Blease et al., 2010; Bonanno et al., 2010; Furr et al., 2010; Masten & Narayan, 2012; Masten & Obradovi , 2008; Masten & Osofsky, 2010; Pine, Costello, & Masten, 2005).

Theoretical Perspectives that Inform Disaster Research

Contemporary research on child development in the context of disasters has emerged from a confluence of dynamic systems theories emphasizing the interplay among individual characteristics, the context, and the developmental history that shapes adaptation (Masten & Narayan, 2012). Disaster research is informed by developmental systems theory (Gottlieb, 2007; Thelen & Smith, 1998), which describes individual children as continually developing, self-organizing, and active agents in their own lives, shaping and being shaped by many interactions between the organism and context across diverse circumstances. It is also informed by ecological systems theory, which delineates the role of nested contexts, such as family, school, community, and society, and the transactions among them, as additional systems that encompass children (Bronfenbrenner, 1979; Lerner, 1998). These theories emphasize the interdependence of children's individual adaptation and context, suggesting that perturbations in any part of the system— through disaster-related injury, separation from caregivers, loss of community ties, or threatening environments—have the power to disrupt development.

Additionally, most contemporary approaches assume that adaptive and mal-adaptive postdisaster development are best understood in the context of a child's individual history of development in interaction with the particular circum-stances of the disaster experience. Key elements of developmental history expected to influence children's adaptation to disaster include the individual's history of attachment relationships, which influence the expectations of warmth and security from caregivers that children bring to a traumatic experience (Sroufe, Carlson, Levy, & Egeland, 1999). Another element is the developmental history of the stress-response systems, which influences how an organism responds to stress and is shaped and tuned by experience and includes biologi-cal responses, subjective perceptions of threat, ability to cope, and self-efficacy (Gunnar & Quevedo, 2007; Yehuda, MacFarlane, & Shalev, 1998).

Disasters, war, and terrorism can influence the course of development in many ways. These include direct exposure to threats, witnessing atrocities and horrors, exposures mediated by parents or the media, migration or acculturation, and loss of hope for the future (APA, 2010; Comer & Kendall, 2007; Masten & Narayan, 2012; Norris, Friedman, Watson, et al., 2002). The interaction between the devel-opmental legacy of the child and the threats encountered shapes adaptation to adversity in many ways. This "co-action" (Gottlieb, 2007) of multiple influences and interactions can result in diverse or similar effects in the context of disaster. Different children might have different outcomes in response to very similar disaster experiences, reflecting multifinality (Cicchetti & Rogosch, 1996; Franks, 2011). Different children might also have comparable outcomes following differ-ent disaster exposures, such as similar symptom patterns (e.g., trauma symptoms or distress) or positive adaptation (e.g., competence in school), reflecting equifi-nality or converging pathways (Cicchetti & Rogosch, 1996; Layne et al., 2010).

Disasters and the regularity with which they reoccur in the lives of children around the globe provide powerful motivations for understanding resilience, with the goal of informing efforts to ameliorate disaster effects and promote recovery. Resilience research is focused on understanding the processes by which individuals and other systems (e.g., families, communities) respond and recover effectively from severe threats to adaptation or development (Cicchetti, 2010; Luthar, 2006; Masten & Narayan, 2012; Masten & Obradović 2008). From a systems perspective, resilience refers to *the capacity of a dynamic system to with-stand or recover from significant challenges that threaten its stability, viability, or development* (Masten, 2011). Disasters were of great interest in the early litera-ture on resilience (Garmezy, 1983) and this interest has persisted (e.g., Masten & Narayan, 2012; Masten & Obradović 2008).

There also has been recent attention to the possibility of spreading effects of disaster over time in individual development, discussed in terms of *developmen-tal cascades* (Masten & Cicchetti, 2010). Developmental cascades are the processes by which effects from one level or domain of functioning spread to affect other levels or domains over time. This concept has been applied to disaster research in recent reviews and empirical studies that discuss the possible ways for disaster effects to spread over time, within and across domains of functioning, with progressive, expanding, transactional, and intergenerational effects (La Greca, Silverman, Lai, & Jaccard, 2010; Masten & Narayan, 2012; Pine et al., 2005). Through these processes, exposure to trauma can activate cascading pathways that change the course of development for worse or better. For example, disasters could permanently alter the stress response, instill epigenetic change, or reduce academic success, with long-term consequences for health and function in later life and in subsequent generations (Meaney, 2010; Pratchett & Yehuda, 2011; Silverman & La Greca, 2002). Conversely, disasters could result in improved function with lasting consequences, for example, by uniting communities and activating post-traumatic growth (Kilmer & Gil-Rivas, 2010; Qouta et al., 2008).

Mass trauma has the power to disrupt interdependent systems at multiple levels of functioning (e.g., terrorism attempts to devastate a maximum number of human beings in one event), which taxes or overwhelms normative functioning and mobilizes multisystem resilience processes (Masten & Narayan, 2012). Interventions that have the potential to deter negative cascades and promote dynamic, self-propelling change have applications in effective postdisaster recovery (discussed more below).

Together, systems and ecology theories and developmental psychopathology and resilience frameworks have informed empirical efforts designed to aid in the understanding of children's responses to disasters, motivating the shift toward multiple-levels-of-analysis research paradigms (Cicchetti, 2010; Feder, Nestler, & Charney, 2009; Kim-Cohen & Gold, 2009; Sapienza & Masten, 2011). Studies that not only incorporate behavioral and family factors influencing children's functioning but also examine the neuroendocrine response, neural correlates of trauma exposure, and genetic moderators for pre- and postdisaster functioning are better equipped to explain the complex ways that disasters, war, and terrorism shape adaptive or maladaptive development, as well as individual differences in response to these events. Exemplary studies that contribute to an understanding of such complexity are highlighted below.

Factors Affecting the Impact of Exposure and Process of Recovery

Children are active, dynamic systems who develop from the interplay of individual and environmental factors; these processes also influence the nature of exposure to disasters and the potential for and processes of recovery. Moreover, reviews of the literature suggest that factors that exert risk or protective effects for exposure to disasters might also exert similar effects for resilience

(Furr et al., 2010; Norris, Friedman, Watson, et al., 2002; Silverman & La Greca, 2002). For example, impoverished children and families are disproportionately more likely to experience disasters and to be more strongly impacted in their aftermath, quite possibly because disadvantaged children and adults have a greater biological vulnerability to stress; fewer resources for recovery; and less effective protective systems at the biological, family, or community level (Masten & Narayan, 2012). There are numerous other examples of factors that predict both the extent of predisaster exposure and postdisaster functioning, such as high socioeconomic status and individual self-regulation skills, either of which can buffer disaster exposure and promote recovery (Kithakye, Morris, Terranova, & Myers, 2010; Klasen et al., 2010). This section highlights examples of factors that influence children's experiences in disasters and their recovery processes, namely, dose of exposure, age and developmental timing of exposure, sex differences, and parent–child relationships.

Dose of Exposure

Although children's development in the context of disasters is complex and multidetermined, it is widely observed that a greater dose of exposure to disasters leads to worse outcomes, a phenomenon long described as a "dose-response gradient" (Garmezy, 1983; Garmezy & Rutter, 1985; Masten & Narayan, 2012). The concept of "dose," however, can refer to different aspects of exposure severity, including objective proximity or degree of threat, subjective proximity or threat, repeated exposures, and a piling up of traumatic experiences or cumulative adversities within a specified time window. Thus, "dose" could reflect a multitude of factors, such as the degree of proximity, the extent of injury endured or witnessed, cumulative exposure such as disasters that occur during preexisting trauma or adversity, or experiences that also fracture relationships or ecological systems that encompass the child (Masten & Narayan, 2012).

Empirical studies of the effects of disasters on children have documented examples of dose-response relationships. Children who directly experienced the tsunami in Sri Lanka and those with concurrent exposure to war or family violence fared worse than those with more minimal exposure (Catani et al., 2010). Presumably, these children had a higher cumulative exposure or "dose." Similarly, in regard to proximity of exposure, children who were trapped inside the World Trade Center during the September 11 terrorist attacks experienced more post-traumatic stress and separation anxiety than those outside the buildings (Comer & Kendall, 2007). Additionally, children who were more severely exposed to September 11 (e.g., multiple instances of witnessing trauma, being injured or evacuated) were at higher risk for mood and anxiety disorders than those less severely exposed, and their risk was highest if a family member was exposed, even if the children were not directly exposed themselves (Hoven et al.,

2005). These findings illustrate how cumulative or concurrent exposure to trauma, proximity to the event, and the degree of perceived personal threat can shape children's experiences at the time of the disaster and predict the extent of postdisaster functioning. These findings also suggest that indirect but traumatic effects on children via parental exposure might be equally if not more harmful, perhaps particularly if they disrupt the attachment system.

The processes by which the dose of exposure impacts children's acute impairment and postdisaster adaptation are contingent on capacities spread throughout dynamic systems (Masten & Narayan, 2012). Accordingly, the relationships of exposure and dose with children's subsequent functioning are likely complex and nonlinear. Experiences that are beyond the range of acceptable exposure for any human being, such as rape and killing associated with being a child soldier and chronic, life-threatening violence or torture directed at the self or the family, are regarded as "toxic" experiences that can fundamentally compromise adaptive functioning (Betancourt et al., 2010; Klasen et al., 2010; Layne et al., 2010; Montgomery & Foldspang, 2005). Conversely, the degree of exposure does not affect all children similarly, suggesting the presence of moderators and potential resilience processes. For example, characteristics of parent–child relationships (described below) can buffer the risks associated with exposure or exacerbate postdisaster functioning if children's perceived security is compromised at the time of exposure (Masten & Obradovi , 2008; Qouta et al., 2008). Biological predispositions to stress reactivity, prenatal vulnerability to stress, specific genetic variants, and chronic neuroendocrine dysregulation from previous stress can also mediate or moderate the impact of dose on children's capacity to withstand the effects of disasters (Delahanty & Nugent, 2006; Kim-Cohen & Gold, 2009; Nugent, Tyrka, Carpenter, & Price, 2011; Pluess & Belsky, 2011; Yehuda et al., 2005).

In sum, multiple determinants of exposure likely interact in concert to influence postdisaster outcomes. Based on their meta-analysis of 96 studies, Furr et al. (2010) concluded that the most harmful "doses" for children were closer physical proximity, high overall death toll, greater perceived danger, and death of loved ones. Lower dose effects were observed with parental reports than with children's self-reports of symptoms, suggesting that parent and child perspectives on how children are doing might differ, or that parents are not fully aware of children's symptoms (Furr et al., 2010). Also, lower effects of dose were found when more time had lapsed since the disaster, suggesting that dose effects are dynamic and time sensitive and also likely interwoven with recovery processes (Furr et al., 2010; Gershoff, Aber, Ware, & Kotler, 2010).

Age and Developmental Timing

The nature of exposure and the effects of disasters on children and adolescents are also contingent, in part, on the developmental stage during which the disaster strikes. The age and developmental status of the child can influence the impact of exposure; the capacity of the child to perceive, interpret, and respond to the event; the child's capacity to manage fear or take self-protective action; the capacity of the child to elicit help and the nature of help adults offer; the expectations for recovery or the nature of disillusionment; and access to resources (APA, 2010; Franks, 2011; Layne et al., 2010; Masten & Narayan, 2012).

Generally, older children experience more severe exposure during disasters and war. In the Developmental Victimization Survey of more than 2,000 U.S. children aged 2–17 years who faced disasters and maltreatment, age was positively related both to disaster exposure and to victimization (Becker-Blease et al., 2010). Older children and adolescents might be less reliant on caregivers, separated from family at the time of exposure, or perceived by family members to have more responsibility to confront danger, or they might have a greater understanding of the meaning of the threat based on direct or media exposure (Comer, Furr, Beidas, Weiner, & Kendall, 2008; Layne et al., 2010; Masten & Osofsky, 2010). Additionally, older children might be more likely to be recruited to mobilize against political violence or kidnapped and made to serve as child soldiers (Betancourt et al., 2010; Qouta et al., 2008), and they might also have a broader social network of peers and teachers, making interpersonal losses more devastating (Pine et al., 2005). On the other hand, older children and youth might have more capabilities for responding to the threats of disasters or war (discussed further below).

Age differences have also been observed in relation to children's recovery and the nature of postdisaster impairment or psychopathology. Younger children have been reported to exhibit more stress reactions and dysregulation, such as increased hypervigilance and hyperarousal, bed-wetting, emotional detachment and dissociation, and separation anxiety from parents (APA, 2010; Comer & Kendall, 2007; Kronenberg et al., 2010; Pratchett & Yehuda, 2011; Yelland et al., 2010). As a result, some studies have reported that younger children experience more post-traumatic stress (PTS) symptoms and overall psychopathology after exposure to experiences such as September 11, wildfire disasters, and Hurricane Katrina (Hoven et al., 2005; McDermott, Lee, Judd, & Gibbon, 2005; Otto et al., 2007; Weems et al., 2010; Yelland et al., 2010), whereas older children might experience higher rates of depression (Thienruka et al., 2006). However, these findings are mixed, and age of exposure likely interacts with dose of exposure, available support, and history of prior exposure and psychopathology. One interpretation that integrates the effects of age on exposure and recovery is that older children are more likely to experience severe exposures, but when younger children do experience severe exposures, the effects on their functioning are more harmful.

The impact of exposure and the nature of recovery also depend on the current developmental stage of the child and his or her past record of adaptive functioning. Throughout development, children are faced with normative tasks to accomplish, such as the formation of positive attachment relationships and self-regulation in early childhood, behavior management and the development of peer relationships in middle childhood, and intimacy in adolescence (Masten, Burt, & Coatsworth, 2006; Sroufe, 1979). Accordingly, disasters could impair competent functioning at any of these points and confer risk for future maladaptive development. For example, one reason that some studies report younger children's increased rates of PTS symptoms relative to those of older children might be that younger children do not have adequate coping strategies or the cognitive capacity to understand and process the event, or they might have underdeveloped neural structures that regulate fear, anxiety, and arousal, all of which could contribute to heightened PTS symptoms in some contexts (Masten & Narayan, 2012; Pine et al., 2005; Toth & Cicchetti, 1999).

Conversely, cognitive immaturity could also be construed as protective if it shields young children from grasping the extent of horrors experienced, or if "younger" brain regions that suffer insult or injury from trauma have more plasticity for recovery (Cicchetti, 2010; Franks, 2011; Pratchett & Yehuda, 2011). For these reasons, although younger children might show more acute stress or impairment in the immediate aftermath, they might have a better capacity for resilience in the long run (Bonanno et al., 2010). Taken together, these findings suggest that age interacts with many exposure- and recovery-related factors. In a recent review, Franks (2011) urged investigators to adopt a developmental approach to study the effects of disasters on children and to consider the effect of developmental factors, such as existing emotional and behavioral difficulties and age-related appraisals, on pathways of psychopathology or resilience.

Sex Differences

Child sex also plays a role in determining the unique ways in which children are exposed to disasters; how they perceive, report, and internalize horrific events; and the extent to which their experiences are embedded within family and community systems. The type of exposure and the nature of the disaster also matter. For example, boys might be more likely to be recruited into armed conflict and thus might directly witness more bloodshed, whereas girls might be more likely to assume caregiving roles and observe long-term suffering (APA, 2010). In a study of child soldiers, girls were more likely than boys to be sexually assaulted during captivity and faced greater stigma on returning to the community if they were assaulted, whereas boys were more involved in perpetrating violence as child soldiers (Betancourt et al., 2010). These findings illustrate the importance of disparate experiences and community or cultural perceptions in influencing the risks for boys' versus girls' exposure and recovery. Additionally, family relationships might determine gender roles. In war-torn regions, girls perceived relationships with parents as more supportive but were treated more punitively, which contributed to girls' being more shielded from violence, whereas boys perceived parents as rejecting and were raised to be more independent, which facilitated their active roles in military violence (Qouta et al., 2008).

Patterns in the literature have also revealed sex differences in the nature of impairment and psychological problems experienced by boys versus girls. Generally, boys are observed to show more aggression and externalizing problems than girls as a result of exposure, whereas girls show or report more mood and anxiety symptoms (APA, 2010). A recent meta-analysis of PTS studies also found more PTS symptomatology and distress in female children exposed to disasters (Furr et al., 2010). For example, after an industrial disaster in Toulouse, both preadolescent and adolescent girls displayed higher rates of post-traumatic stress disorder (PTSD) than boys in either age group (Godeau et al., 2005), and girls generally displayed more PTSD than boys after the Oklahoma City bombing (Pfefferbaum et al., 2002). Six months after September 11, girls' likelihood of developing PTSD was higher than that of males (Hoven et al., 2005), and girls' rates of PTSD and internalizing problems, as well as their recovery, were worse than males' rates two to three years after Hurricane Katrina (Kronenberg et al., 2010; Weems et al., 2010). Additional studies delineate more specific sex differences, such as increased reproductive impairment in girls facing sexual violence, more alcohol problems in males as a coping mechanism (Norris, Friedman, Watson, et al., 2002), and more feelings of worthlessness and shame related to low self-efficacy in boys (Kar & Bastia, 2006; Vigil, Geary, Granger, & Flinn, 2010).

These findings on sex differences and psychopathology are complicated by evidence suggesting that there are also differences in the perceptions and reporting of threats and symptoms by boys and girls. Girls might perceive more threat, report elevated symptoms, have a greater tendency to share their emotions and experiences following disasters, and be more likely to internalize rather than externalize adverse events (Bonanno et al., 2010; Crick & Zahn-Waxler, 2003; Masten & Osofsky, 2010; Norris, Friedman, Watson, et al., 2002). For example, girls were found to report more distress after September 11 (Comer & Kendall, 2007; Lengua, Long, Smith, & Meltzoff, 2005) and more perceived threat after a wildfire disaster than boys, but there were no actual differences in PTSD symptoms (McDermott et al., 2005). These studies and comprehensive reviews (e.g., Norris, Friedman, Watson, et al., 2002) suggest that actual and perceived impairment from disasters might be confounded.

Other reports suggest further complexity. One study conducted on children in terrorist attacks found that although girls reported a wider range of PTSD symptoms, boys' symptoms were more severe (Laufer & Solomon, 2009). Additionally, research employing a multiple-levels-of-analysis perspective to illustrate sex differences in neuroendocrine regulation has found that in certain contexts of disaster, there might be different relationships among cortisol, distress, and subsequent impairment for boys than for girls (Delahanty & Nugent, 2006; Vigil et al., 2010). Together, these findings indicate that although patterns in the literature might suggest that girls are more prone to PTSD and internalizing problems, perceived distress might be amplifying these effects, and methodological issues such as reporter bias and the length of time that has elapsed since the disaster should also be considered. Additionally, given that we know that sex differences exist in normative emotions, behavior, and neurohormonal functioning across development and in transitions to puberty, it is likely that timing, biological predispositions, and chemical changes also affect how girls and boys differentially experience disasters.

Parenting and Attachment Relationships

Parent–child relationships play a pivotal role in children's exposure to disasters and their recovery patterns. Children form expectations about trust and safety based on their experiences in relationships with caregivers, and parents serve as reference points during threats to children's basic safety (Ainsworth, Bell, & Stayton, 1991; Sroufe et al., 1999). Through a process generally called "social referencing," children gauge their safety based on parental cues (see Masten, Best, & Garmezy, 1990); signals from parents to mobilize and prepare for threat are evolutionarily adaptive (Bowlby, 1969; Meaney, 2010). Thus, it is not surprising that research with animal models indicates that the loss of caregivers is one of the most powerful and broad stressors to an organism's functioning, because it can cause profound and permanent changes across multiple adaptive systems, including behavioral, emotional, and physiological dysregulation and disruptions in homeostasis (Gunnar & Quevedo, 2007; Hofer, 2006).

In the context of disasters, parent–child relationships are critically important for safety and protection, especially for younger children who cannot survive independently (Pine et al., 2005). Warm and supportive parent–child relationships can buffer the risks associated with traumatic exposure and promote resilience (Masten & Obradovi , 2008). During the tsunami in Thailand, positive parent–child relationships buffered the risk for children's PTSD symptoms (Wickrama & Kaspar, 2007). Amidst military violence in Palestine, the extent of exposure to violence was a predictor for psychopathology, but the amount of nurturing and warmth in the parent–child relationship predicted resilience (Qouta et al., 2008).

Conversely, disruptions in positive parent–child relationships and parents who are physically or psychologically compromised at the time of exposure pose a serious risk to children's ability to cope. Parenting that is overprotective or insensitive to children's needs has been reported to compromise children's functioning after natural disasters (Bokszczanin, 2008) and terrorist attacks

(Finzi-Dottan, Dekel, Lavi, & Su'ali, 2006). For adolescents exposed to war in Afghanistan, it was the extent of family violence concurrently perpetuated against children and their mothers that most strongly predicted psychopathology over time, even though many adolescents were resilient to war-related and socioeconomic stressors (Panter-Brick, Goodman, Tol, & Egerman, 2011). As noted above, it was the severity of parents' exposure, rather than children's direct exposure, that was the strongest predictor of children's psychopathology after September 11 (Hoven et al., 2005). Together these findings suggest that determinants of resilience or maladaptive outcomes after exposure to disasters extend well beyond children's individual characteristics to relationships with caregivers and other attachment figures.

Parenting and attachment relationships also serve as powerful mediators and moderators between children's exposure and their recovery. In Ugandan child soldiers returning home, parental support and family connectedness soothed the extent of children's emotional distress (Annan, Blattman, & Horton, 2006). Parent–child relationships that were high in emotional communication were correlated with decreases in children's PTSD symptoms following exposure to the September 11 attacks (Otto et al., 2007). Additionally, supportive relationships moderated the correlation between children's experiences of a California earthquake and chronic distress, but at high levels of exposure and high distress, the buffering effects of positive relationships were not as strong (Proctor et al., 2007). This finding suggests that parent–child relationships are powerful factors in guarding children against exposure, but disasters can still be overwhelming to the family system, and the impact on parents also matters. Preschool-aged children of parents who had higher levels of both PTSD and depression after September 11, as opposed to parents with only depression or those who were psychologically well, displayed more aggressive behavior and higher emotional reactivity (Chemtob et al., 2010). These findings illustrate that parental psychopathology and impairment could affect children's well-being.

Research to date suggests that both children's perceptions of their parents' ability to provide safety and parents' attunement to their children are vital for children's survival. However, positive relationships alone might not guarantee children's resilience in the face of severe adversity. Individual differences at multiple levels of functioning might also play a moderating or mediating role.

Individual Differences in Pathways to Psychopathology or Resilience

The preceding sections discuss mediators and moderators of exposure to disasters and children's recovery at a broad level and consider the effects of dose of exposure, child characteristics, and family relationships on children's vulnerability and resilience. However, at the level of the individual adaptive system, a complex system of biological predispositions, genetic underpinnings, and capacities of neuroendocrine regulation networks interact to influence children's responses to stressful events.

For example, one of the core determinants of children's adaptation after disasters or trauma involves the capacities of the stress regulation system. Under normative conditions, the hippocampal-pituitary-adrenal (HPA) axis responds to stress by triggering corticotropin-releasing hormones and adrenocorticotropic hormones to release cortisol, a steroid hormone. These components work in tandem to efficiently counter stress and dampen the release of subsequent steroid hormones, which are taxing at high and chronic concentrations (Fisher, Gunnar, Dozier, Bruce, & Pears, 2006; Gunnar & Quevedo, 2007; Shonkoff, Boyce, & McEwen, 2009). However, conditions of acute or chronic stress, such as disasters or ongoing trauma, can disrupt the efficiency and effectiveness of the coordinated stress response and weaken the body's ability to counter subsequent stress.

Additionally, genetic variants can directly or indirectly influence HPA functioning via variations in cortico-releasing hormones (CRH1) that stimulate and inhibit cortisol secretion, proteins involved in binding receptors for cortisol (FKBP5), and neurotransmitters such as the serotonin transporter polymorphism (5-HTTLRP), which is implicated in amydgala reactivity, sensitivity to stress, and internalizing problems (Cicchetti, 2010; Nugent et al., 2011). Moreover, variations in brain structures and functions, such as frontal cortex abnormalities and asymmetry, might also differentially affect children's responses to traumatic events (Carrion, Weems, & Bradley, 2010). Thus, a multiple-levels-of-analysis perspective that considers variation in neuroendocrine functioning, genes, neural correlates, and past history of life stress can best inform our understanding of the individual differences that characterize children's psychopathology or resilience following disasters.

Sensitivity and Vulnerability in the Context of Disasters

Developmental and dynamic systems perspectives emphasize that the effects of stress, disasters, and trauma on children's biological and regulatory functioning are not linear but rather vary as a function of children's predispositions and the nature and timing of exposure. Although the HPA axis functions to coordinate the activation and dampening of cortisol released to combat stress, perturbations to the axis as a result of overwhelming stress have been documented to have mixed effects, leading in some cases to hypoactivation and in some cases to hyperactivation of the stress response (Pratchett & Yehuda, 2011). For example, exposure to life stress, trauma, or abuse in childhood can contribute to up-regulation of stress responses during acute stress, but chronic stress might reverse these processes toward down-regulation in order to protect against the toxicity and allostatic load imposed by repeated cascades of stress hormones (Gunnar & Quevedo, 2007; MacFarlane, 2010; Nugent et al., 2011). These processes have been observed in children exposed to maltreatment and trauma across development (Cicchetti & Cannon, 1999; Pratchett & Yehuda, 2011).

Further, some children who are exposed to disasters or trauma in early childhood are more vulnerable to the effects of subsequent trauma, a sensitization effect sometimes referred to as "kindling" or "scarring" that manifests as increased susceptibility to PTSD in adulthood in individuals with a history of abuse or early life stress (Delahanty & Nugent, 2006; Pervanidou, 2008; Yehuda et al., 2010). However, other individuals appear to become less susceptible to subsequent PTSD, suggesting what has been called "steeling effects" or "stress inoculation" (Rutter, 1983, 2006). Consensus has not been reached about when the up- or down-regulations discussed above occur, under what contexts, and what individual characteristics are driving them. However, there is good evidence indicating that chronic down-regulation of cortisol responsiveness is a risk factor for later PTSD because the body is underprepared to adequately respond to subsequent trauma (Delahanty & Nugent, 2006; MacFarlane, 2010; Yehuda et al., 2010). Additionally, recent research has also outlined a multitude of intervening factors along the pathway from initial trauma exposure to later onset of PTSD, including disruptions in the HPA axis, processing errors that render fragmented memories vulnerable to intrusion and flashbacks, changes in behavior and expectations about encounters with others and the environment, and increased chances of revictimization (Delahanty & Nugent, 2006; Pratchett & Yehuda, 2011; Yehuda & Harvey, 1997; Yehuda et al., 1998). Further, as noted above, outcomes also are likely to vary as a function of exposure dose, developmental timing, or protective factors available to the individual.

The preceding sections emphasize that many intertwined systems operate in tandem to influence children's responses to stress, which are grounded in developmental history and previous experiences with stress. Rather than a linear relationship between dose and response, it is likely that integrated networks operate together to influence to pre- and postdisaster adaptation, leading to nonlinear relations between disaster exposure and child outcomes. Specific, emerging theoretical frameworks, such as differential susceptibility to the environment and the adaptive calibration model of stress reactivity (e.g., Belsky & Pluess, 2009; Del Giudice, Ellis, & Shirtcliff, 2010; Ellis & Boyce, 2011), are helpful in disentangling these nonlinear relationships. These theories propose that experiences tune biological systems or predispositions for adaptive or maladaptive responses to adversity in the expected environment, with room for recalibration as life unfolds. As a result, children's adaptation in the face of disasters is contingent on their functioning across coordinated systems, their prior capacity to manage adversity, and qualities of the environment struck by the disaster.

Further, their adaptation can wax and wane over time as a function of strengths, deficits, and new experiences. Additionally, children might be born prepared with capacities to encounter the environments that their parents have endured (Pluess & Belsky, 2011; Yehuda et al., 2005), or qualities of the early rearing environment might lead to changes in gene expression, reflecting epigenetic programming (Cicchetti, 2010; Meaney, 2010).

These theoretical frameworks can be applied to children prenatally exposed to trauma via maternal exposure (discussed below) and to those who face early and chronic trauma, such as ongoing wars, or experiences of natural disasters superimposed on existing conditions of family violence. It is likely that these children's stress regulation patterns and subsequent recalibration would be different from those of children who face a single-event trauma. Future research is needed in order to decipher how children's stress response patterns differ as a function of severity, chronicity, or cumulative exposure to disastrous events.

Prenatal Programming of the Stress Response

Recent research has revealed that aspects of experience can "program" genetic changes, suggesting that stress reactivity and regulation could change throughout development as a function of changes in gene expression or programming effects (Meaney, 2010; Pluess & Belsky, 2011). For example, the landmark studies by Meaney and colleagues (e.g., Meaney, Aitken, Viau, Sharma, & Sarrieau, 1989) on the role of maternal licking and grooming of rat pups in initiating hormone cascades for adaptive stress regulation emphasized the roles of early experiences, social experiences, and timing in programming future adaptation. One important extension of this research, with applications for research on the effects of disasters on child development, is that the timing of the exposure to trauma matters in programming the stress response and the risk for later psychopathology (Gunnar & Quevedo, 2007; Meaney, 2010; Pratchett & Yehuda, 2011). For example, pregnant mothers who were exposed to September 11 and developed PTSD had lower levels of cortisol than exposed well mothers, and their infants also had lower cortisol levels. Further, the severity of the exposure was inversely related to infants' cortisol levels and was strongest during third-trimester exposure (Yehuda et al., 2005). These findings suggest that the stress response system adjusts to protect against prenatal exposure to overwhelming stress and that children's capacities to manage stress can be programmed by parents' experiences.

Transgenerational programming effects have also been found in situations of chronic trauma, such as the Holocaust. Parents who developed PTSD in the aftermath of the Holocaust were more likely to have children with lower levels of cortisol, even though their children were never directly exposed, and this effect was true only for mothers, not fathers (Yehuda, Bell, Bierer, & Schmiedler,

2008; Yehuda et al., 2007). Children with low cortisol levels might be born at risk for PTSD as a result of disruptions in their stress response systems from parents' exposures that occurred before they were conceived. More broadly, these findings also emphasize that children encounter their environments and respond to disasters armed with their developmental histories. Thus, development does not begin at conception; it also has roots in the experiences of past generations.

Interventions

The identification of robust predictors of children's vulnerability or resilience in the face of disasters, terrorism, or war has implications for intervention. Efforts have been made to target processes hypothesized to play a key role in worsening or improving adaptation during or following severe adversities. These include efforts to reduce exposure or risk, increase access to resources, and mobilize protective systems (Masten & Obradovi , 2008; Masten & Osofsky, 2010).

Investigators committed to studying children's resilience after disasters have identified a constellation of factors that might predict children's functioning in the longer term, such as the degree of social support available, effective or counterproductive coping strategies, the presence of predisaster emotional or behavioral problems, parental reactions, and fractures in the family system (Bonanno et al., 2010; La Greca & Silverman, 2009; Masten & Obradovi , 2008; Norris, Friedman, & Watson, 2002). Such factors have been used to generate resilience checklists in order to identify and predict children's postdisaster adjustment (Silverman, La Greca, & Ortiz, 2004). Additionally, one of the most important considerations for interventions is that children's adaptive capacity for resilience depends on their functioning at multiple levels, including biological, family, and contextual influences (APA, 2010; Betancourt & Khan, 2008; Cicchetti, 2010; Sapienza & Masten, 2011; Williams, Alexander, Bolsover, & Bakke, 2008).

Interventions that target the systems in which children are nested are likely to have the most optimal effects. For example, a randomized controlled trial (RCT) that targeted both mothers and children in war-torn Bosnia in an effort to promote positive and supportive relationships found that both groups experienced improvements in psychological functioning and quality of life, and children also improved in weight gain (Dybdahl, 2001). These findings underscore the potential for an intervention that targets attachment relationships to promote children's functioning at both psychological and biological levels, a complement to past findings that maternal loss can compromise an organism's fitness at multiple levels (Gunnar & Quevedo, 2007; Hofer, 2006) and that family relationships weigh heavily on children's functioning during disasters and war (Catani et al., 2010; Panter-Brick et al., 2011).

Another intervention that targeted children's social systems—an RCT to promote coping, cognitive skills, and social support in children exposed to political violence—found that peer support mediated the effects of the intervention on decreased PTSD symptoms (Tol et al., 2010). This finding emphasizes the role of the social context in children's recovery after trauma. School-based RCTs have been effective arenas for interventions through fostering adaptive grief reactions, meaning-making, and facilitating supportive groups for students who might have experienced disasters or trauma together (Layne et al., 2008; Murray, Cohen, Ellis, & Manarino, 2008).

At the biological level, few studies to date have targeted stress dysregulation after disasters as a point of intervention, but research has documented changes in children's cortisol levels after disasters (Vigil et al., 2010). Research has also found that attachment-based interventions can buffer cortisol dysregulation and neurobiological impairment in other conditions of trauma, such as institutional deprivation (Zeanah et al., 2003), foster care (Dozier, Peloso, Lewis, Laurenceau, & Levine, 2008; Fisher et al., 2006), or maltreatment (Cicchetti, Rogosch, Toth, & Sturge-Apple, 2011). Taken together, these findings suggest that it might be fruitful to consider interventions for children in disaster that target multiple systems, including neurobiological processes and family relationships.

Successful interventions also need to consider age and developmental timing in efforts to reduce exposure and promote recovery. Disasters and trauma have the power to overwhelm children's emotional, cognitive, and self-regulatory capacity, which might still be underdeveloped; thus, efforts should be made to restore parent–child relationships, school and community support, and daily routines with predictable structure as soon as possible (Betancourt & Khan, 2008; Masten & Obradovi , 2008; Norris, Steven, Pfefferbaum, Wyche, & Pfefferbaum, 2008). Interventions for children and adolescents might also need to consider the timing and pace of implementation, as well as the multitude of issues and emotions that children experience. In some cases, such as severe or mass trauma, children might need to gradually process traumatic memories, or they might experience secondary reactions to trauma such as anger, sadness, and externalizing behavior (La Greca, 2001; Norris, Friedman, & Watson, 2002).

Some treatment paradigms created for adults have been adapted for children. For example, narrative exposure therapy (NET), an exposure- and testimony-based treatment originally developed for adult torture survivors, has been tailored for children (KIDNET) with a focus on creative expression and narratives that aid children in retrieving and processing memories of trauma and disasters (Neuner et al., 2008). Examples of populations targeted for KIDNET implementation have included refugee children and those exposed to war and genocide, with evidence of lasting improvements in symptoms of PTSD and depression (Onyut et al., 2005; Ruf et al., 2010). Although KIDNET shows a promising ability to curb impairment in children, more empirical evidence is needed across children of different ages and different disaster contexts.

Although intervention research on disasters has made significant gains in identifying targets for intervention and implementing effective treatments, research remains very limited on prevention efforts to prepare children for exposure to disasters before they occur (Bonanno et al., 2010; Masten & Obradovi , 2008). A recent report provides an example of an experiment to promote resilience in advance of community violence. A school-based stress inoculation training (SIT) program was implemented for Israeli children living in high-conflict areas. Subsequently, following a three-week period of severe exposure to traumatic rocket attacks, children who had received SIT displayed less distress and fewer PTSD symptoms than control children matched for dose of exposure from non-SIT-trained schools (Wolmer, Hamiel, & Laor, 2011). This study offers encouraging evidence that children living in contexts with high risk for exposure to conflict or natural disasters could be prepared in ways that would promote resilience.

This type of research is rare, however. Most of the research conducted in areas of disaster does not meet the methodological rigor of RCTs because of the challenges associated with implementation during ongoing conflict or aftermath, securing control groups, and keeping field investigators blind to experimental conditions (Masten & Narayan, 2012; Peltonen & Punamäki, 2010). Additionally, basic longitudinal research on the long-term effects of disasters on children's developmental pathways is scarce (Betancourt, 2011); thus translational research on interventions that deter long-term maladaptation is severely lacking.

Despite the current challenges that investigators face in studying development in disasters, experts on children's resilience in extreme adversity have proposed a series of consensus guidelines to promote optimal child outcomes in disasters. Such preparedness guidelines include boosting safety through predisaster preparation, formulating and practicing crisis plans in the event of disasters, and securing competent first responders who are knowledgeable about the developmental capacities and vulnerabilities of children (Markenson & Redlener, 2004; Masten & Narayan, 2012; Masten & Osofsky, 2010; NCCD, 2010). In addition, Hobfoll et al. (2007) proposed five general principles for mass-trauma interventions based on the extant adult and child disaster literature, focused on promoting safety, calmness, self- and collective efficacy, connectedness, and hope. These principles are highly compatible with the need to promote recovery and resilience at multiple levels of children's functioning and in the contexts in which children are nested (Masten, 2001). Finally, when formulating effective interventions that reach large groups of children, it is critically important to remain aware of individual differences in children's experiences of disasters, as well as moderators of exposure and recovery that predict resilience. Such moderators include genetic variations, quality of attachment, children's individual skills, and cultural differences in the meaning of the events and the conflict and suffering that ensue (Barber, 2008; Kim-Cohen & Gold, 2009).

Conclusions

Disaster research from multiple disciplines—including child development, clinical sciences, community studies, neuroendocrinology, neuroscience, and ecology—has contributed to dramatic advancements in knowledge and theory about child development in relation to disasters, war, and terrorism over the past few decades. This progress has been propelled by both theoretical integration and empirical rigor. Theoretical frameworks that embrace the complexities of dynamic systems and studies that focus on multiple-level processes offer great promise for enhancing understanding of risk and resilience and its applications to improve practice and policy.

These frameworks have been valuable in delineating the risk or protective processes that predict postdisaster adaptation depending on the developmental capacities of the child, his or her previous experiences and expectations, and the resources available to the individual or family when the disaster strikes. Grounded in these theories, empirical research is beginning to elucidate the layers of complexity involved in children's responses to disasters, with growing attention to the roles of genetic variation; neural correlates; emotional, physiological, and neuroendocrine regulation; behavioral functioning; and family and community networks. This integrative and interdisciplinary research holds the potential for continued advances in understanding the effects of disasters on development.

Although the complexities of this science can be daunting, recent reviews and empirical studies have emphasized patterns and consistencies that sharpen and deepen our understanding of children's pre- and postdisaster functioning, delineating the meaning and influence of dose, developmental timing, sex and cultural differences, attachment relationships, community resources, and individual differences (APA, 2010; Bonanno et al., 2010; Franks, 2011; Furr et al., 2010; Masten & Narayan, 2012; Norris, Friedman, & Watson, 2002; Norris, Friedman, Watson, et al., 2002; Qouta et al., 2008). For example, the derived meaning, subjective experiences, and risk for long-term impairment or recovery after disasters and mass trauma might be widely disparate for younger versus older children or males versus females. Differences might depend on cognitive maturity and ability to comprehend the level of devastation, the amount of protection available from parents, gender roles or sex differences that dictate the level of exposure or perceived threat, or biological differences in genetic or neurohormonal variations. Additionally, recent research on the neurobiological effects of trauma on development emphasizes patterns in stress reactivity and regulation that can be predicted from developmental histories of stress, prenatal exposure to trauma, or changes in the parental environment or context that have programming effects on the epigenome (MacFarlane, 2010; Nugent et al., 2011; Pratchett & Yehuda, 2011).

On the whole, findings indicate that there has been significant research progress, particularly through increasing the understanding that factors influencing child development in disasters are dynamic and multidetermined, and by beginning to delineate *which factors matter* for psychopathology or resilience. Now, efforts are needed to clarify the roles of these factors, how they matter for exposure and recovery in different contexts; how they affect individual differences in adjustment, resilience, and competence; the variation in response that results from interplay between and among factors; and how they change as a function of the nature, timing, severity, and chronicity of disasters.

More research is also needed in order to refine prevention efforts to bolster the adaptive capacity of children at risk for exposure to disasters, to intervene to promote resilience, and to restore competent functioning in the aftermath. There are widely acknowledged gaps in the methodology available for assessing psychopathology and resilience in the contexts of disasters, particularly in the areas of predisaster assessment, representative sampling, experimental versus control groups, and long-term follow-ups. However, notable advancements have also been made in assessments of multiple dimensions of adaptation following disasters, identification of biological markers that moderate outcomes of risk or resilience, outcome measures that focus on competence and well-being along with vulnerability and psychopathology, and increasingly sophisticated statistical techniques such as developmental cascades and analyses of pediatric neuroimaging data in children exposed to trauma (Betancourt & Khan, 2008; Carrion et al., 2010; La Greca et al., 2010; Masten & Obradovi , 2008; Nugent et al., 2011). Moving forward, increased emphasis on methodology that captures the developmental span of children from predisaster status to exposure and postdisaster functioning will inform understanding of the developmental processes of vulnerability and recovery.

Models that conceptualize normative development and its vicissitudes as multidetermined, dynamic, and nonlinear are revolutionizing theory and research in order to explain the complexities of development after disaster strikes (Cicchetti, 2010; Feder et al., 2009; Masten & Narayan, 2012; Pine et al., 2005). Emerging themes reflecting this new wave of work include epigenetic programming, differential susceptibility to context, prenatal programming of stress reactivity and regulation, and pathway models of risk and recovery (Ellis & Boyce, 2011; Masten & Cicchetti, 2010; Meaney, 2010; Pluess & Belsky, 2011). Emerging models suggest that designing and implementing effective and efficient ways to address disruptions in multiple systems will be contingent on collaboration among scientists, practitioners, front-line responders, and policy makers. Masten (2011) has noted that collaborative strategies might well result in better science, as well as better preparation or response to trauma or disaster, producing "translational synergy." Realizing the potential of emerging models for both application and theory will require continued emphasis on empirical rigor, interdisciplinary collaboration, multiple levels of analysis, thoughtful interpretation, careful dissemination, and a deep appreciation of the dynamic nature of human adaptation and development in the context of disaster, war, terrorism, and other extreme experiences.

Disclosure Statement

Preparation of this chapter was supported in part by a predoctoral fellowship awarded to A.J.N. by the National Institute of Mental Health (Award No. 5T32MH015755). A.S.M. has no conflicts of interest to disclose.

References

Ainsworth, M. D. S., Bell, S. M., & Stayton, D. J. (1991). Infant-mother attachment and social development: "Socialisation" as a product of reciprocal responsiveness to signals. In M. Woodhead, R. Carr, & P. Light (Eds.), *Becoming a person: Child development in social context* (Vol. 1, pp. 30–55). Florence, KY: Taylor and Frances Routledge.

American Psychological Association. (2010). *Resilience and recovery after war: Refugee children and families in the United States.* Washington, DC: Author.

Annan, J., Blattman, C., & Horton, R. (2006). The state of youth and youth protection in Northern Uganda: Findings from the Survey for War Affected Youth. Retrieved August 2, 2011, from http://reliefweb.int/sites/reliefweb.int/files/resources/6110A06A7120 D7FBC12576570033752B-Full_Report.pdf

Barber, B. K. (2008). Contrasting portraits of war: Youths' varied experiences with political violence in Bosnia and Palestine. *International Journal of Behavior Development,* 32(4), 298–309.

Becker-Blease, K. A., Turner, H. A., & Finkelhor, D. (2010). Disasters, victimization and children's mental health. *Child Development,* 81(4), 1040–1052.

Belsky, J., & Pluess, M. (2009). Beyond diathesis stress: Differential susceptibility to environmental influences. *Psychological Bulletin,* 135(6), 885–908.

Betancourt, T. S. (2011). Attending to the mental health of war-affected children: The need for longitudinal and developmental research perspectives. *Journal of the American Academy of Child and Adolescent Psychiatry,* 50(4), 323–325.

Betancourt, T. S., Borisova, I. I., Williams, T. P., Brennan, R. T., Whitfield, T. H., de la Soudiere, M., et al. (2010). Sierra Leone's former child soldiers: A follow-up study of psychosocial adjustment and community reintegration. *Child Development,* 81(4), 1076–1094.

Betancourt, T. S., & Khan, K. T. (2008). The mental health of children affected by armed conflict: Protective processes and pathways to resilience. *International Review of Psychiatry*, 20(3), 317–328.

Bokszczanin, A. (2008). Parental support, family conflict, and overprotectiveness: Predicting PTSD symptom levels of adolescents 28 months after a natural disaster. *Anxiety Stress and Coping*, 21(4), 325–335.

Bonanno, G. A., Brewin, C. R., Kaniasty, K., & La Greca, A. M. (2010). Weighing the costs of disaster: Consequences, risks, and resilience in individuals, families and communities. *Psychological Science in the Public Interest*, 11(1), 1–49.

Bowlby, J. (1969). *Attachment and loss: Vol. 1. Attachment*. London: Hogarth.

Bronfenbrenner, U. (1979). *The ecology of human development: Experiments by nature and design*. Cambridge, MA: Harvard University Press.

Carrion, V. G., Weems, C. F., & Bradley, T. (2010). Natural disasters and the neurodevelopmental response to trauma in childhood: A brief overview and call to action. *Future Neurology*, 5(5), 667–674.

Catani, C., Gewirtz, A. H., Wieling, E., Schauer, E., Elbert, T., & Neuner, F. (2010). Tsunami, war, and cumulative risk in the lives of Sri Lankan school children. *Child Development*, 81(4), 1175–1190.

Chemtob, C. M., Nomura, Y., Rajendran, K., Yehuda, R., Schwartz, D., & Abramovitz, R. (2010). Impact of maternal posttraumatic stress disorder and depression following exposure to the September 11 attacks on preschool children's behavior. *Child Development*, 81(4), 1128–1140.

Cicchetti, D. (2010). Resilience under conditions of extreme stress: A multilevel perspective. *World Psychiatry*, 9(3), 145–154.

Cicchetti, D., & Cannon, T. D. (1999). Neurodevelopmental processes in the ontogenesis and epigenesis of psychopathology. *Development and Psychopathology*, 11, 375–393.

Cicchetti, D., & Rogosch, F. (1996). Equifinality and multifinality in developmental psychopathology. *Development and Psychopathology*, 8(4), 597–600.

Cicchetti, D., Rogosch, F., Toth, S. L., & Sturge-Apple, M. L. (2011). Normalizing the development of cortisol regulation in maltreated infants through preventative interventions. *Development and Psychopathology*, 23(3), 789–800.

Comer, J. S., Furr, J. M., Beidas, R. S., Weiner, C. L., & Kendall, P. C. (2008). Children and terrorism-related news: Training parents in coping and media literacy. *Journal of Consulting and Clinical Psychology*, 76(4), 568–578.

Comer, J. S., & Kendall, P. C. (2007). Terrorism: The psychological impact on youth. *Clinical Psychology: Science & Practice*, 14(3), 182–212.

Crick, N. R., & Zahn-Waxler, C. (2003). The development of psychopathology in females and males: Current progress and future challenges. *Development and Psychopathology*, 15(3), 719–742.

Delahanty, D. L., & Nugent, N. R. (2006). Predicting PTSD prospectively based on prior trauma history and immediate biological responses. *Annals of the New York Academy of Science*, 1071, 27–40.

Del Giudice, M., Ellis, B. J., & Shirtcliff, E. A. (2010). The Adaptive Calibration Model of stress responsivity. *Neuroscience and Behavioral Reviews*, 35(7), 1562–1592.

Dozier, M., Peloso, E., Lewis, E., Laurenceau, J.-P., & Levine, S. (2008). Effects of an attachment-based intervention on the cortisol production of infants and toddlers in foster care. *Development and Psychopathology*, 20(3), 845–859.

Dybdahl, R. (2001). Children and mothers in war: An outcome study of a psychosocial intervention program. *Child Development*, 72(4), 1214–1230.

Ellis, B. J., & Boyce, W. T. (2011). Differential susceptibility to the environment: Toward an understanding of sensitivity to developmental experiences and context. *Development and Psychopathology*, 23(1), 1–5.

Feder, A., Nestler, E. J., & Charney, D. S. (2009). Psychobiology and molecular genetics of resilience. *Nature Reviews Neuroscience*, 10(6), 446–457.

Finzi-Dottan, R., Dekel, R., Lavi, T., & Su'ali, T. (2006). Posttraumatic stress disorder reactions among children with learning disabilities exposed to terrorist attacks. *Comprehensive Psychiatry*, 47(2), 144–151.

Fisher, P. A., Gunnar, M. R., Dozier, M., Bruce, J., & Pears, C. (2006). Effects of therapeutic interventions for foster children on behavioral problems, caregiver attachment, and stress regulatory neural systems. *Annals of the New York Academy of Science*, 1094, 215–225.

Franks, B. A. (2011). Moving targets: A developmental framework for understanding children's changes following disasters. *Journal of Applied Developmental Psychology*, 32(2), 58–69.

Freud, A., & Dann, S. (1951). An experiment in group upbringing. *Psychoanalytic Study of the Child*, 6, 127–168.

Furr, J. M., Comer, J. S., Edmunds, J. M., & Kendall, P. C. (2010). Disasters and youth: A meta-analytic examine of posttraumatic stress. *Journal of Consulting and Clinical Psychology*, 78(6), 765–780.

Garmezy, N. (1983). Stressors of childhood. In N. Garmezy & M. Rutter (Eds.), *Stress, coping, and development* (pp. 43–84). New York: McGraw Hill.

Garmezy, N., & Rutter, M. (1985). Acute reactions to stress. In M. Rutter & L. Hersov (Eds.), *Child and adolescent psychiatry: Modern approaches* (2nd ed., pp. 152–176). Oxford, UK: Blackwell Scientific.

Gershoff, E., Aber, J. L., Ware, A., & Kotler, J. (2010). Exposure to 9/11 among youth and their mothers in New York City: Enduring associations with mental health and sociopolitical attitudes. *Child Development*, 81(4), 1141–1159.

Godeau, E., Vignes, C., Navarro, F., Iachan, R., Ross, J., Pasquier, C., et al. (2005). Effects of a large-scale industrial disaster on rates of symptoms consistent with posttraumatic stress disorders among schoolchildren in Toulouse. *Archives of Pediatric and Adolescent Medicine*, 159(6), 579–584.

Gottlieb, G. (2007). Probabilistic epigenesis. *Developmental Science*, 10(1), 1–11.

Gunnar, M., & Quevedo, K. (2007). The neurobiology of stress and development. *Annual Review of Psychology*, 58, 145–173.

Hobfoll, S. E., Watson, P., Bell, C. C., Bryant, R. A., Brymer, M. J, Friedman, M. J., et al. (2007). Five essential elements of immediate and mid-term mass trauma intervention: Empirical evidence. *Psychiatry*, 70(4), 283–315.

Hofer, M. A. (2006). Psychobiological roots of early attachment. *Current Directions in Psychological Science*, 15(2), 84–88.

Hoven, C. W., Duarte, C. S., Lucas, C. P., Wu, P., Mandell, D. J., Goodwin, R. D., et al. (2005). Psychopathology among New York City public school children 6 months after September 11. *Archives of General Psychiatry*, 62, 545–552.

Kar, N., & Bastia, B. K. (2006). Post-traumatic stress disorder, depression and generalised anxiety disorder in adolescents after a natural disaster: A study of comorbidity. *Clinical Practice and Epidemiology in Mental Health*, 2, 17–23.

Kilmer, R., & Gil-Rivas, V. (2010). Exploring posttraumatic growth in children impacted by Hurricane Katrina: Correlates of the phenomenon and developmental considerations. *Child Development*, 81(4), 1210–1226.

Kim-Cohen, J., & Gold, A. L. (2009). Measured gene-environment interactions and mechanisms promoting resilient development. *Current Directions in Psychological Science*, 18(3), 138–142.

Kithakye, M., Morris, A. S., Terranova, A. M., & Myers, S. S. (2010). The Kenyan political conflict and children's adjustment. *Child Development*, 81(4), 1113–1127.

Klasen, F., Oettingen, G., Daniels, J., Post, M., Hoyer, C., & Adam, H. (2010). Posttraumtic resilience in former Ugandan child soldiers. *Child Development*, 81(4), 1095–1112.

Korol, M., Kramer, T. L., Grace, M. C., & Green, B. L. (2002). Dam break: Long-term follow-up of children exposed to the Buffalo Creek disaster. In A. M. La Greca, W. K. Silverman, E. M. Vernberg, & M. C. Roberts (Eds.), *Helping children cope with disasters and terrorism* (pp. 241–257). Washington, DC: American Psychological Association.

Kronenberg, M. E., Hansel, T. C., Brennan, A. M., Lawrason, B., Osofsky, H. J., & Osofsky, J. D. (2010). Children of Katrina: Lessons learned about post-disaster symptoms and recovery patterns. *Child Development*, 81(4), 1240–1258.

La Greca, A. M. (2001). Children experiencing disasters: Prevention and intervention. In J. Hughes, A. La Greca, & J. Conley (Eds.), *Handbook of psychological services for children and adolescents*. London: Oxford University Press.

La Greca, A. M., & Silverman, W. K. (2009). Treatment and prevention of posttraumatic stress reactions in children and adolescents exposed to disasters and terrorism: What is the evidence? *Child Development Perspectives*, 3(1), 4–10.

La Greca, A. M., Silverman, W. K., Lai, B., & Jaccard, J. (2010). Hurricane-related exposure experiences and stressors, other life events, and social support: Concurrent and prospective impact on children's persistent posttraumatic stress symptoms. *Journal of Consulting and Clinical Psychology*, 78(6), 794–805.

Laufer, A., & Solomon, Z. (2009). Gender differences in PTSD in Israeli youth exposed to terror attacks. *Journal of Interpersonal Violence*, 24(6), 959–976.

Layne, C. M., Olsen, J. A., Baker, A., Legerski, J.-P., Isakson, B., Pasali , A., et al. (2010). Unpacking trauma exposure risk factors and differential pathways of influence: Predicting post-war mental distress in Bosnian adolescents. *Child Development*, 81(4), 1053–1075.

Layne, C. M., Saltzman, W. R., Poppleton, L., Burlingame, G. M., Pasali , A., Durakovi , E., et al. (2008). Effectiveness of a school-based group psychotherapy program for war-exposed adolescents: A randomized controlled trial. *Journal of the American Academy of Child and Adolescent Psychiatry*, 47(9), 1048–1062.

Lengua, L. J., Long, A. C., Smith, K. I., & Meltzoff, A. N. (2005). Pre-attack symptomatology and temperament as predictors of children's responses to the September 11 terrorist attacks. *Journal of Child Psychology and Psychiatry*, 46(6), 631–645.

Lerner, R. L. (1998). Theories of human development: Contemporary perspectives. In W. Damon & R. Lerner (Eds.), *Handbook of child psychology Volume 1: Theoretical models of human development* (pp. 1–24). New York: John Wiley & Sons.

Luthar, S. S. (2006). Resilience in development: A synthesis of research across five decades. In D. Cicchetti & J. Cohen (Eds.), *Developmental psychopathology, Volume 3: Risk, disorder, and adaptation* (2nd ed., pp. 739–795). Hoboken, NJ: Wiley and Sons.

MacFarlane, A. C. (2010). The long-term costs of traumatic stress: Intertwined physical and psychological consequences. *World Psychiatry*, 9, 3–10.

MacFarlane, A. C., & Van Hooff, M. (2009). Impact of child exposure to disaster on adult mental health: 20-year longitudinal follow-up study. *British Journal of Psychiatry*, 195, 142–148.

Markenson, D., & Redlener, I. (2004). Pediatric terrorism preparedness national guidelines and recommendations: Findings of an evidence-based consensus process. *Biosecurity and Bioterrorism: Biodefense Strategy, Practice, and Science*, 2(4), 301–319.

Masten, A. S. (2001.) Ordinary magic: Resilience processes in development. *American Psychologist*, 56(3), 227–238.

Masten, A. S. (2011). Resilience in children threatened by extreme adversity: Frameworks for research, practice, and translational synergy. *Development and Psychopathology*, 23(2), 141–154.

Masten, A. S., Best, K. M., & Garmezy, N. (1990). Resilience and development: Contributions from the study of children who overcome adversity. *Development and Psychopathology*, 2(4), 425–444.

Masten, A. S., Burt, K. B., & Coatsworth, J. D. (2006). Competence and psychopathology in development. In D. Cicchetti & D. Cohen (Eds.), *Developmental psychopathology, Volume 3, Risk, disorder and psychopathology* (2nd ed., pp. 696–738). New York: Wiley.

Masten, A. S., & Cicchetti, D. (2010). Editorial: Developmental cascades (Special Issue, Part 1). *Development and Psychopathology*, 22(3), 491–495.

Masten, A. S., & Narayan, A. J. (2012). Child development in the context of disasters, war and terrorism: Pathways to risk and resilience. *Annual Review of Psychology*, 63, 227–257.

Masten, A. S., & Obradovi , J. (2008). Disaster preparation and recovery: Lessons from research on resilience in human development. *Ecology and Sociology*, 13(1), 9–24.

Masten, A. S., & Osofsky, J. D. (2010). Disasters and their impact on child development: Introduction to the special section. *Child Development*, 81(4), 1029–1039.

McDermott, B. M., Lee, E. M., Judd, M., & Gibbon, P. (2005). Posttraumatic stress disorder and general psychopathology in children and adolescents following a wildfire disaster. *Canadian Journal of Psychiatry*, 50(3), 137–143.

Meaney, M. J. (2010). Epigenetics and the biological definition of gene x environment interactions. *Child Development*, 81(1), 41–79.

Meaney, M. J., Aitken, D. H., Viau, V., Sharma, S., & Sarrieau, A. (1989). Neonatal handling alters adrenocortical negative feedback sensitivity and hippocampal type II glucocorticoid receptor binding in the rat. *Neuroendocrinology*, 50, 597–604.

Montgomery, E., & Foldspang, A. (2005). Seeking asylum in Denmark: Refugee children's mental health and exposure to violence. *European Journal of Public Health*, 15(3), 233–237.

Murray, L. K., Cohen, J. A., Ellis, B. H., & Mannarino, A. (2008). Cognitive behavioral therapy for symptoms of trauma and traumatic grief in refugee youth. *Child and Adolescent Psychiatry Clinics of North America*, 17, 585–604.

National Commission on Children in Disasters. (2010). 2010 *report to the president and Congress*. Rockville, MD: Agency for Healthcare and Research Quality.

Neuner, F., Catani, C., Ruf, M., Schauer, E., Schauer, M., & Elbert, T. (2008). Narrative exposure therapy for the treatment of traumatized children and adolescents (KIDNET): From neurocognitive theory to field intervention. *Child and Adolescent Psychiatry Clinics of North America*, 17, 641–664.

Norris, F. H., Friedman, M. J., & Watson, P. J. (2002). 60,000 disaster victims speak: Part II. Summary and implications of the disaster mental health research. *Psychiatry*, 65(3), 240–260.

Norris, F. H., Friedman, M. J., Watson, P. J., Byrne, C. M., Diaz, E., & Kaniasty, K. (2002). 60,000 disaster victims speak: Part I. An empirical review of the empirical literature, 1981–2001. *Psychiatry*, 65(3), 207–239.

Norris, F. H., Steven, S. P., Pfefferbaum, B., Wyche, K. F., & Pfefferbaum, R. L. (2008). Community resilience as a metaphor, theory, set of capacities, and strategy for disaster readiness. *American Journal of Community Psychology*, 41(1), 127–150.

Nugent, N. R., Tyrka, A. R., Carpenter, L. L., & Price, L. H. (2011). Gene-environment interactions: Early life stress and risk for depressive and anxiety disorders. *Psychopharmacology*, 214(1), 175–196.

Onyut, L. P., Neuner, F., Schauer, E., Ertl, V., Odenwald, M., Schauer, M., et al. (2005). Narrative exposure therapy as a treatment for child war survivors with posttraumatic stress disorder: Two case reports and a pilot study in an African refugee settlement. *BMC Psychiatry*, 5, 7–15.

Otto, M. W., Henin, A., Hirshfeld-Becker, D. R., Pollack, M. H., Biederman, J., & Rosenbaum, J. (2007). Posttraumatic stress disorder symptoms following media exposure to tragic events: Impact of 9/11 on children at risk for anxiety disorders. *Journal of Anxiety Disorders*, 21(7), 888–902.

Panter-Brick, C., Goodman, A., Tol, W., & Eggerman, M. (2011). Mental health and childhood adversities: A longitudinal study in Kabul, Afghanistan. *Journal of the American Academy of Child and Adolescent Psychiatry*, 50(4), 349–363.

Peltonen, K., & Punamäki, R.-L. (2010). Preventative interventions among children exposed to trauma of armed conflict: A literature review. *Aggressive Behavior*, 36, 95–116.

Pervanidou, P. (2008). Biology of post-traumatic stress disorder in childhood and adolescence. *Journal of Neuroendocrinolgy*, 20(5), 632–638.

Pfefferbaum, B., Doughty, D. E., Reddy, C., Patel, N., Gurwitch, R. H., Nixon, S. J., et al. (2002). Exposure and peritraumatic response as predictors of posttraumatic stress in children following the 1995 Oklahoma City bombing. *Journal of Urban Health*, 79(3), 354–363.

Pine, D. S., Costello, J., & Masten, A. S. (2005). Trauma, proximity, and developmental psychopathology: The effects of war and terrorism on children. *Neuropsychopharmacology*, 30(10), 1781–1792.

Pluess, M., & Belsky, J. (2011). Prenatal programming of postnatal plasticity? *Development and Psychopathology*, 23(1), 29–38.

Pratchett, L. C., & Yehuda, R. (2011). Foundations of posttraumatic stress disorder: Does early life stress lead to adult posttraumatic stress disorder? *Development and Psychopathology*, 23(2), 477–491.

Proctor, L. J., Fauchier, A., Oliver, P. H., Ramos, M. C., Rios, M. A., & Margolin, G. (2007). Family context and young children's responses to earthquake. *Journal of Child Psychology and Psychiatry*, 48(9), 941–949.

Qouta, S., Punamäki, R.-L., & El Sarraj, E. (2008). Child development and family mental health in war and military violence: The Palestinian experience. *International Journal of Behavior Development*, 32(4), 310–321.

Ruf, M., Schauer, M., Neuner, F., Catani, C., Schauer, E., & Elbert, T. (2010). Narrative exposure therapy for 7–16-year-olds: A randomized control trial with traumatized refugee children. *Journal of Traumatic Stress*, 23(4), 437–445.

Rutter, M. (1983). Stress, coping, and development: Some issues and some questions. In N. Garmezy & M. Rutter (Eds.), *Stress, coping and development in children* (pp. 1–41). New York: McGraw-Hill.

Rutter, M. (2006). Implications of resilience concepts for scientific understanding. *Annals of the New York Academy of Science*, 1094(1), 1–12.

Sapienza, J. K., & Masten, A. S. (2011). Understanding and promoting resilience in children and youth. *Current Opinions in Psychiatry*, 24(4), 267–273.

Shonkoff, J. P., Boyce, W. T., & McEwen, B. S. (2009). Neuroscience, molecular biology, and the childhood roots of health disparities. *Journal of the American Medical Association*, 301(21), 2252–2259.

Silverman, W. K., & La Greca, A. M. (2002). Children experiencing disasters: Definitions, reactions, and predictors of outcomes. In A. M. La Greca, W. K. Silverman, E. M. Vernberg, & M. C. Roberts (Eds.), *Helping children cope with disasters and terrorism* (pp. 11–33). Washington, DC: American Psychological Association.

Silverman, W. K., La Greca, A. M., & Ortiz, C. D. (2004, July). Resilience building in children prior to traumatic exposure: Screening considerations. In R. H. Gurwitch (Chair), *Trauma, risk factors, and resilience: Making connections.* Symposium presented at the annual meeting of the American Psychological Association, Honolulu, HI.

Sroufe, L. A. (1979). The coherence of individual development: Early care, attachment, and subsequent developmental issues. *American Psychologist*, 34(10), 834–841.

Sroufe, L. A., Carlson, E. A., Levy, A. K., & Egeland, B. (1999). Implications of attachment theory for developmental psychopathology. *Development and Psychopathology*, 11(1), 1–13.

Thelen, E., & Smith, L. (1998). Dynamic systems theories. In R. M. Lerner (Ed.), *Handbook of child psychology. Volume 1: Theoretical models of human development* (5th ed., pp. 563–634). New York: Wiley.

Thienruka, W., Cardozo, B. L., Somchai-Chakkraband, M. L., Pengjuntr, W., Tantipiwatanaskul, P., Sakornsatian, S., et al. (2006). Symptoms of posttraumatic stress disorder and depression among children in tsunami-affected areas in Southern Thailand. *Journal of the American Medical Association*, 296(5), 549–559.

Tol, W. A., Komproe, I. H., Jordans, M. J. D., Gross, A. L., Susanty, D., Macy, R. D., et al. (2010). Mediators and moderators of a psychosocial intervention for children affected by political violence. *Journal of Consulting and Clinical Psychology*, 78(6), 818–828.

Toth, S. L., & Cicchetti, D. (1999). Psychopathology and child psychotherapy. In S. W. Russ & T. H. Ollendick (Eds.), *Handbook of psychotherapy with children and families* (pp. 15–44). New York: Kluwer Academic/Plenum.

Vigil, J. M., Geary, D. C., Granger, D. A., & Flinn, M. V. (2010). Sex differences in salivary cortisol, alpha-amylase, and psychological functioning following Hurricane Katrina. *Child Development*, 81(4), 1227–1239.

Weems, C. F., Taylor, L. K., Cannon, M. F., Marino, R. C., Romano, D. M., Scott, B. G., et al. (2010). Posttraumatic stress, context, and the lingering effects of the Hurricane Katrina disaster among ethnic minority youth. *Journal of Abnormal Child Psychology*, 38(1), 49–56.

Wickrama, K. A. S., & Kaspar, V. (2007). Family context of mental health risk in Tsunami-exposed adolescents: Findings from a pilot study in Sri Lanka. *Social Science and Medicine*, 64(3), 713–723.

Williams, R., Alexander, D. A., Bolsover, D., & Bakke, F. K. (2008). Children, resilience, and disasters: Recent evidence that should influence a model of psychosocial care. *Current Opinions in Psychiatry*, 21(4), 338–344.

Wolmer, L., Hamiel, D., & Laor, N. (2011). Preventing children's posttraumatic stress after disaster with teacher-based intervention: A controlled study. *Journal of the American Academy of Child and Adolescent Psychiatry*, 50(4), 340–348.

Yehuda, R., Bell, A., Bierer, L. M., & Schmiedler, J. (2008). Maternal, not paternal, PTSD related to increased risk for PTSD in offspring of Holocaust survivors. *Journal of Psychiatric Research*, 42(13), 1104–1111.

Yehuda, R., Engel, S. M., Brand, S. R., Seckl, J., Marcus, S. M., & Berkowitz, G. S. (2005). Transgenerational effects of posttraumatic stress disorder in babies of mothers exposed to the World Trade Center attacks during pregnancy. *Journal of Clinical Endocrinology and Metabolism*, 90(7), 4115–4118.

Yehuda, R., Flory, J. D., Pratchett, L. C., Buxbaum, J., Ising, M., & Holsboer, F. (2010). Putative biological mechanisms for the association between early life adversity and the subsequent development of PTSD. *Psychopharmacology, 212*(3), 405–417.

Yehuda, R., & Harvey, P. (1997). Relevance of neuroendocrine alterations in PTSD to memory-related impairments of trauma survivors. In D. J. Read & S. D. Lindsay (Eds.), *Recollections of trauma* (pp. 221–252). New York: Plenum.

Yehuda, R., McFarlane, A. C., & Shalev, A. Y. (1998). Predicting the development of post-traumatic stress disorder from the acute response to a traumatic event. *Biological Psychiatry, 44*(12), 1305–1313.

Yehuda, R., Teicher, M. H., Seckl, J., Grossman, R. A., Morris, A., & Bierer, L. M. (2007). Parental posttraumatic stress disorder as a vulnerability factor for low cortisol trait in offspring of Holocaust survivors. *Archives of General Psychiatry, 64*(9), 1040–1048.

Yelland, C., Robinson, P., Lock, C., La Greca, A. M., Kokegei, B., Ridgeway, V., et al. (2010). Bushfire impact on youth. *Journal of Traumatic Stress, 23*(2), 274–277.

Zeanah, C. H., Nelson, C. A., Fox, N. A., Smyke, A. T., Marshall, P., Parker, S. W., et al. (2003). Designing research to study the effects of institutionalization on brain and behavioral development: The Bucharest Early Intervention Project. *Development and Psychopathology, 15*, 885–907.

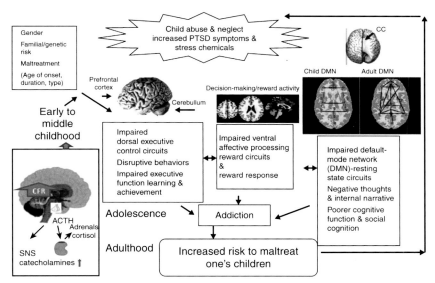

Figure 4.1 The developmental traumatology model of the neurobiology of the intergenerational transmission of child abuse and neglect. In this model, child maltreatment increases baseline levels of stress chemicals (e.g., cortisol from the hypothalamic-pituitary-adrenal [HPA] axis and catecholamines from the locus coeruleus and sympathetic nervous system [SNS]), which in turn adversely affect the development of prefrontal and cerebellar executive brain circuits, lead to immaturity of control and reward inhibitory brain regions, and disrupt the development of the brain default mode network (DMN). The DMN is connected through myelinated circuits in the corpus callosum (CC). These adverse effects lead to psychopathology (e.g., anxiety, depression, PTSD symptoms) and addiction. Parental psychopathology and addiction, in turn, lead to the intergenerational transmission of child maltreatment.

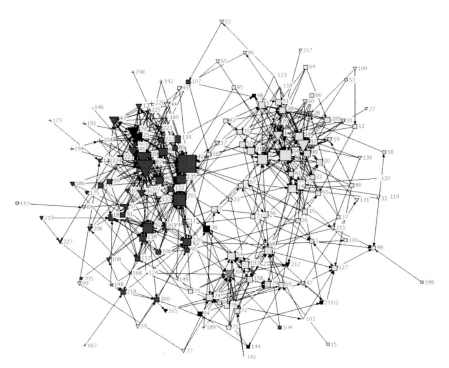

Figure 7.1 Social network of 224 adult family members of children enrolled in the ABC Day Care Center at the time of the fire. Blue = child died; yellow = child injured; black = two or more children injured; green = one child died, one injured. Square = mother; triangle = father; + = other caretaker. The size of the symbol is proportional to the degree of network participation, measured by both the number of persons the respondent named and the number of times he or she was named by others.

PART IV

Culture and Community Context in Understanding Trauma, Psychopathology, and Violence

7

Four Meanings of "Community" in Disaster

FRAN H. NORRIS

Disasters, by definition, happen to whole communities. Thus, in order to understand the effects of disasters, we need to consider carefully how communities influence the course of disaster recovery and are themselves modified by the experience. This is challenging for many reasons, not the least of which being that "community" has a variety of meanings. Although communities are changing rapidly due to contemporary patterns of life (commuting) and modern technologies (social media), in the disaster field, we still largely think of them as entities that have geographic boundaries and a shared fate (Norris, 2006). At least implicitly, disaster research reflects the ecological premise that organisms of all kinds survive, thrive, or decline in interdependence with their environments, and people are no exception (Harvey & Narra, 2007). It is equally important, however, to recognize community as a psychological construct that imbues disaster survivors with a sense of connectedness to others.

Presented here more or less in temporal sequence, the following four meanings of "community" appear most critical for understanding the consequences of disasters:

(1) *Context of response:* Disaster-stricken communities can be characterized by varying levels of pre-event adaptive capacities and resources that influence the effectiveness of response and recovery efforts.

(2) *Zone of impact:* Disaster-stricken communities can also be characterized by shared impacts (destruction or disruption of infrastructure, symbols, places, and services) that influence mental health over and above the effects of personal loss and trauma.

(3) *Frame for recovery:* For quite some time after disaster strikes, communities evolve or even emerge to meet collective needs, provide meaning to survivors, and achieve shared aims. Of the four meanings of "community," this one is most subjective and most likely to transcend spatial considerations.

(4) *Place of intervention:* It is widely agreed that postdisaster interventions must be provided by local people in the communities where people work and live; a smaller but important body of literature argues that community should be the *focus* of intervention, rather than simply the setting in which more traditional therapies are delivered.

In this chapter, I aim to consider each of these four meanings in some depth, with the goal of providing a reasonably comprehensive picture of the intersection between community and disaster. These are questions that have intrigued me for many years, and thus I rely heavily on my own work, including some recent findings of studies that are now in process. The chapter is roughly organized in the order suggested by the above list, beginning with a discussion of how preexisting attributes of communities are thought to influence population and individual resilience during and after disasters, and then shifting to the implications of disasters for mental health, with an emphasis on the consequences of the physical damages and social disruption shared by the community at large. Then, I consider how community can be generated by events and might serve as a vehicle for making sense of them. Finally, I touch upon the topic of community as the setting or focus of intervention efforts.

Community as the Context of Response

The first meaning of community in the disaster arena is the *context* in which response and recovery occur. An individual's resilience is inextricably linked to his or her community's ability to prepare for, respond to, and adapt to adverse conditions. In recognition of such interdependencies, "community resilience" has emerged as a key concept for disaster readiness (Norris, Stevens, Pfefferbaum, Wyche, & Pfefferbaum, 2008).

The concept of resilience appears in a variety of disciplines, including physics/engineering, biology/ecology, sociology, and psychology. Across domains of concern, most definitions of resilience emphasize a capacity for successful adaptation in the face of a disturbance, stress, or adversity. What we primarily seek to discover in resilience research is the capacity for resilience, that is, those preexisting and emergent resources that increase the likelihood of adaptation, as is manifest in psychological or population wellness. On the basis of their review of the interdisciplinary literature, Norris et al. (2008) identified four primary sets of resources thought to yield community resilience: economic development, social capital, information and communication, and community competence. Primary points are summarized below, but the reader is referred to the earlier review for greater detail and discussion.

Economic development encompasses the community's level of economic resources, the diversity of those resources, and the equity of their distribution.

Land and raw materials, physical capital, accessible housing, health services, schools, and employment opportunities create the essential resource base of a resilient community (Godschalk, 2003; Pfefferbaum, Reissman, Pfefferbaum, Klomp, & Gurwitch, 2005). However, community resilience depends not only on the volume of resources but also on their diversity. Communities that are dependent on a narrow range of resources are less able to cope with change that involves the depletion of that resource, a state that is sometimes referred to as "resource dependency" (Adger, 2000). For example, Cutter et al. (2006) described one community that was especially devastated by Hurricane Katrina in August 2005 because residents were almost totally reliant on the shrimping industry, on which the storm's impact was tremendous. Poor communities are often considered the weakest links in hazard mitigation (Cutter et al., 2006; Godschalk, 2003). Not only are they at greater risk for death and severe damage, but they often are less successful in mobilizing support after disasters (Finch, Emrich, & Cutter, 2010; Kaniasty & Norris, 1995).

The second set of adaptive capacities for community resilience, *social capital*, results from the fact that individuals invest in, access, and use resources embedded in social networks in order to gain returns (Bourdieu, 1985). For crisis response, an important dimension of social capital is the presence of interorganizational networks that are characterized by reciprocal links, frequent supportive interactions, and cooperative decision-making processes (Goodman et al., 1998). Longstaff (2005) highlighted the importance of "keystones" or "hubs," "super-connected" network members who link one network to another (see also Fullilove & Saul, 2006).

Social capital encompasses the familiar concept of social support, which usually refers to interpersonal relationships perceived as loving, caring, and readily available in times of need (Barrera, 1986). For the most part, social support entails helping behaviors within family and friendship networks, but social capital also encompasses relationships between individuals and their larger neighborhoods and communities (Perkins, Hughey, & Speer, 2002). Three fundamental social psychological dimensions of social capital are sense of community, place attachment, and citizen participation. "Sense of community" is an attitude of bonding (trust and belonging) with other members of one's group or locale, including mutual concerns and shared values. "Place attachment" implies an emotional connection to one's neighborhood or city, somewhat apart from connections to the specific people who live there; it often underlies citizens' efforts to revitalize a community (Perkins et al., 2002). Citizen participation is the engagement of community members in formal organizations, including religious congregations, school and resident associations, neighborhood watches, and self-help groups (Goodman et al., 1998; Pfefferbaum et al., 2005). Empowering community settings are characterized by inspired, committed leadership and by opportunities for members to play meaningful roles.

The third set of capacities for community resilience, *information and communication*, is vital for disaster preparedness. In an emergency, people need accurate information about the danger and behavioral options, and they need it quickly. To be effective, information must be correct, and the sender must be trusted (Longstaff, 2005). Closer, local sources of information are more likely to be relied upon than unfamiliar, distant sources. The Working Group on Governance Dilemmas in Bioterrorism Response (2004) concluded that trusted communication treats the public as a capable ally, invests in public outreach, and reflects the values and priorities of local populations.

Community competence, the final set of capacities outlined by Norris et al. (2008), is the capacity for meaningful, intentional action (Brown & Kulig, 1996). There appears to be high consensus that critical reflection and problem solving are fundamental prerequisites for community resilience (Goodman et al., 1998; Pfefferbaum et al., 2005). Endangered communities must be able to learn about their risks and options and work together flexibly and creatively to solve problems. The capacity to acquire information, to reflect on that information critically, and to solve emerging problems is far more important for community resilience than is a detailed security plan that rarely foresees all contingencies (Longstaff, 2005).

Collective action can depend heavily on the presence of collective efficacy, that is, community members' trust in the effectiveness of organized community action. Sampson, Raudenbush, and Earl (1997) defined collective efficacy as a composite of mutual trust and shared willingness to work for the common good. Paton and Johnston (2001) proposed that an initial focus on promoting collective efficacy would increase the likelihood of achieving success in working with a community to adopt mitigation strategies. Collective efficacy is highly related to empowerment (Perkins et al., 2002), a process through which people lacking an equal share of valued resources gain greater access to and control over those resources. Rich, Edelstein, Hallman, and Wandersman (1995) examined the dynamics of community empowerment after the discovery of environmental hazards and concluded that the effectiveness of a community's response is shaped by a combination of resources (e.g., sufficient education to understand the technical issues, money to hire lawyers or scientific advisors), a culture that permits challenges to authority, institutions that provide a basis for coordinating a response, and political mechanisms that involve citizens in decision making.

To date, research on the effects of community resources on postdisaster outcomes is meager. Some studies have examined how individual-level perceptions of community resilience (Kimhi & Shamai, 2004), sense of community (Paton, Millar, & Johnston, 2001), or collective efficacy (Benight, 2004) correlate with individual-level outcomes, but the question of whether independently assessed community resources influence the postdisaster wellness of constituent populations has not been thoroughly researched. I examine this question in a subsequent section.

A focus on community as the context, if not the cause, of resilience has critical implications for public health policy. Representing a paradigm shift compared to earlier disaster mitigation approaches, community preparedness calls for the use and integration of all the community's resources into disaster planning, including those that exist outside government as well as inside. Our work in identifying the adaptive capacities that underlie community resilience is consistent with this approach. The translation of findings into policy recommendations involves a discussion of changes in the socioeconomic structure of at-risk communities.

Community as the Zone of Impact

Past reviews of the disaster research literature (Bonanno, Brewin, Kaniasty, & LaGreca, 2010; Galea, Nandi, & Vlahov, 2005; Norris et al., 2002) have concluded unequivocally that disasters cause substantial and widespread distress in community populations and more lasting psychological problems in a minority of persons who were either severely exposed or especially vulnerable because of past psychopathology or weak psychosocial resources. The range of consequences experienced by disaster survivors is broad, including various *psychological problems*, such as depression, anxiety, and, most notably, post-traumatic stress disorder (PTSD); *physical health problems*, such as sleep disruption, somatic complaints, and impaired immune function; *chronic problems in living*, such as troubled interpersonal relationships and financial stress; and *resource loss*, such as declines in perceived control and perceived social support (Norris et al., 2002). Community-wide effects are usually expressed in terms of the population prevalence of specific conditions, such as PTSD. For example, on the basis of their review, Galea et al. (2005) concluded that the prevalence of postdisaster PTSD is typically in the range of 5–10% in the general population, although it is higher (30% to 40%) among victims with significant personal exposure.

Prevalence alone, however, does little to distinguish individual from collective aspects of disaster exposure, as rates of disorder in the population can be expected to vary most strongly along with the extensiveness of trauma and personal loss (Norris & Wind, 2009). A somewhat different question is whether individuals are affected only by their own losses or are affected additionally by the severity of losses experienced by the community at large. Certainly, past research has focused on personal loss, which is the extent to which a given individual has experienced trauma (e.g., injury, life threat, bereavement) or loss (e.g., property damage, disaster-related unemployment). Notwithstanding the importance of individual differences in the severity of exposure, many losses are shared by all members of the community. Hurricane Katrina, for example, destroyed 350 buildings listed in the National Register of Historic Places, as well as two major bridges on the Mississippi Gulf Coast (Scurfield, 2008). Destruction of a "keystone" neighborhood, such as a central business district, might challenge an entire city or region (Fullilove & Saul, 2006). I personally remember my own overwhelming sadness when I first viewed what had been the most beautiful park in Louisville, Kentucky, after it was stripped bare by a tornado in 1974. To ignore losses like these in our research would seem to miss the point of what it means to be a victim of disaster.

Community-wide losses are not confined to built and natural environments but extend to the social environment. These impacts were eloquently described by Erikson (1976) in his ethnography of the Buffalo Creek, West Virginia, dam collapse that caused heavy loss of life and massive displacement in a small mining town. The loss of social connections was severe, leaving survivors feeling isolated and alone. More recently, Scurfield (2008) shared his observation that hundreds of thousands of Katrina survivors in Mississippi experienced profound grief over their lost sense of place on the Mississippi Gulf Coast. Kaniasty and Norris (1993) tested a more specific "social support deterioration model," which posited that the impact of disasters on mental health occurs in part because of disruptions of social networks and declines in perceptions of support availability. Many things can lead to postdisaster declines in social support, including displacement and death of significant others, loss of routine opportunities for companionship and leisure, community conflicts about the causes of the disaster and appropriate responses, and violated expectations of aid (Kaniasty & Norris, 2004).

Assessing Community-Level Effects

More than 25 years ago, Bolin (1985) observed that there are two broad categories of disaster victims. *Primary victims* are those who directly experience physical, material, or personal losses, and *secondary victims* are others who live in the affected area. Although they sustain no personal injuries or property damage, secondary victims do experience a variety of inconveniences and the potential for economic, environmental, governmental, social, and cultural disruptions ranging from mild to severe. Primary and secondary victims alike might experience declines in opportunities for companionship and leisure, and both might be party to community conflicts about the causes of the disaster and appropriate responses. From this conceptualization, it can be inferred that disasters have potential psychological consequences even for those persons who experience no trauma or loss (Norris, 2006). These impacts are sometimes characterized as direct and indirect effects.

In an early study of indirect effects, Smith, Robins, Przybec, Goldring, and Solomon (1986) studied residents of areas in and around Times Beach, Missouri, who had been flooded or exposed to toxic contaminations, or both. They categorized study participants as direct victims (n = 139), indirect victims (persons who were exposed via the experiences of relatives and close friends; $n = 215$), or nonvictims ($n = 189$). The investigators found little evidence of indirect effects in their study, as generally the direct victims differed from both the indirect victims and nonvictims, who did not differ significantly from one another.

In contrast, Norris, Phifer, and Kaniasty (1994) did find evidence of indirect effects in their study of floods in eastern Kentucky (Appalachia). The 220 respondents in their study were all participating in a larger panel study of older adult mental health and had been interviewed three months before, as well as four times after the floods. The study spanned 10 flooded and 5 adjacent nonflooded counties, and archival data were used to capture county-level damages independently of the self-report measures of personal loss. This measure of "community destruction" explained significant variance in psychological well-being, physical health, and perceived social support over and above that explained by personal loss. The pattern of findings was instructive. Only primary victims (those with personal loss) showed increases in negative affect from before to after the flood, but both primary and secondary victims showed decreases in positive affect. Only primary victims showed increases in medical conditions and symptoms, but both primary and secondary victims showed increases in fatigue. Only primary victims showed declines in perceptions of kin support, but both primary and secondary victims showed declines in nonkin support. Together, the various findings appeared to reflect community-wide tendencies of residents to feel less positive about their surroundings, less energetic, and less able to enjoy life in the aftermath of the disaster. No one would suggest that such consequences constitute psychopathology, but they do indicate that disasters might impair the quality of life in the community for quite some time. Personal loss and community destruction interacted; victims who fared most poorly were those who experienced both high personal loss and high community destruction.

Recently, my colleagues participating in the National Center for Disaster Mental Health Research (especially Sandro Galea and Melissa Tracy) and I examined community impacts using more advanced statistical approaches than were widely available at the time of the Kentucky study. The Galveston Bay Recovery Study (GBRS) was launched approximately two months after Hurricane Ike, while effects were still acute. Hurricane Ike was a strong Category 2 storm (maximum winds were 1 mph below Category 3 status) when it struck Galveston, Texas, on September 13, 2008. The GBRS sample was composed of 658 adults who were representative of the population 18 years and older living in Galveston and Chambers counties (the most severely damaged counties) on the date when Hurricane Ike hit Galveston Bay and who had been living in the area for at least one month prior to the event. Interviews were performed using a computer-assisted interview system; 88% were conducted via telephone, and 12% were conducted in person. All interviews took place between November 7, 2008, and March 24, 2009, and lasted an average of 70 minutes (see Norris, Sherrieb, and Galea [2010] for further details).

Participants were asked a series of questions about their experiences during and after Hurricane Ike. A measure of personal exposure was created by counting experiences such as personal injury, threat to life, property damage, and financial loss. Community damages were assessed with a six-item measure regarding the level of damages and disruption to (1) area schools, churches, or hospitals; (2) streets and highways; and (3) places for recreation. Sizable percentages reported that the hurricane had damaged area schools, churches, hospitals, streets, and recreational settings in their areas "a lot." PTSD symptoms related specifically to Hurricane Ike were measured via a modified version of the PTSD Checklist, Civilian Version (Blanchard, Jones-Alexander, Buckley, & Forneris, 1996). Collective efficacy was measured with a 10-item scale of social control and social cohesion (Sampson et al., 1997).

We examined the effects of *community-level* damage/disruption and collective efficacy using generalized estimating equations and software that corrected for clustering in the sample selection. We aggregated individual reports of area damage/disruption and collective efficacy to the zip code level, thereby making them community-level (objective), rather than individual-level (subjective), measures. There were 21 zip codes in the data, with an average of 33 participants each. Although zip code is not a measure of neighborhood, it is an objective measure of area, and preliminary analyses showed that key variables varied across these geographic units. Reasonably, in order for a variable to be considered as potentially community-level, the between-community variance must be significantly greater than the within-community variance, and this was the case for PTSD symptoms, community damage, and collective efficacy.

Consistent with our expectations, the measure of community-level damage/disruption explained significant variance in disaster-related distress (PTSD symptoms) over and above that explained by the severity of personal hurricane exposure. Although the effects of the individual- and community-level exposure measures were solely additive (i.e., there was no interaction), it was nonetheless true that the greatest distress was reported by individuals who experienced both high personal loss and high community destruction. Contrary to our expectations, collective efficacy (also aggregated by area) did not modify the effects of community-level damage/disruption on distress, but it did buffer (lessen) the effects of personal exposure. We found a similar buffering effect of average community income. In other words, individuals in higher resource communities were able to withstand greater amounts of personal loss.

Community Impacts of Mass Violence

The potential of disasters to have indirect or community-wide effects on mental health is particularly salient in the context of mass violence. Palinkas, Prussing,

Reznik, and Landsverk (2004) studied the consequences of two high school shootings in San Diego using a community-based research approach. The researchers interviewed 85 key informants representing the experiences of students, teachers and school administrators, service providers, parents, and community leaders. Distress at exposure to media was very common and was accompanied by considerable resentment of the media for uncritically assuming that bullying led to the shooters' behavior and for intruding into their lives. Many expressed the desire to forget about the shooting, to return to a normal life. Interest in school activities diminished, and absenteeism rose. There was widespread reluctance to discuss the shootings and guilt over this very reluctance. Anger was common, although not usually directed at the shooters themselves, who sometimes were viewed with some sympathy and regret. Many students were unusually irritable with one another, and parents sometimes expressed anger at the school district for failing to prevent the incident. Faculty were fragmented over the issue. Palinkas and colleagues noted that these community reactions might hinder the implementation of effective prevention and treatment strategies. Likewise, the consequences of the Columbine high school shootings went far beyond the school itself. Lawrence and Birkland (2004) provided a fascinating glimpse into the various ways in which the problem was framed in the media, including themes of inadequate gun control, inadequate school security, inadequate parental involvement, and "pop culture" issues such as violent content in movies and video games. Columbine generated the most intense period of legislative activity on school violence ever.

The issue of direct and indirect effects of disasters has intrigued a number of researchers in the aftermath of terrorist attacks. With particular emphasis on research following the September 11 attacks on the World Trade Center in New York City, Galea and Resnick (2005) provided a thoughtful discussion of why psychopathology might emerge in some portion of the general population in the case of terrorism. In the New York example, the prevalence of PTSD was far lower among persons exposed only indirectly, but because they composed a large proportion of the population, there were almost as many indirect cases as direct cases. As the authors noted, the findings from New York raised questions about "what constitutes exposure for PTSD, and by extension, what constitutes PTSD itself" (p. 113). Throughout the New York metropolitan area, people felt terror, helplessness, or horror (PTSD Criterion A2) even if they were not directly affected by the September 11 attacks.

Most severe of all might be the example of war. On the basis of his observations of war-torn communities in Croatia, Bosnia, and Herzegovina, Adjukovic (2004) argued that terms such as "social trauma," "collective trauma," or "mass trauma" should replace "psychological trauma" in order to capture the pervasive and long-lasting effects of war on communities, including fragmentation, mistrust, breakdown of social institutions, and economic and political instability.

Population Impacts and Indicators

Taken together, these various studies and perspectives should make it clear that the effects of disaster and mass trauma on the community are potentially far-reaching. Traditional research methods (predominantly epidemiologic surveys) provide only a limited view of community-level effects, suggesting that we should experiment with research approaches that make use of vital statistics, administrative information, and other sources of community-level data. Several examples of this approach can be found in the literature: Curtis, Miller, and Berry (2000) found that reports and confirmations of child abuse were higher 3, 6, and 11 months after Hurricane Hugo relative to the same months in the previous year, and results for the Loma Prieta earthquake were similar. Cohan and Cole (2002) found that divorce rates increased after Hurricane Hugo in the 24 disaster-declared counties in South Carolina as opposed to the other 22 counties; conversely, Nakonezny, Reddick, and Rodgers (2004) found that divorce rates decreased in Oklahoma after the 1995 bombing, a finding they attributed to terror management theory, which suggests that when mortality becomes salient, people increasingly behave according to traditional values. While studying the community-wide consequences of the James Byrd murder (a notorious hate crime that occurred in Jasper, Texas), Wicke and Silver (2009) found a postevent increase in violent crime in Jasper despite a decrease in violence in the control community (Center, Texas). Su, Tran, Wirtz, Langteau, and Rothman (2009) found an increase in traffic fatalities and in alcohol/drug-related driving citations in the Northeast United States (and only in the Northeast) in the last three months of 2001 (after the September 11 terrorist attacks) that could not be accounted for by an increase in miles driven.

Whereas most past efforts to assess community-wide impacts have focused on one or two selected indicators of social stress (e.g., divorce, child maltreatment), Roxane Silver and I are currently collaborating to develop an index that simultaneously captures multiple domains of a community's quality of life (QoL). We aim to capture three primary domains of psychosocial QoL: public health, civil society, and public trust. Each domain encompasses multiple subdomains: *health/disability, mortality, mental health, natality,* and *health behavior* in the domain of public health; *child-family welfare, bonds/attachments,* and *crime/safety* in the domain of civil society; and *confidence in government, service/citizenship,* and *political engagement* in the domain of public trust. The domains are latent constructs (abstractions) and not directly measurable. However, each subdomain is manifest in multiple observable (measurable) conditions or characteristics (e.g., incidence of preterm births in the domain/subdomain of public health/natality; property crime rate in the domain/subdomain of civil society/crime and safety, and voting behavior in the domain/subdomain of public trust/political engagement). There are potentially numerous measures for each subdomain. "Impact" is defined as change in QoL from before to after an event. Within regions affected by a disaster, objective county-level measures of disaster impact (mortality, damages in dollars, proportion of families applying for individual assistance from the Federal Emergency Management Agency [FEMA]) should correlate with changes in psychosocial QoL (psychosocial impacts). Our hope in this research is to create a uniform metric that can be used at the policy level to incorporate human factors into assessments of risk and event impacts. Currently, the U.S. Department of Homeland Security measures the consequences of an event in terms of casualties and economic losses but does not take into account an event's effects on the public's psychosocial well-being, because such impacts have been difficult to quantify. A theory-informed and validated index that can be derived from routinely collected data would allow psychosocial impacts to be considered in future risk assessments.

Community as the Frame for Recovery

Not all presumed causes of community postdisaster resilience are preexisting attributes, such as those described previously. In fact, it is possible that one of the most important factors is the preservation or generation of community after the event. Communal narratives give survivors of a trauma shared meaning and purpose (Sonn & Fisher, 1998). Couto (1989) described how "group formulations" (narratives and symbols) became a mechanism for empowerment in Aberfan, South Wales, after a horrific environmental disaster took the lives of 104 schoolchildren and 20 adults. Writing about their own experiences in the aftermath of the September 11 terrorist attacks in lower Manhattan, Landau and Saul (2004) concluded that community recovery depends partly on collectively telling the story of the community's experience and response. In an anthropological study of six Guinean communities attacked by Sierra Leonean and Liberian forces (Abramowitz, 2005), symptoms of post-traumatic stress were much higher in three of the communities than in the others. In the three more distressed communities, respondents shared the feeling that government and nongovernmental organizations had neglected them. Social rituals and practices, including reciprocity and charity, were abandoned. There was widespread belief that some community members had prospered at the expense of others. In the three less distressed communities, residents shared a belief that customs and social practices would return to normal as soon as economic conditions improved. Most important, they had created a collective story that emphasized their resistance to the violence.

An interesting exposition of community as a frame for making sense of events was provided by Ryan and Hawdon (2008) in their account of the aftermath of the mass shooting at Virginia Tech that occurred on April 16, 2007. Ryan and Hawdon noted that by the afternoon of the shooting, a "master frame" had emerged in the university community about what happened, who had been harmed, and who was responsible. Although competing frames emerged over time, the original one endured. Ryan and Hawdon argued that individual and collective frames are mutually reinforcing—that is, social rituals that celebrate the collective's frame reinforce the individual's frame. They noted further (p. 47) that displays of solidarity create and maintain the frame that "we are a good community who suffered a tragedy that was not of our doing and that we did not deserve." The authors concluded that university communities like Virginia Tech might be especially likely to create post-disaster frames that emphasize solidarity because they also possess a strong collective identity. This is consistent with the premise that a preexisting sense of community (an element of social capital) facilitates community resilience.

A particularly intriguing facet of the meaning of community as a frame or narrative is that sometimes new communities of survivors emerge after mass trauma. The consequences of being embedded, to varying degrees, in an emergent community of grief are not known but are likely to be a complex mixture of positive and negative forces. Many possibilities were captured in the observations of clinicians who worked with the mothers of children killed in the 1995 bombing of the Murrah Federal Building in Oklahoma City, which housed a daycare center (Allen, Whittlesey, Pfefferbaum, & Ondersma, 1999). These mothers coalesced into a "community of suffering, healing, and celebrity." As Allen et al. described them, their connection to similar others might have increased social support for some mothers, but tensions, rivalries, conflicts, and dependencies within the group caused some mothers to feel less valued and inadequately supported.

There are also historical accounts of survivor groups that formed specifically for the purpose of seeking justice. Perhaps the best-known example is the group known as "Mothers of Plaza de Mayo," which emerged following the notorious "disappearances" during the Argentine dictatorship of the mid- to late 1970s. Wearing white kerchiefs and carrying photos of their missing children (usually adult men), the Mothers persistently marched in the plaza, bravely calling attention to the political repression and "silencing" of their losses and seeking justice and "punishment for the culprits" (Kordon, Edelman, Lagos, Nicoletti, & Bozzolo, 1988). More broadly, Danieli (2009, p. 351) discussed the healing role of reparative justice in the aftermath of mass trauma, noting the "mutually reinforcing context of shared mourning, shared memory, a sense that the memory is preserved, that the nation has transformed it into a part of its global consciousness." Reparative justice is fundamentally a collective process.

Creating Community: The Case of the ABC Day Care Fire

With the lack of research on survivor communities, we know very little about what draws people together and what the long-term functional consequences are of finding meaning via the creation of community after public tragedies. As part of a larger study of grief and PTSD, my colleagues (Art Murphy, Eric Jones, Kathleen Sherrieb, and Holly Prigerson) and I are presently conducting research relevant to this question. On June 5, 2009, a fire in a federally funded, privately operated day care center in Hermosillo, Sonora, Mexico, left 49 children dead and 40 others hospitalized for serious burns and smoke inhalation. An estimated 142 infants and toddlers were being cared for at the time of the blaze. Although the center had recently passed safety inspections, there were no water sprinklers in the building, fire alarms were not working properly, and an emergency exit was bolted shut. The aftermath of the fire has been marked by candlelight vigils, civil unrest, and multiple arrests for negligent homicide (see http://en.wikipedia.org/wiki/2009_Hermosillo_daycare_center_fire for more information).

The impact of this fire on Hermosillo is evident everywhere. There are three formal memorials to the children, one at the site of the fire and two others in major public plazas. At each memorial, 49 crosses each include a child's name, often accompanied by a large poster-size photo of the child's face. Many of the children were buried side by side in elaborate graves in the local cemetery. Even more striking are the billboards around the city with a deceased child's photo and a call for justice. Marches and demonstrations have been commonplace, and the event has caused Mexico to reconsider its policy of "franchising" its federally funded day care centers. On the day of our departure from a visit to Hermosillo in September 2010, a group of mothers holding placards depicting children's faces and the word "justice" blocked the entrance to the airport. Parents of injured children have been active as well, seeking ongoing medical help and compensation.

Approximately eight months postdisaster (January–March 2010), we interviewed 224 mothers, fathers, and other family members (such as grandparents) who had significant caretaking roles related to the children who either died (33 mothers, 23 fathers, 42 caretakers) or were injured (58 mothers, 34 fathers, 34 caretakers) in the fire. Not surprisingly, the sample was highly distressed, with 37% of parents/caretakers of injured children and 75% of parents/caretakers of deceased children meeting criteria for PTSD. Almost half (46%) of the bereaved sample also met criteria for prolonged grief disorder. As of this writing, we are in the field collecting the second wave of data (20 months postevent).

In this study, we are using social network analysis to capture the interdependence of survivors and the emerging "community of parents." We will need the Wave 2 data before we can fully assess the functional consequences of participation in this network, but a few observations can be shared now. Two pieces of background information are important for the consideration of these results. First, these parents had no meaningful relationships with one another before the fire. They largely dropped children off and picked them up at this day care center, which they had chosen mainly because of its convenience relative to their work.

Second, child outcomes were virtually random; whether a child lived or died was determined by chance, and was wholly undetermined by parent factors.

The network analyses yielded several interesting findings relevant to understanding the emergence of community in the aftermath of mass trauma. First, by the time of the interview eight months postfire, the parents were highly interconnected. Most parents easily named other ABC parents that they were in contact with and/or were included in other parents' lists. In generalized estimating equations predicting the extent of network participation for the total sample, significant effects emerged for child outcome (a family-level variable) and relationship to child (a person-level variable), and there was also significant interaction between the two variables. Families of children who died became more deeply embedded in the community than families of injured children. Both mothers and fathers participated more than other caretakers, but the effect of being a mother was approximately twice as strong as the effect of being a father. The interaction suggested that mothers and fathers of deceased children participated in the community of parents equally, but fathers were less involved than mothers when the child was injured but survived. The participation of men was more variable than that of women, with a few fathers being named by other parents very often, suggesting they played leadership roles in the parent groups.

Second, two distinctly separate groups of parents emerged (see Fig. 7.1), and these were almost perfectly determined by child outcome. Parents of children who died formed one group of relationships, and parents of injured children formed another. Network analysis also yields a measure of "betweenness," which has to do with the extent to which an individual links other individuals or groups to each other. Controlling for the number of ties (the primary predictor of all other network measures), bereavement was inversely related to betweenness, suggesting that bereaved parents/caretakers were especially likely to stick solely to their own. Mothers played a greater role than others in linking network participants together.

Third, network participation was significantly and positively associated with distress. When we controlled for child outcome and relationship, the severity of PTSD symptoms was a significant predictor of embeddedness in the total sample, as was grief in a more specific analysis of parents and caretakers of children who died. We cannot say at this point whether this was cause or effect, but we suspect that it was more the former than the latter (i.e., that it was the severity of their distress that drew individuals into the community as one way of coping).

Fourth, somewhat to our surprise, network participation was completely unrelated to perceptions of social support or social constraints. Previous research suggests that social support from family and friends is one factor that can help to alleviate bereavement-related distress, but the research also shows that

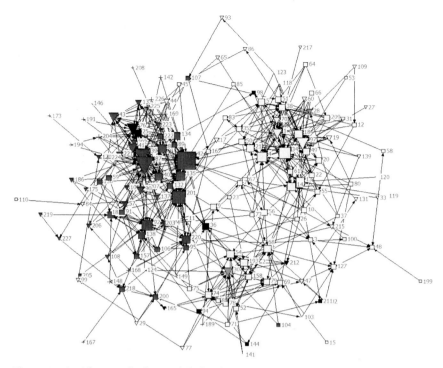

Figure 7.1 Social network of 224 adult family members of children enrolled in the ABC Day Care Center at the time of the fire. Blue = child died; yellow = child injured; black = two or more children injured; green = one child died, one injured. Square = mother; triangle = father; + = other caretaker. The size of the symbol is proportional to the degree of network participation, measured by both the number of persons the respondent named and the number of times he or she was named by others. (See color insert.)

bereaved persons often confront "social constraints" and "social ineptitudes" that can heighten or maintain their distress (e.g., Lepore, Silver, Wortman, & Wayment, 1996). Often unintentionally, people who would normally provide emotional support to the parent fail to do so in the case of a child's death because of their own discomfort. Thus we anticipated that participation in a network of people who shared and understood their experience would afford a support advantage. When the second wave of data are available, we can explore this puzzling finding in more depth by examining changes over time in social support and other measures of psychosocial well-being as a function of community participation.

In closing this section, I should note that disasters are not always followed by community solidarity. Residents of areas afflicted by technological accidents often bitterly debate the severity of the threat, and antagonisms can yield high levels of anger, alienation, and mistrust (Kaniasty & Norris, 2004). In a study of a railroad chemical spill (Bowler, Mergler, Huel, & Cone, 1994), for example, 69% of respondents believed that their community was divided between persons who felt they suffered from the accident and others who claimed there were no adverse consequences, and 36% believed they personally suffered because their own sense of victimization was minimized by friends and neighbors. The divisiveness has numerous implications, not yet fully understood, for what a disaster means for one's sense of community. As the world witnessed following Hurricane Katrina, survivors might legitimately perceive neglect and injustices in disaster response that can fundamentally undermine the relationship between citizen and state.

Community as the Place of Intervention

Disaster mental health practice has been written about extensively, and I will not attempt to summarize the whole of this body of work. Suffice it to say that numerous authors have called attention to the challenges in providing disaster mental health services, the difficulties in conducting controlled intervention research, and the consequent paucity of empirical evidence supporting the efficacy of potential approaches to preventing or treating postdisaster psychological disorders (e.g., Hamblen, Barnett, & Norris, in press; Litz & Gibson, 2006; National Institute of Mental Health, 2002).

Noting the lack of empirical evidence, Hobfoll and colleagues (2007) tackled the formidable challenge of developing a set of evidence-informed principles that can guide psychosocial interventions in the aftermath of disasters and mass trauma. Hobfoll et al. touched upon various components of cognitive behavioral and other psychological interventions that have been shown to be efficacious for treating PTSD or, more generally, for enhancing persons' skills and assets for managing stress. The authors' emphasis on "essential elements" rather than on particular treatments was a useful way of conceptualizing and extending the interventions' evidence base. In brief, they argued that safety, calmness, efficacy, hope, and connectedness are the five essential elements of mass trauma interventions.

Most relevant to the aims of this chapter is the subset of the disaster mental health literature that has emphasized community as the place or focus of disaster-related interventions. Often, when writers advocate for community-based interventions, they continue to be concerned with the provision of fairly traditional one-on-one treatments but are aware that, in the aftermath of disasters, providers cannot sit back and wait for persons with mental health needs to approach them. People to be served by disaster mental health programs are often new constituents who do not see themselves as "mentally ill" (Wang et al., 2007). It has long been recognized that disaster mental health services must be provided in the heart of the affected community, and that service providers need to be proactive in their efforts to identify and reach out to persons in need (Flynn, 1994; Hodgkinson & Stewart, 1998). These goals have been addressed in different ways: by exploring mechanisms for screening the public and referring appropriate persons to treatment (e.g., Brewin et al., 2008; Norris et al., 2006); by developing approaches for the wide-scale training of community-based therapists in order to increase the local capacity to provide evidence-based treatments (Hamblen, Norris, Gibson, & Lee, 2010; Marshall, Amsel, Neria, & Suh, 2006); and by developing treatments specifically targeting the types of distress commonly associated with disasters, regardless of whether this distress precisely matches standard diagnostic categories, which it often does not (Hamblen et al., 2009).

Notwithstanding the need to disseminate evidence-based treatments, providing disaster-related mental health services in the community often requires a "public health approach" that differs sharply from traditional treatment models. While introducing the conclusions of a task force co-convened by the United Nations and the International Society of Traumatic Stress Studies, Susan Solomon (2003) summarized this viewpoint well: "Although professionals working in the mental health arena are seldom trained or prepared to work at a broader community level, the scale of these emergences may require abandoning dyadic interventions for those that can be implemented via community action using a public health approach. (p. 12)"

Two well-known examples of a public health approach are psychological first aid (PFA) and crisis counseling. PFA has rapidly become the most commonly recommended approach for the immediate aftermath of disasters. It is a brief intervention designed to be used in shelters, family assistance centers, and other places where survivors gather (Brymer et al., 2006). PFA aims to help individuals feel safe and secure, reduce their acute stress reactions, and connect them to social supports and ongoing services, as needed. PFA's stated aim is to enhance natural resilience rather than to prevent psychopathology. To my knowledge, PFA has not yet been formally evaluated. Evaluating PFA will be quite challenging given its rapid implementation and intentional lack of formal assessment protocols.

Crisis counseling, the most commonly used approach over the months following a disaster, is usually associated with projects funded by FEMA's Crisis Counseling Assistance and Training Program. Crisis counseling programs (CCPs) aim to address the short-term mental health needs of individuals and communities affected by disasters (Flynn, 1994). Based on the assumption that most disaster survivors are naturally resilient, CCPs emphasize outreach, supportive counseling, education, consultation, and linkages to other services. The program relies on a mix of local professional and paraprofessional crisis counselors. Crisis counseling services are usually brief, rarely involving more than one or two visits.

Despite its 30-year history, the evidence base on the reach and effectiveness of CCPs is small. The urgency of getting new programs planned and implemented in the context of disaster leaves little time or energy for thinking about research, but progress is being made. A standardized "cross-site" evaluation plan was implemented in the fall of 2005, and the results so far reveal several clear strengths (Jones, Allen, Norris, & Miller, 2009; Norris & Bellamy, 2009; Norris, Hamblen, & Rosen, 2009). For the community at large, crisis counseling might well be the "right" amount of intervention in the aftermath of disaster.

It has been argued that community should be the *focus* of intervention, rather than merely the place (e.g., Ajdukovic, 2004; Harvey & Narra, 2007; Landau & Saul, 2004; Norris & Thompson, 1995; van den Eynde & Veno, 1999). From a community perspective, no element of mass trauma intervention is potentially more far-reaching than the goal of augmenting and protecting social relationships (Ajdukovic, 2004). The pattern of help utilization after disasters resembles a pyramid, with its broad foundation being the family, followed by other primary support groups such as friends, neighbors, and co-workers (Kaniasty & Norris, 2004), and finally formal agencies and other persons outside of the victim's immediate circle. Proportionately few trauma victims turn to professionals for emotional, informational, or tangible support. Thus every effort should be made to boost and protect community members' capacity to help and care for one another. Norris and Alegria (2005) argued that postdisaster interventions that address socially engaged emotions, social support, and social functioning would be especially appropriate for many ethnic minority groups.

Approaches that work directly with communities to enhance their resilience are only minimally represented in the research literature. Although research is needed before they can claim an evidence base, interventions that promote community resilience appear to hold considerable promise for promoting safety, calmness, efficacy, hope, and connectedness in the aftermath of disasters. As Norris et al. (2008) discussed in greater detail, if their aim is to build collective resilience, communities must develop economic resources, reduce risk and resource inequities, and attend conscientiously to their areas of greatest social vulnerability. They must engage local people in every step of the mitigation process, create organizational linkages, and boost and protect social supports. They must plan for the unexpected, which means that community organizations must develop decision-making skills and cultivate trusted sources of information. In a nutshell, disaster readiness is about social change.

An exciting community-focused intervention that is now being evaluated is the Communities Advancing Resilience Toolkit (CART) developed by Pfefferbaum and colleagues (2011). CART is an integrated system for community assessment and strategic planning designed to enhance community resilience to terrorism and disasters. CART is a community intervention process that provides tools and models to facilitate assessment and strategic planning by community groups. In earlier phases, CART developers focused on creating, applying, and testing community resilience assessment tools. The CART developers are now working with Community Emergency Response Teams to demonstrate that affiliated volunteer disaster responders and local neighborhood associations can use the CART Integrated System to enhance community resilience. The long-term goal is to provide a set of Web-available, stand-alone tools and models that can be applied in order to better enable organizations and communities to prepare for, respond effectively to, and recover from catastrophes.

Closing

In closing this chapter on the meanings of community, I must acknowledge that I have discussed the influence of culture very little. The concepts I have described here have nothing and everything to do with culture. On the one hand, the work and writings informing my understanding of the four meanings of community spanned the continents of Asia; Africa; Australia; and South, Central, and North America. I cannot envision a human culture or society in which the basic concepts of resilience, disaster impacts, and meaning making do not apply. I cannot imagine a human culture or society in which economic development, social capital, communication, and competence are irrelevant. On the other hand, the manifestations and collaterals of these constructs are undoubtedly culture specific. Mechanisms for assuring economic and social security are often based on long-held traditions, such as the relative degree of filial responsibility (de Vries, 1995). Social support is universally relevant, but facets such as reciprocity norms, relative comfort with kin and nonkin, and modes of expressing emotional support vary substantially across cultures (de Vries, 1995; Oliver-Smith, 1986). Local meanings of community strongly influence openness to change (Oliver-Smith, 1986), and grassroots action is facilitated by cultures that permit challenges to authority (Rich et al., 1995). Any earnest attempt to enhance disaster resilience and recovery in a particular community will feature local culture and mores prominently.

In summary, I have argued that "community" has four key meanings that are important for understanding disaster impact and recovery. Indeed, it might be that nothing is more fundamental to our nation's security than the strength of its communities. When disaster strikes, the capacity of communities to respond effectively and recover swiftly resides in the people themselves—in their sense of competence and self-sufficiency, in the strengths of their social networks and bonds, in their ability to access and use information, in their capacity to mobilize and distribute resources, and in their efforts to recognize and reduce the social vulnerabilities that impede collective response and recovery.

I have also tried to show that communities are not static; they can be transformed, destroyed, or created by disaster. In the aftermath of disaster, we must be continually mindful that the community itself must take ownership of problems, solutions, and the direction of change (Landau & Saul, 2004; van den Eynde & Veno, 1999). Interventionists from outside the community can enhance a community's capacity to make informed choices, but they must recognize that the choices remain the community's own.

Disclosure Statement

The work in this chapter was supported by several funded projects, as follows: Department of Homeland Security (DHS), National Consortium for the Study of Terrorism and Responses to Terrorism (START), N00140510629, G. LaFree, Center Director, F. Norris, Dartmouth, PI (community resilience); National Institute of Mental Health (NIMH), P60 MH082598, F. Norris, PI (Galveston Bay Recovery Study); DHS, 2010-ST-108-LR0001, R. Silver, PI (quantitative index of impacts); and NIMH, R21 MH090703-02, F. Norris, PI (ABC Day Care Study).

References

Abramowitz, S. (2005). The poor have become rich, and the rich have become poor: Collective trauma in the Guinean Languette. *Social Science and Medicine, 61,* 2106–2118.

Adger, W. (2000). Social and ecological resilience: Are they related? *Progress in Human Geography, 24,* 347–364.

Ajdukovic, D. (2004). Social contexts of trauma and healing. *Medicine, Conflict and Survival, 20,* 120–135.

Allen, J., Whittlesey, S., Pfefferbaum, B., & Ondersma, M. (1999). Community and coping of mothers and grandmothers of children killed in a human-caused disaster. *Psychiatric Annals, 29,* 85–91.

Barrera, M. (1986). Distinctions between social support concepts, measures, and models. *American Journal of Community Psychology, 14,* 413–445.

Benight, C. (2004). Collective efficacy following a series of natural disasters. *Anxiety, Stress, and Coping, 17,* 401–420.

Blanchard, E., Jones-Alexander, J., Buckley, T., & Forneris, C. (1996). Psychometric properties of the PTSD Checklist (PCL). *Behavioral Research and Therapy, 34,* 669–673.

Bolin, R. (1985). Disaster characteristics and psychosocial impacts. In B. Sowder (Ed.), *Disasters and mental health: Selected contemporary perspectives* (pp. 3–28). Rockville, MD: National Institute of Mental Health.

Bonanno, G., Brewin, C., Kaniasty, K., & LaGreca, A. (2010). Weighing the costs of disaster: Consequences, risks, and resilience in individuals, families, and communities. *Psychological Science, 11*, 1–49.

Bourdieu, P. (1985). The forms of capital. In J. Richardson (Ed.), *Handbook of theory and research for the sociology of education* (p. 248). New York: Greenwood.

Bowler, R., Mergler, D., Huel, G., & Cone, J. (1994). Psychological, psychosocial and psychophysiological sequelae in a community affected by a railroad chemical disaster. *Journal of Traumatic Stress, 7*, 601–624.

Brewin, C., Scragg, P., Robertson, M., Thompson, M., d'Ardenne, P., & Ehlers, A. (2008). Promoting mental health following the London Bombings: A screen and treat approach. *Journal of Traumatic Stress, 21*, 3–8.

Brown, D., & Kulig, J. (1996/1997). The concept of resiliency: Theoretical lessons from community research. *Health and Canadian Society, 4*, 29–52.

Brymer, M., Layne, C., Jacobs, A., Pynoos, R., Ruzek, J., Steinberg, A., et al. (2006). Psychological first aid field operations guide (2nd ed.). Los Angeles: National Child Traumatic Stress Network and National Center for PTSD.

Cohan, C., & Cole, S. (2002). Life course transitions and natural disaster: Marriage, birth, and divorce following Hurricane Hugo. *Journal of Family Psychology, 16*, 14–25.

Couto, R. (1989). Catastrophe and community empowerment: The group formulations of Aberfan's survivors. *Journal of Community Psychology, 17*, 236–248.

Curtis, T., Miller, B., & Berry, E. (2000). Changes in reports and incidence of child abuse following natural disasters. *Child Abuse & Neglect, 24*, 1151–1162.

Cutter, S., Emrich, C., Mitchell, J., Boruff, B., Gall, M., Schmidtlein, M., et al. (2006). The long road home: Race, class, and recovery from Hurricane Katrina. *Environment, 48*, 10–20.

Danieli, Y. (2009). Massive trauma and the healing role of reparative justice. *Journal of Traumatic Stress, 22*, 351–357.

de Vries, M. (1995). Culture, community and catastrophe. Issues in understanding communities under difficult conditions. In S. Hobfoll & M. de Vries (Eds.), *Extreme stress and communities: Impact and intervention* (pp. 375–393). Dordrecht, the Netherlands: Kluwer.

Erikson, K. (1976). Loss of communality at Buffalo Creek. *American Journal of Psychiatry, 133*, 302–305.

Finch, C., Emrich, C., & Cutter, S. (2010). Disaster disparities and differential recovery in New Orleans. *Population and Environment, 31*, 179–202.

Flynn, B. (1994). Mental health services in large scale disasters: An overview of the Crisis Counseling Program. *NCPTSD Clinical Quarterly, 4*, 11–12.

Fullilove, M., & Saul, J. (2006). Rebuilding communities post-disaster in New York. In Y. Neria, R. Gross, R. Marshall, & E. Susser (Eds.), *9/11: Mental health in the wake of terrorist attacks* (pp. 164–177). New York: Cambridge University Press.

Galea, S., Nandi, A., & Vlahov, D. (2005). The epidemiology of post-traumatic stress disorder after disasters. *Epidemiology Reviews, 27*, 78–91.

Galea, S., & Resnick, H. (2005). Psychological consequences of mass trauma in the general population. *CNS Spectrums, 10*, 107–115.

Godschalk, D. (2003). Urban hazard mitigation: Creating resilient cities. *Natural Hazards Review, 4*, 136–143.

Goodman, R., Speers, M., McLeroy, K., Fawcett, S., Kegler, M., Parker, E., et al. (1998). Identifying and defining the dimensions of community capacity to provide a basis for measurement. *Health Education & Behavior, 25*, 258–278.

Hamblen, J., Barnett, E., & Norris, F. (in press). Long term mental health treatment for adult disaster survivors. In J. Framingham and M. Teasley (Eds.), *Behavioral health response to disasters*. Boca Raton, FL: CRC Press.

Hamblen, J., Norris, F., Gibson, L., & Lee, L. (2010) Training community therapists to deliver cognitive behavioral therapy in the aftermath of disaster. *International Journal of Emergency Mental Health, 12,* 33–40.

Hamblen, J., Norris, F., Pietruszkiewicz, S., Gibson, L., Naturale, A., & Louis, C. (2009). Cognitive behavioral therapy for postdisaster distress: A community based treatment program for survivors of Hurricane Katrina. *Administration and Policy in Mental Health and Mental Health Services Research, 36,* 206–214.

Harvey, M., & Narra, P. (2007). Sources and expression of resilience in trauma survivors: Ecological theory, multicultural perspectives. *Journal of Aggression, Maltreatment, & Trauma, 14,* 1–7.

Hobfoll, S., Watson, P., Bell, C., Bryant, R., Brymer, M., Friedman, M., et al. (2007). Five essential elements of immediate and mid-term mass trauma intervention: Empirical evidence. *Psychiatry, 70,* 283–315.

Hodgkinson, P., & Stewart, M. (1998). *Coping with catastrophe: A handbook of post-disaster psychosocial aftercare* (2nd ed.). London: Routledge.

Jones, K., Allen, M., Norris, F., & Miller, C. (2009). Piloting a new model of crisis counseling: Specialized crisis counseling services in Mississippi after Hurricane Katrina. *Administration and Policy in Mental Health and Mental Health Services Research, 36,* 195–205.

Kaniasty, K., & Norris, F. (1993). A test of the support deterioration model in the context of natural disaster. *Journal of Personality and Social Psychology, 64,* 395–408.

Kaniasty, K., & Norris, F. (1995). In search of altruistic community: Patterns of social support mobilization following Hurricane Hugo. *American Journal of Community Psychology, 23,* 447–477.

Kaniasty, K., & Norris, F. (2004). Social support in the aftermath of disasters, catastrophes, and acts of terrorism: Altruistic, overwhelmed, uncertain, antagonistic, and patriotic communities. In R. Ursano, A. Norwood, & C. Fullerton (Eds.), *Bioterrorism: Psychological and public health interventions* (pp. 200–229). Cambridge, UK: Cambridge University Press.

Kimhi, S., & Shamai, M. (2004). Community resilience and the impact of stress: Adult response to Israel's withdrawal from Lebanon. *Journal of Community Psychology, 32,* 439–451.

Kordon, D., Edelman, L., Lagos, D., Nicoletti, E., & Bozzolo, R. (1988). *Psychological effects of political repression.* Buenos Aires, Argentina: Sudamericana/Planeta.

Landau, J., & Saul, J. (2004). Facilitating family and community resilience in response to major disaster. In F. Walsh & M. McGoldrick (Eds.), *Living beyond loss: Death in the family* (pp. 285–309). New York: Norton.

Lawrence, R., & Birkland, T. (2004). Guns, Hollywood, and school safety: Defining the school-shooting problem across public arenas. *Social Science Quarterly, 85,* 1193–1207.

Lepore, S., Silver, R., Wortman, C., & Wayment, C. (1996). Social constraints, intrusive thoughts, and depressive symptoms among bereaved mothers. *Journal of Personality and Social Psychology, 70,* 271–282.

Litz, B., & Gibson, L. (2006). Conducting research on mental health interventions. In E. C. Ritchie, P. Watson, & M. Friedman (Eds.), *Interventions following mass violence and disasters: Strategies for mental health practice* (pp. 387–404). New York: Guilford.

Longstaff, P. (2005). *Security, resilience, and communication in unpredictable environments such as terrorism, natural disasters, and complex technology.* Syracuse, New York: Author.

Marshall, R. D., Amsel, L., Neria, Y., & Jung Suh, E. (2006). Strategies for determination of evidence-based treatments: Training clinicians after large-scale disasters. In F. Norris, S. Galea, M. Friedman, & P. Watson (Eds.), *Research methods for studying mental health after disasters and terrorism* (pp. 226–242). New York: Guilford.

Nakonezny, P., Reddick, R., & Rodgers, J. (2004). Did divorces decline after the Oklahoma City Bombing? *Journal of Marriage and the Family, 66,* 90–100.

National Institute of Mental Health (2002). *Mental health and mass violence: Evidence based early psychological intervention for victims/survivors of mass violence: A workshop to reach consensus on best practices.* NIH Publication Office No. 02–5138. Washington, DC: U.S. Government Printing Office.

Norris, F. (2006). Community and ecological approaches to understanding and alleviating postdisaster distress. In Y. Neria, R. Gross, R. Marshall, & E. Susser (Eds.), *September 11, 2001: Treatment, research, and public mental health in the wake of a terrorist attack* (pp. 141–156). New York: Cambridge University Press.

Norris, F., & Alegria, M. (2005). Mental health care for ethnic minority individuals and communities in the aftermath of disasters and mass violence. *CNS Spectrums, 10,* 132–140.

Norris, F., & Bellamy, N. (2009). Evaluation of a national effort to reach Hurricane Katrina survivors and evacuees: The Crisis Counseling Assistance and Training Program. *Administration and Policy in Mental Health and Mental Health Services Research, 36,* 165–175.

Norris, F., Donahue, S., Felton, C., Watson, P., Hamblen, J., & Marshall, R. (2006). A psychometric analysis of Project Liberty's Adult Enhanced Services Referral Tool. *Psychiatric Services, 57,* 1328–1334.

Norris, F., Friedman, M., Watson, P., Byrne, C., Diaz, E., & Kaniasty, K. (2002). 60,000 disaster victims speak, Part I: An empirical review of the empirical literature, 1981–2001. *Psychiatry, 65,* 207–239.

Norris, F., Hamblen, J., & Rosen, C. (2009). Service characteristics and counseling outcomes: Lessons from a cross-site evaluation of crisis counseling after Hurricanes Katrina, Rita, and Wilma. *Administration and Policy in Mental Health and Mental Health Services Research, 36,* 176–185.

Norris, F., Phifer, J., & Kaniasty, K. (1994). Individual and community reactions to the Kentucky floods: Findings from a longitudinal study of older adults. In R. Ursano, B. McCaughey, & C. Fullerton (Eds.), *Individual and community responses to trauma and disaster: The structure of human chaos* (pp. 378–400). Cambridge, UK: Cambridge University Press.

Norris, F., Sherrieb, K., & Galea, S. (2010). Prevalence and consequences of disaster-related illness and injury from Hurricane Ike. *Rehabilitation Psychology, 55,* 221–230.

Norris, F., Stevens, S., Pfefferbaum, B., Wyche, K., & Pfefferbaum, R. (2008). Community resilience as a metaphor, theory, set of capacities, and strategy for disaster readiness. *American Journal of Community Psychology, 41,* 127–150.

Norris, F., & Thompson, M. (1995). Applying community psychology to the prevention of trauma and traumatic life events. In J. Freedy & S. Hobfoll (Eds.), *Traumatic stress: From theory to practice* (pp. 49–71). New York: Plenum.

Norris, F., & Wind, L. (2009). The experience of disaster: Trauma, loss, adversities, and community effects. In Y. Neria, S. Galea, & F. Norris (Eds.), *Mental health consequences of disasters* (pp. 29–44). New York: Cambridge University Press.

Oliver-Smith, A. (1986). *The martyred city*. Albuquerque: University of New Mexico Press.

Palinkas, L., Prussing, E., Reznik, V., & Landsverk, J. (2004). The San Diego East County School shootings: A qualitative study of community level post-traumatic stress. *Prehospital and Disaster Medicine, 19,* 113–121.

Paton, D., & Johnston, D. (2001). Disasters and communities: Vulnerability, resilience, and preparedness. *Disaster Prevention and Management, 10,* 270–277.

Paton, D., Millar, M., & Johnston, D. (2001). Community resilience to volcanic hazard consequences. *Natural Hazards, 24,* 157–169.

Perkins, D., Hughey, J., & Speer, P. (2002). Community psychology perspectives on social capital theory and community development practice. *Journal of the Community Development Society, 33,* 33–52.

Pfefferbaum, B., Reissman, D., Pfefferbaum, R., Klomp, R., & Gurwitch, R. (2005). Building resilience to mass trauma events. In L. Doll, S. Bonzo, J. Mercy, & D. Sleet (Eds.), *Handbook on injury and violence prevention interventions*. New York: Kluwer Academic.

Pfefferbaum, R., Pffefferbaum, B., Van Horn, R., Neas, B., Klomp, R., Norris, F., et al. (2011). *The Communities Advancing Resilience Toolkit (CART): An intervention to build community resilience to disasters*. Manuscript submitted for publication.

Rich, R., Edelstein, M., Hallman, W., & Wandersman, A. (1995). Citizen participation and empowerment: The case of local environmental hazards. *American Journal of Community Psychology, 23,* 657–676.

Ryan, J., & Hawdon, J. (2008). From individual to community: The "framing" of 4–16 and the display of social solidarity. *Traumatology, 14,* 43–51.

Sampson, R., Raudenbush, S., & Earls, F. (1997). Neighborhoods and violent crime: A multilevel study of collective efficacy. *Science, 277,* 918–924.

Scurfield, R. (2008). Post-Katrina storm disorder and recovery in Mississippi more than 2 years later. *Traumatology, 14,* 88–106.

Smith, E. M., Robins, L. N., Przybeck, T. R., Goldring, E., & Solomon, S. D. (1986). Psychosocial consequences of a disaster. In J. H. Shore (Ed.), *Disaster stress studies: New methods and findings* (pp. 49–76). Washington, DC: American Psychiatric Press.

Solomon, S. (2003). Introduction. In B. Green, M. Friedman, J. De Jong, S. Solomon, T. Keane, J. Fairbank, et al. (Eds.), *Trauma in war and peace: Prevention, practice, and policy* (pp. 3–16). New York: Kluwer Academic/Plenum.

Sonn, C., & Fisher, A. (1998). Sense of community: Community resilient responses to oppression and change. *Journal of Community Psychology, 26,* 457–472.

Su, J., Tran, A., Wirtz, J., Langteau, R., & Rothman, A. (2009). Driving under the influence (of stress): Evidence of a regional increase in impaired driving and traffic fatalities after the September 11 terrorist attacks. *Psychological Science, 20,* 59–65.

van den Eynde, J., & Veno, A. (1999). Coping with disastrous events: An empowerment model of community healing. In R. Gist & B. Lubin (Eds.), *Response to disaster: Psychosocial, community, and ecological approaches* (pp. 167–192). Philadelphia: Bruner/ Mazel.

Wang, P. S., Gruber, M. J., Powers, R. E., Schoenbaum, M., Speier, A. H., Wells, K. B., et al. (2007). Mental health service use among Hurricane Katrina survivors in the eight months after the disaster. *Psychiatric Services, 58,* 1403–1411.

Wicke, T., & Silver, R. C. (2009). A community responds to collective trauma: An ecological analysis of the James Byrd murder in Jasper, Texas. *American Journal of Community Psychology, 44,* 233–248.

Working Group on Governance Dilemmas in Bioterrorism Response. (2004). Leading during bioattacks and epidemics with the public's trust and help. *Biosecurity and Bioterrorism: Biodefense Stategy, Practice, and Science, 2,* 25–39.

8

Epidemiology of Violence Exposure in the Home and Community and Children's Physical Health Risk

The Urban Asthma/Allergy Paradigm

ROSALIND J. WRIGHT

Over the past four decades, there has been increasing interest in the role of violence exposure, a specific traumatic stressor, on children's development and
health. In part this is because epidemiologic studies have demonstrated that
children's exposure to such traumatic events is more prevalent than was once
believed (Briggs-Gowan, Ford, Fraleigh, McCarthy, & Carter, 2010; Fairbank &
Fairbank, 2009). Data suggest that the exposure prevalence in the general population ranges between 10% and 80%, depending on the country being studied,
urban versus rural sampling, age, gender, race/ethnicity, socioeconomic status
(SES), and how violence exposure was classified.

Earlier research on the health effects of violence centered on the direct exposure of individuals to violent acts (e.g., child abuse). More recent investigations
have also focused on indirect exposures due to either witnessing violence in
various contexts or the effect of living in a violent environment, with a chronic
pervasive atmosphere of fear and the perceived threat of violence, on children's
development. The scope of violence exposure examined in epidemiology has
thus broadened to include child maltreatment (i.e., direct victimization), witnessing violence in the home (domestic or family violence), and direct victimization and/or witnessing violence in the communities in which the children
live, as well as in specialized contexts such as political violence or warfare.
Children often experience more than one type of violence, and these might have
both independent and interrelated effects (Bogat, et al., 2005; Margolin & Gordis,
2000).

Our understanding of the full scope of the potential health effects continues
to expand as well. Much of the earlier work focused on the effects of violence on
behavioral and psychological problems in children and adolescents (Bradshaw
& Garbarino, 2004; Cooley-Quille, Boyd, Frantz, & Walsh, 2001; Cummings,

El-Sheikh, Kouros, & Buckhalt, 2009; Cummings, Goeke-Morey, Schemerhorn, Merrilees, & Cairns, 2009; Henning, Leitenberg, Coffey, Bennett, & Jankowski, 1997; Holt, Buckley, & Whelan, 2008; Trickett, Duran, & Horn, 2003; Williams, 2007). The growing body of research documenting long-term physiological disturbances in children growing up in violent neighborhoods and homes (Bremner, 2003; Cicchetti & Rogosch, 2001; Kliewer, 2006; McCrory, De Brito, & Viding, 2010; Saltzman, Holden, & Holahan, 2005) suggests even broader health effects. My group, as well as others, have documented links between adverse childhood experiences including abuse and increased psychological morbidity in adulthood (Arnow, 2004; Rich-Edwards, Spiegelman, et al., 2010), as well as chronic physical disorders including cardiovascular disease, diabetes, and obesity (Boynton-Jarrett, Rich-Edwards, Jun, Hibert, & Wright 2011; Felitti, 2009; Rich-Edwards, et al., 2010; Riley, Wright, Jun, Hibert, & Rich-Edwards, 2010; Wegman & Stetler, 2009). A number of models framed within life course theory have been proposed to explain the relationship between early life trauma (including intergenerational effects) and adult physical health (Braveman & Barclay, 2009; Springer, 2009), but a leading hypothesis for the enduring impact of traumatic stressors is related to the programming of key physiologic stress pathways during vulnerable early life periods of development (e.g., prenatal development, early childhood) (Bremner, 2003). Despite increased focus on the importance of trauma experiences in early development, little research has focused on how these effects manifest in early childhood, particularly in relation to physical health, and on the underlying biological mechanisms that might be operating.

Studies examining the influence of violence exposure in early life on asthma expression in urban high-risk populations begin to address some of the existing gaps in our understanding. This overview reviews epidemiologic evidence from prospective population-based studies examining associations between violence exposure among both mothers and their infants and early childhood asthma expression. These studies consider violence exposure at both the family and the community level within a framework that explores the complex mechanisms underlying these associations.

Stress and Asthma Paradigm

The rationale for conducting this work within the asthma and allergy paradigm is briefly outlined here. Most asthma cases begin in early childhood, with half diagnosed by age 3 years and two-thirds by age 5 (Gelfand, 2009). Immune and lung development occur largely in utero and during early childhood (Wright, 2007, 2010). Regulatory pathways that involve the collaboration of innate and adaptive immune responses are involved. The influence of factors outside the immune system (i.e., neurohormonal and autonomic nervous system functioning) is also important. An important step toward identifying children at risk for costly respiratory (i.e., asthma, reduced lung function) and allergic disorders is characterizing important exposures during critical periods of development and the mechanisms that lead to and maintain early predisposition. This developmental framework presupposes that adverse early life experiences, including prenatal exposures, might negatively influence neuroendocrine and immune developmental processes relevant to asthma risk.

At the same time there has been accumulating evidence that psychological stress is an important factor contributing to asthma expression. My group has taken advantage of existing data sets and developed a number of cohort studies in order to examine the influence of a host of psychosocial stressors examined in the perinatal period on childhood asthma expression. In large part, these efforts have been aimed at understanding determinants of asthma disparities that disproportionately impact urban, lower-income, and ethnic minority populations (Gold & Wright, 2005; Wright & Subramanian, 2007). As with any epidemiologic study, the first challenge was to characterize the relevant stressor(s). Important considerations included the prevalence of the stressor(s) of interest in these particular populations. The decision was also theoretically guided through an empirical understanding of how certain stressor characteristics influence behavioral and physiological correlates that might have a particular pathogenic effect. Such correlates can vary based on the condition being considered—in this case, allergic sensitization and asthma. Traumatic stressors, including violence exposure, warrant particular consideration in this context for many reasons, as discussed below (Wright & Bosquet Enlow, 2008).

Low-income women, especially ethnic minorities, report greater and more frequent exposure to negative life events and chronic stress, and greater psychological distress as a result. For example, in a study examining stressors immediately before or during pregnancy among a sample of 143,452 women (Braveman, et al., 2010), stress exposure increased as income decreased, with 57% of low-income women experiencing at least one chronic stressor (e.g., economic hardship [37%], job loss [19%], separation or divorce [15%], incarceration of partner [8%], and domestic violence [5%]); 29% experienced multiple stressors concurrently. The effects of these stress exposures might be compounded among minorities by racism-related stressors (Myers, 2009), which some researchers also conceptualize as a form of violence.

Trauma, like other stress, occurs at increased rates among low-income minority populations (Holman, Silver, & Waitzkin, 2000; Kessler, Sonnega, Bromet, Hughes, & Nelson, 1995). Holman and colleagues (2000) examined the rates of trauma in an ethnically diverse, community-based sample (N = 1,456). Nearly 10% of respondents had experienced a trauma in the past year; 57% reported at least one lifetime event including interpersonal violence occurring outside the family (21%), acute losses or accidents (17%), witnessing death or violence (13%), and/or domestic violence (12%). Hien and Bukszpan (1999) examined lifetime interpersonal violence among a "control" group of urban low-income women, predominantly Latinas or blacks, who had been screened for the absence of psychopathology. Almost 28% of these urban women reported a history of childhood abuse, compared to general population estimates of 10%. Urban minority women also experience heightened levels of community violence (Brown, Hill, et al., 2005; Clark, et al., 2007).

Compared to other forms of stress, trauma is more likely to result in psychological morbidity (e.g., post-traumatic stress disorder [PTSD], depression) and persistent psychophysiological changes (hypothalamic-pituitary-adrenal [HPA] axis, sympathetic-adrenal-medullary [SAM] system). These effects often persist years after the exposure, particularly when the exposure occurs during a critical developmental window (e.g., when stress regulatory systems are becoming consolidated in the mother as well as the next generation) (Aardal-Eriksson, Eriksson, Thorell, 2001; Heim, et al., 2000; King, Mandansky, King, Fletcher, & Brewer, 2001; Yehuda, 2001). For example, a recent study on adults demonstrated that a cumulative measure of child trauma, but not adult trauma, predicted psychiatric symptom complexity in adulthood, highlighting the persistent effects of multiple trauma exposures specifically in childhood on adult functioning (Cloitre, et al., 2009). Moreover, it seems reasonable to focus on more extreme stressors (i.e., traumatic stressors, violence), given that these stressors are more typically associated with blunted HPA (e.g., cortisol) reactivity—a profile more likely related to immune diseases (Eskandari, Webster, & Sternberg, 2003) and respiratory illnesses in children (Beijers, Jansen, Riksen-Walraven, & de Weerth, 2010). Finally, existing studies provide evidence supporting the intergenerational transmission of psychophysiological vulnerability in traumatized populations (Yehuda & Bierer, 2008). That is, the effects of trauma exposure in mothers might have implications for the developing child, even starting in pregnancy.

Critical Periods of Development and Perinatal Programming

Plasticity is a consequence of environmental exposures in critical periods that affect key physiological systems involved in developmental processes (Feinberg, 2007). Although both asthma and lung function are polygenic traits (Holberg, Morgan, Wright, & Martinez, 1998; Kumar & Ghosh, 2009), maternal factors in particular contribute to the intergenerational correlation (Bjerg, et al., 2007; Holberg et al., 1998; Litonjua, Carey, Burge, Weiss, & Gold, 1998). The risk of developing atopic disorders is particularly increased if a positive parental history of atopy is present, with effects being strongest for maternal history (Bjerg et al., 2007; Litonjua et al., 1998). Studies have also shown a greater correlation in forced expiratory volume in one second and other lung function parameters between mothers (compared with fathers) and offspring (Holberg et al., 1998). In addition to heritable traits, this might be due to perinatal programming, the influence of nongenetic or environmental factors during the perinatal period that organize or imprint physiological systems in the child (Wright, 2007). This includes stress responses in the mothers.

Stressors are thought to influence pathogenesis by causing dysregulated biobehavioral states (e.g., depression, PTSD) that in turn exert lasting effects on physiological processes that influence disease risk (Cacioppo, et al., 1998; Cohen & Herbert, 1996; Cohen, Janicki-Deverts, & Miller, 2007). In response to stress, physiological systems might operate at higher or lower levels than in normal homeostasis. The disturbed balance of these systems is most relevant to disease. Immune and neural defensive biological responses important for the short-term response to stress might produce long-term damage if not checked and terminated (McEwen, 2002). The detrimental cost of such accommodation is conceptualized as "allostatic load" (i.e., wear and tear from chronic under- or overactivity). Disturbed regulation of stress systems (e.g., HPA, SAM) in the mother consequent to her own stress history (remote and contemporaneous) might modulate offspring immune function beginning in utero (Arck, Knackstedt, & Blois, 2006; de Weerth & Buitelaar, 2005; Yehuda & Bierer, 2008). Such transgenerational effects might occur through biological mechanisms operating in utero (e.g., epigenetic effects, altered maternal-fetal HPA functioning) (see Chapter 2). Another pathway might be through trauma-elicited effects on maternal psychological functioning that then may influence parenting behaviors (Whitelaw & Whitelaw, 2009; Yehuda & Bierer, 2008). Trauma history might also influence other maternal health behaviors (e.g., cigarette smoking) that have implications for asthma risk in the child. Figure 8.1 summarizes one conceptual model of how violence exposure in both mothers and their infants might influence childhood asthma risk, as well as lung function growth and development.

Programming of the HPA Axis

Prenatal stress has been associated with early and long-term developmental effects resulting in part from altered maternal and/or fetal glucocorticoid (GC) exposure. Maternal and fetal stress stimulate placental secretion of corticotropin-releasing hormone, which in turn might be elevated in neonatal circulation (Goland, et al., 1993; Reinisch, Simon, Karow, & Gandelman, 1978; Seckl, 1997, 2001). This might stimulate the fetal HPA axis to amplify fetal GC excess and activate additional elements of the fetal stress response (i.e., catecholamines) that influence the developing immune and autonomic nervous systems (Arck et al., 2006). Alterations in stress-induced maternal cortisol might influence fetal immune system development and Th2 cell predominance,

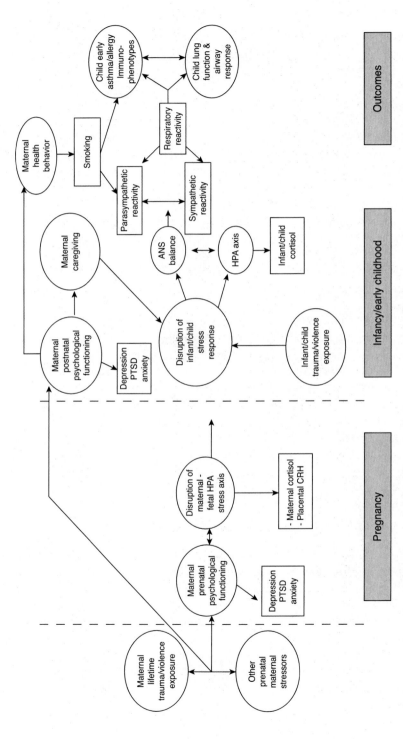

Figure 8.1 Conceptual model for pathways linking violence in mothers and infants to childhood allergic disorders and respiratory outcomes.

perhaps through the direct influence of stress hormones on cytokine production (von Hertzen, 2002; Wonnacott & Bonneau, 2002; Wright, Cohen, & Cohen, 2005). This might induce selective suppression of Th1-mediated cellular immunity and trigger a shift toward Th2-mediated humoral immunity (Elenkov & Chrousos, 1999; Elenkov, Iezzoni, Daly, Harris, & Chrousos, 2005).

The HPA system remains highly reactive and labile in early infancy and starts to become organized when the individual is between 2 and 6 months of age. Sensitive caregiving that is responsive to the signals and needs of the child buffers the reactivity of the HPA axis, programming it to become an effective physiological regulator. Insensitive caregiving, conversely, might promote hyper- or hyporeactive HPA systems (Lyons-Ruth & Block, 1996). Increased stress has been associated with lower levels of parenting sensitivity and higher levels of negative parenting behaviors (e.g., abuse, hostility). These associations are thought to be mediated through stress's negative effects on individuals' psychological resources and mental health. Furthermore, under conditions of extreme stress, the interdependence among parenting experiences, interactive behavior, infant temperament, and developmental outcomes tends to increase (Belsky, 1984). Maternal stress has been associated with poor stress regulation and other negative outcomes in both animal and human offspring (Caldji, Diorio, & Meaney, 2000; Coplan, et al., 1996; Francis, Caldji, Champagne, Plotsky, Meaney, 1999). Studies of human HPA functioning suggest that altered reactivity of the HPA system is associated with early life trauma (Cicchetti & Rogosch, 2001; De Bellis, et al., 1999; Heim et al., 2000; Kaufman, et al., 1997), severe deprivation (Gunnar, Bruce, & Hickman, 2001), and maternal depression (Hessl, Dawson, & Frey, 1998). Other studies directly correlate children's cortisol levels with various maternal social stressors (Essex, Klein, Cho, & Kraemer, 2002; Lupien, King, Meaney, & McEwen, 2000; Schmidt, et al., 1997; Tout, de Haan, Campbell, & Gunnar, 1998).

Programming of Autonomic Reactivity

Several animal models, as well as human studies, support the connection between an adverse intrauterine environment (including cortisol disruption) and experiences in early postnatal life and alterations of autonomic nervous system (ANS) balance (e.g., sympathovagal balance) (Card, Levitt, Gluhovsky, & Rinaman., 2005; Herlenius & Lagercrantz, 2004; Pryce, Ruedi-Bettschen, Dettling, & Feldon, 2002). Experimental rat models have shown that prenatal stress is associated with exaggerated cardiovascular reactivity to restraint stress (Igosheva, Klimova, Anishchenko, & Glover, 2004). In human studies, lower gestational age—a marker of adverse intrauterine conditions, including stress—has been associated with increased blood pressure reactivity in later life (Feldt, et al., 2007; Ward, et al., 2004).

In humans, infants' autonomic responses show developmental changes, with relative stability starting between 6 and 12 months of age (Alkon, et al., 2006). Some have proposed that the fetal ANS is dysregulated by exposure to increased levels of maternal cortisol during pregnancy (Field, Diego, Hernandez-Reif, 2006). In the postnatal period, studies have demonstrated that infants provided with sensitive caregiving show increases in vagal regulation over the first year. Infants of depressed mothers have been found not to show this increase; this is attributed to the insensitive nature of the caregiving characteristic of depressed mothers, which fails to support the development of autonomic regulation (Field & Diego, 2008). Other research links domestic violence exposure and child abuse, as well as other childhood adversities (e.g., foster care), to disrupted ANS functioning in children (Fainsilber Katz, 2007; Oosterman, De Schipper, Fisher, Dozier, & Schuengel, 2010; Rigterink, Fainsilber Katz, & Hessler, 2010; Shenk, Noll, Putnam, & Trickett, 2010). The balance between functional parasympathetic and sympathetic activity in relation to stress, emotional stimuli, and immune function might be important for the expression of allergic sensitization and atopic disorders, as well as early airway obstruction (Bienenstock, Goetzl, & Blennerhassett., 2003; Undem, Kajekar, Hunter, & Myers, 2000; Undem & Weinreich, 2003; Wright et al., 2005).

Violence exposure across the life course has been shown to result in changes in physiology (e.g., autonomic response, HPA axis disruption as indexed by shifts in the circadian rhythm of cortisol) previously linked to inflammatory disease risk in both adult women and children. This includes those exposed to child abuse (Ford, Fraleigh, Albert, & Connor, 2010; Neigh, Gillespie, & Nemeroff, 2009), domestic violence (Rigterink et al., 2010), and violence in the communities in which they live (Suglia, Staudenmayer, Cohen, & Wright, 2010; Kliewer, 2006). Although there are inconsistencies in the literature with regard to the physiological changes (e.g., hormonal disruption) that are associated with various disease outcomes, a blunted HPA axis (more typically characterized by lower morning cortisol levels or flattening of the diurnal slope) has been specifically associated with increased susceptibility to autoimmune/inflammatory diseases (Eskandari et al., 2003; Raison & Miller, 2003). This is also a pattern frequently described in the setting of extreme chronic stress that includes traumatic stressors (even those occurring remotely relative to the timing of study) and cumulative stressors that are chronic or which co-occur (Shimomitsu & Odagiri, 2001; Wright, Rodriguez, & Cohen, 1998). Extreme stressor effects that are more likely to be associated with a blunted prenatal maternal cortisol response might be especially relevant given data from animal models and human studies linking this pattern of HPA axis disruption to increased susceptibility to immune disorders (Eskandari et al., 2003; Raison & Miller, 2003).

Maternal Psychological Functioning

The presence of maternal PTSD and/or depression, a marker for biobehavioral dysregulation in the mother, might contribute to the development of disrupted stress regulatory systems in children starting in utero. PTSD is characterized by dysfunctional patterns of reactivity and regulation of the HPA system and the ANS (Butler, Braff, et al., 1990; Charney, Deutch, Krystal, Southwick, & Davis, 1993; Lipschitz, Rasmusson, & Southwick 1998; Mason, Kosten, Southwick, & Gille, 1990; Orr, Lasko, Shalev, & Pitman, 1995; Paige, Reid, Allen, & Newton, 1990; Perry, Pollard, Blakley, Baker, & Vigilante, 1995; Yehuda, 2001). Maternal trauma exposure, including exposure during pregnancy or in the years prior to pregnancy, and related psychopathology (PTSD, depression) have been associated with altered HPA axis reactivity in offspring that presents as early as the neonatal period. For example, Seng and colleagues found that pregnant women with higher PTSD symptoms had lower peak basal salivary cortisol levels and worse perinatal outcomes (Seng, Low, Ben-Ami, & Liberzon, 2005). Blunted cortisol levels have also been noted among nontraumatized adult offspring of parents with PTSD who survived the Holocaust (Yehuda, et al., 2007). Recently, Yehuda and colleagues found lower cortisol levels in mothers who had developed PTSD during pregnancy in response to the World Trade Center attacks and in the 9-month-old infants of those mothers (Yehuda & Bierer, 2008; Yehuda, et al., 2005), supporting prenatal programming effects. Notably, lower cortisol levels were most apparent in babies born to mothers with PTSD subsequent to trauma exposure in the third trimester. Neonates might mimic their mother's late-pregnancy hormonal patterns, which are disrupted in the presence of psychopathology (Field, et al., 2006; Jolley, Elmore, Barnard, & Carr, 2007; Nierop, Bartsikas, Zimmermann, & Ehler, 2006; Rich-Edwards, et al., 2008). Newborns of depressed mothers also demonstrate low vagal tone at rest and during interactions with their mothers, suggesting ANS dysregulation, as well as characteristics suggestive of dysfunctional neuroregulatory mechanisms (e.g., poorer responsiveness to stimuli, increased crying and inconsolability, and more difficult temperament) (Dawson, et al., 1994; Field, et al., 2004; Field, Hernandez-Reif, Diego, Schanberg, & Kuhn, 2006; Goodman & Gotlib, 1999; Jones, et al., 1998; Monk, Sloan, et al., 2004; Sheridan & Nelson, 2009).

Maternal Psychological Functioning and
Postnatal Caregiving

Self-regulation, fundamental to the ability to form relationships, including the parent–child relationship, is disrupted in both PTSD and depression (Hien, Cohen, & Campbell, 2005). PTSD involves heightened reactivity (e.g., irritability, outbursts of anger) and an inability to modulate reactivity. Regulation difficulties associated with PTSD are likely associated with withdrawn, intrusive, irritable, and unresponsive parenting behaviors (Schechter, 2004). Such behaviors are associated with dysregulation of the HPA axis (Hertsgaard, Gunnar, Larson, Brodersen, & Lehman, 1995) and with disruptions to young children's ability to self-regulate and manage stress (Benoit & Parker, 1994; Carlson, Cicchetti, et al., 1989; Ogawa, Sroufe, Weingield, Carlson, & Egeland, 1997; Schuder & Lyons-Ruth, 2004; True, Pisani, & Oumar, 2001; van Ijzendoorn, Schuengel, & Bakermans-Kranenburg, 1999; Ward & Carlson, 1995). Depression is characterized by sadness, irritability, hostility, and low levels of positive affect (Goodman & Gotlib, 1999; Gotlib & Goodman, 1999). Depressed mothers might engage in a host of parenting behaviors linked to poor child self-regulation, including low amounts and quality of stimulation, slow response to infant cues, and irritable behaviors hypothesized to mediate the link between maternal depression and child difficulties (Goodman & Gotlib, 1999). Because infants of traumatized mothers might exhibit stress regulation difficulties from birth due to the prenatal programming processes, traumatized mothers might face additional challenges in providing sensitive care. Highly reactive infants who receive insensitive care might be at especially high risk (Campos, Frankel, & Camras, 2004; Keenan, Grace, & Gunthorpe, 2003; Robinson & Acevedo, 2001). Insensitive caregiving might impact the postnatal development of stress regulatory systems (Alpern & Lyons-Ruth, 1993; Bogat, DeJonghe, Levendosky, Davidson, & von Eye., 2006; Cicchetti & Cohen, 2006; Dawson et al., 1994).

Testing Components of the Model in Epidemiological Research

Violence Exposure and Maternal Mental Health

We examined associations between lifetime exposure to physical and sexual abuse and prenatal depression in two sociodemographically distinct populations in the Boston area designed in parallel in order to facilitate data merging. The study included 2,128 participants recruited from a large urban and suburban managed care organization (Project Viva) and 1,509 women recruited primarily from prenatal clinics in urban community health centers Asthma Coalition on Community, Environment, and Social Stress (ACCESS) Project. Questionnaires administered in midpregnancy ascertained information on lifetime violence exposure using the Conflicts Tactics Scale (Straus, 1996) and on depressive symptoms ascertained with the Edinburgh Depression Scale, using a cutoff of >13 to indicate probable prenatal depression (Cox, Chapman, Murray, & Jones, 1996). Project Viva consisted largely of white, college-educated, married women >30 years of age who were primarily U.S. born and who reported an annual household income over $70,000; Project ACCESS participants were younger, more likely foreign born, and Latino or black, and the majority lived in households earning less than $20,000 per year. Project ACCESS participants were twice as likely as those in Project Viva to report symptoms consistent with prenatal depression (22% versus 11%), and 57% of women in Project ACCESS and 46% in Project Viva reported lifetime physical and/or sexual abuse. In merged analysis, women reporting lifetime physical or sexual abuse had an odds ratio (OR) for prenatal depression of 1.6 (95% confidence interval [CI] = 1.3–2.1), adjusting for age and race/ethnicity. Lifetime physical (OR = 1.5 [1.2–1.9]) and sexual abuse (OR = 1.7 [1.2–2.3]) independently predicted prenatal depression. When simultaneously considering abuse occurring in different developmental periods in these pregnant women (child/teen, prepregnancy adult, and pregnancy life periods), all were independently predictive of depression: abuse in childhood (OR = 1.2 [1.0–1.6]), prepregnancy adult abuse (OR = 1.7 [1.3–2.2]), and abuse during pregnancy (OR = 1.8 [1.1–2.7]). Adjustment for childhood socioeconomic position did not substantively change observed effects, and there were no clear interactions between abuse and adult socioeconomic position.

In another urban Boston sample of low-income Hispanic and non-Hispanic white women of childbearing age (n = 386), we examined the prevalence and psychological correlates of witnessing community violence on psychological functioning using the Brief Symptom Inventory to assess anxiety and depressive symptoms. Community violence exposure was ascertained with a multi-item survey assessing the witnessing of violence (hearing gunshots; shoving, kicking, or punching fights; knife attacks; and shootings) in self-defined neighborhoods in the past 12 months (recent) and more than 12 months prior to the survey (remote exposure). In analysis adjusted for marital status, educational attainment, and intimate partner violence, we found that women who witnessed violence in their neighborhoods were twice as likely to experience depressive and anxiety symptoms as those who did not report community violence exposure (Clark et al., 2007). Witnessing community violence was associated with increased anxiety or depressive symptoms after adjusting for domestic violence exposure, even among women who were not victims of or participants in neighborhood conflicts. Sixty-six percent of women witnessed at least one violent event: 52% witnessed a fight, 46% heard gunshots in their neighborhood, 10% witnessed knife attacks, and 8% witnessed a shooting in their lifetime. The majority of participants had witnessed violence in their communities more than a year prior to interview (57%), whereas 19% had witnessed events in the preceding 12 months.

Violence Exposure and Maternal Prenatal Physiology

We explored the effects of multiple social stressors on HPA axis functioning in black (n = 68) and Hispanic (n = 132) pregnant women enrolled in the ACCESS study. In mid-pregnancy, these women completed the Revised Conflict Tactics Scale to assess interpersonal violence, the Experiences of Discrimination survey, the Crisis in Family Systems-Revised negative life events survey, and the My Exposure to Violence survey to assess community violence exposure (Suglia, et al., 2010a). Salivary cortisol samples were collected five times per day over three days to enable assessment of area under the curve (AUC), morning change, and basal awakening response in order to characterize diurnal salivary cortisol patterns. Repeated measures mixed models (stratified by race/ethnicity) were performed, adjusting for education level, age, smoking status, body mass index, and weeks pregnant at the time of cortisol sampling. The majority of Hispanic participants (57%) had low cumulative stress exposure, whereas the majority of black participants had intermediate (35%) or high (41%) cumulative stress exposure. Results showed that among black but not Hispanic women, cumulative stress was associated with lower morning cortisol levels, including a flatter waking-to-bedtime rhythm (data shown for black women in Fig. 8.2). These analyses suggest that cumulative stressful experiences are associated with disrupted HPA functioning among these pregnant women, with most of the variance explained by the violence exposures.

Maternal Lifetime Violence Exposure and Infant Immune Function

Immune development and the predisposition to atopy begin during gestation, as noted previously. Research continues to delineate early immunophenotypes

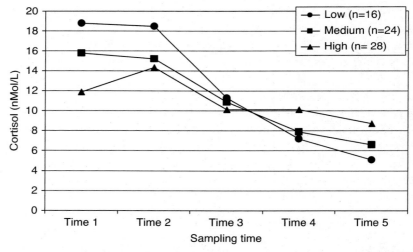

Figure 8.2 Diurnal maternal cortisol by cumulative stress (low, medium, and high) in black women enrolled in Project ACCESS. (Reproduced with the publisher's permission from Suglia et al., [2010]. Cumulative stress and cortisol disruption among Black and Hispanic pregnant women in an urban cohort.*Psychological Trauma* 2(4), 326–334.)

and early airway response outcomes among children predisposed to chronic atopic disorders (Hahn & Bacharier, 2005; Heaton, et al., 2005; Saglani & Bush, 2007; Williams & Flohr, 2006). Mechanisms of inflammation central to the pathophysiology of atopic disorders overlap and include immune-mediated inflammation associated with a Th2-biased response (Mossman & Coffman, 1989; Mossman & Sad, 1996; Robinson, et al., 1992) and a tendency to produce immunoglobulin E (IgE) in response to environmental stimuli (e.g., allergens). These mechanisms have their roots in utero (Devereux, Barker, & Seaton, 2002; Devereux, Seaton, & Barker, 2001; Liao, et al., 1996; Miles, et al., 1996; Peden, 2000; Prescott, et al., 1998). Those with early sensitization to allergens (i.e., start-ing in the first two to three years of life) are at greatest risk of developing chronic atopic disorders, airway inflammation, and obstruction (Halken, 2003; Illi, et al., 2001; Johnke, Norberg, Vach, Host, & Andersen, 2006; Martinez, et al., 1995; Panettieri, Covar, Grant, Hillyer, & Bacharier, 2008). Consequently, researchers have begun to examine in vitro responses of peripheral blood mononuclear cells to allergens or mitogens in order to gain a better understanding of the immunodeviations that facilitate the manifestation of atopy in response to envi-ronmental factors including stress (Chen, Fisher, Bacharier, & Strunk, 2003; Wright, Finn, et al., 2004). Elevated cord blood total IgE is associated with aeroal-lergen sensitization and the development of allergic diseases in children, par-ticularly in those with a maternal history of atopy (Halken, 2003; Odelram, Bjorksten, Leander, & Kjellman, 1995; Tariq, Arshad, Matthews, & Hakim, 1999).

Although studies of maternal stress and infant outcomes typically examine events occurring during the index pregnancy, we examined the relationship between maternal interpersonal trauma (IPT) experienced over the mother's life course and cord blood total IgE, a biomarker of atopic risk at birth, in Project ACCESS (Sternthal, et al., 2009). We hypothesized that maternal IPT might be linked to infant health through more latent effects (i.e., lasting effects from abuse in childhood/adolescence), proximate effects (i.e., trauma experienced in or around the pregnancy), and cumulative life-course effects (i.e., allostatic load of cumulated traumas over the mother's life). Maternal IPT was categorized as unexposed (n = 285), early (childhood and/or teenage years only, n = 107), late (adulthood and/or index pregnancy only, n = 29), or chronic (early and late, n = 57) exposure. Relative to no IPT, early (OR = 1.8, 95% CI = 1.1–3.0) and chronic (OR = 2.3, 95% CI = 1.2–4.2) maternal IPT were independently associated with increased cord blood IgE levels in unadjusted models. When adjusting for maternal age and race, season of birth, child's gender, and the mother's childhood and current SES, early effects became nonsignificant (OR = 1.5, 95% CI = 0.85–2.6). Chronic IPT remained sig-nificant when adjusting for these standard control variables in addition to other current negative life events, allergen exposure in the home, and potential pathway variables (maternal atopy, prenatal smoking, and birth weight) (OR = 2.2, 95% CI 1.1–4.5). Figure 8.3 shows how the predicted probability of the infant's having an

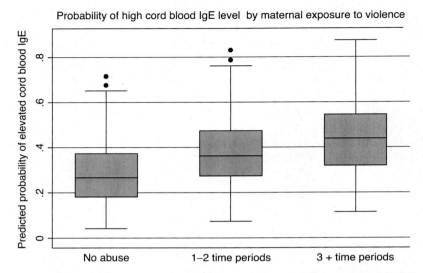

Figure 8.3 Maternal lifetime exposure to interpersonal trauma/violence and the probability of elevated cord blood IgE in her offspring.

elevated cord blood IgE level (upper quartile, 1.08 IU/ml) is associated with an increasing number of life periods in which mothers reported experiencing IPT. These data demonstrate that infants born to mothers with chronic trauma exposure—that is, exposure both early in life and more proximate to the pregnancy—were at the greatest risk of expressing elevated IgE.

Maternal Diurnal Cortisol in Pregnancy and Wheeze Risk in Urban Children

Disruption of the HPA axis might link prenatal maternal stress to childhood chronic diseases, including asthma. Maternal obesity prior to pregnancy has also been associated with increased childhood wheeze risk, although the mechanisms for this are unclear. Associations between obesity and disrupted HPA functioning have been shown in nonpregnant samples (Kumari, Chandola, Brunner, & Kivimaki, 2010; Larsson, Gullberg, Rastam, & Linblad, 2009). We examined associations between prenatal maternal cortisol, maternal obesity, and repeated wheeze at age 2 years in Project ACCESS (n = 261) (Wright, Fisher, Chiu, Cohen, & Coull, 2011). Maternal salivary cortisol was collected five times per day over three days at mean gestational age of 29.0 ± 4.9 weeks in order to characterize diurnal cortisol patterns (timed from awakening), specifically, the cortisol awakening response (CAR) and slope in diurnal secretion. Within-subject cortisol levels were log transformed and averaged across days. Maternal prepregnancy body mass index (BMI) was categorized as obese (BMI > 30 kg/m²) or nonobese

(BMI < 30 kg/m^2). Using logistic regression, we examined whether cortisol metrics (levels at each time point, CAR, diurnal slope) fit in separate models predicted repeated wheeze after adjusting for maternal age, atopy (ever experienced allergy/asthma/eczema), race/ethnicity, education, smoking, obesity, weeks pregnant at cortisol sampling, and child's gender and birthweight for gestational age. Linear mixed models including splines with knots at 30 minutes and at four hours after awakening were performed in order to examine associations between wheezing status and maternal cortisol trajectories by interacting wheezing status with each slope term (slope over first 30 minutes, slope from four hours to bedtime). The majority of mothers were minority (56.5% Hispanic, 24.1% African American); 61% had ≤12 years of education, and 36% had atopy. Repeated wheeze was found in 8.4% of children. An interquartile range increase in log mean cortisol at bedtime (OR = 2.2, 95% CI = 1.2–4.1) and maternal obesity (OR = 2.6, 95% CI = 0.99–6.6) were associated with increased wheeze; a higher CAR was associated with a lower risk of wheeze (OR = 0.7, 95% CI = 0.5–0.98). Linear mixed models revealed an association between a flatter afternoon slope (4 h to bedtime) and repeated wheeze in children of obese mothers (afternoon slope in children with [–0.017] and without [–0.061] repeated wheeze [p = 0.009]), but not in children of nonobese mothers (afternoon slope in children with [–0.050] and without [–0.061] repeated wheeze [p = 0.51]). Disrupted prenatal maternal cortisol rhythms might play a role in programming early childhood wheeze risk. Notably, this pattern of cortisol disruption has been associated with prior trauma history.

Postnatal Caregiving Environment

Postnatally, nonoptimal early childhood environments and caregiving experiences (e.g., maternal psychopathology, insensitivity) might impact the child's emotion regulation development and stress reactivity (Anisman, Zaharia, Meaney, & Merali, 1998; Liu, et al., 1997; Vallee, et al., 1997). Chronic lifetime and more contemporaneous postnatal stress and maternal psychological functioning might negatively influence caregiving quality. Our group and others have shown associations between early caregiver stress and the development of asthmatic phenotypes in early childhood (Mrazek, Klinnert, et al., 1999; Wright, Cohen, Carey, Weiss, & Gold, 2002). We recently demonstrated that maternal ability to maintain positive caregiving processes in the context of even more extreme stress might buffer the effects on child asthma risk. We examined the prospective relationship between maternal intimate partner violence (IPV) and asthma onset in children in the Fragile Families and Child Wellbeing Study (N = 3,117), which is a prospective birth cohort. Maternal report of IPV was assessed after the child's birth and again at 12 and 36 months. Mothers also indicated how many days a week they participated in activities with the child and the amount and type of educational or recreational toys available for the child. Maternal report of physician-diagnosed asthma by age 36 months was the outcome. In adjusted analysis, children of mothers experiencing IPV chronically (at all time periods), compared to those never exposed, had a twofold-increased risk of developing asthma. In stratified analysis, children of mothers experiencing IPV and low levels of mother–child activities (Relative Risk [RR] = 2.7, 95% CI = 1.6–4.7) had a significantly increased risk for asthma. Those exposed to IPV and high levels of mother–child activities had a lower risk for asthma (RR = 1.6, 95% CI = 0.9–3.2).

Community Violence Exposure and Disrupted Physiology in Children

Although community violence has been linked to psychological morbidity in urban youth, data on the physiological correlates of violence and associated post-traumatic stress symptoms are sparse. We examined the influence of child post-traumatic stress symptoms reported in relation to community violence exposure on diurnal salivary cortisol response in a population-based sample of 28 girls and 15 boys ages 7 to 13; 54% self-identified as white, and 46% (Suglia, Staudenmayer, Cohen, & Wright, 2010) as Hispanic. Mothers reported on children's exposure to community violence using the Survey of Children's Exposure to Community Violence and completed the Checklist of Children's Distress Symptoms (CCDS), which captures factors related to post-traumatic stress; children who were 8 years of age or older reported on their own community violence exposure. Saliva samples were obtained from the children four times a day (after awakening, at lunchtime, at dinnertime, and at bedtime) over three days. Mixed models were used to assess the influence of post-traumatic stress symptoms on cortisol expression, examined as diurnal slope and AUC, calculated across the day, adjusting for sociodemographics. In adjusted analyses, higher scores on total traumatic stress symptoms (CCDS) were associated with both greater cortisol AUC and a flatter cortisol waking-to-bedtime rhythm (Fig. 8.4). The associations were primarily attributable to differences on the intrusion, arousal, and avoidance CCDS subscales (Suglia, et al., 2010b). Post-traumatic stress symptomatology reported in response to community violence exposure was associated with diurnal cortisol disruption in these community-dwelling urban children. These findings are strikingly similar to diurnal salivary cortisol patterns reported by Carrion and colleagues (Carrion, et al., 2002) of children in a pediatric clinical sample who met criteria for a diagnosis of PTSD; in that study, a parallel home salivary cortisol collection protocol was used.

Community Violence and Asthma

Indicators of neighborhood disadvantage, characterized by the presence of a number of area-level stressors—including poverty, unemployment/underemployment, a high percentage of unskilled laborers, limited social capital or social

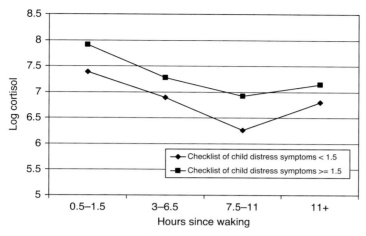

Figure 8.4 Cortisol level (nmol/L) by severity of symptoms on the Checklist of Child Distress Symptoms (low < 1.5 and high ≥ 1.5) and time of collection relative to time of awakening. (Reproduced with the publisher's permission from Suglia et al., [2010]. Posttraumatic stress symptoms related to community violence and children's diurnal cortisol response in an urban community-dwelling sample. *International Journal Behavioral Medicine* 17, 43–50.)

cohesion, substandard housing, and high crime/violence exposure rates—have been investigated in relation to urban children's development (Wright & Subramanian, 2007). Most relevant to this discussion, accumulating evidence suggests that community violence might contribute to the burden of asthma in urban populations (Wright, 2006). Increased exposure is associated with more symptom days (Swahn & Bossarte, 2006), higher hospitalization rates (Wright, Mitchell, et al., 2004), increased asthma prevalence among children living in communities with both elevated crime/violence and other environmental hazards (i.e., ambient air pollutants) (Clougherty et al., 2007), and increased risk of wheezing at ages 2–3 (Berz et al., 2007). Using data from a longitudinal, multi-level study including 2,071 children ages 0 to 9 at enrollment from the Project on Human Development in Chicago Neighborhoods, my group demonstrated a significant association between community violence exposure and increased risk for asthma development in urban children (Sternthal, Jun, Earls, & Wright, 2010). Multilevel logistic regression models estimated the likelihood of asthma, controlling for individual-level (child's age, gender, and race/ethnicity; maternal asthma; SES; and family violence in the home) and neighborhood-level (concentrated disadvantage, collective efficacy, and social disorder) confounders. This association was robust to controlling for these important individual and neighborhood-level confounders as well as pathway variables (maternal smoking, breastfeeding). In adjusted analysis, medium (OR = 1.6, 95% CI = 1.2–2.2) and high (OR = 1.6, 95% CI = 1.1–2.2) levels of community violence were associated with increased asthma risk relative to low levels.

Stress-Enhancing Effects on Physical Environmental Exposures

Because of the covariance across exposures and evidence that social stress and other environmental toxins (e.g., pollutants, tobacco smoke) might influence common physiological pathways (e.g., oxidative stress, proinflammatory immune pathways, autonomic disruption), an understanding of the potential synergistic effects promises to more completely inform assessments of children's asthma risk (Wright, 2009). Epidemiological studies have demonstrated synergistic effects of stress and air pollution on asthma expression among children and adolescents (Chen, Schreier, STrunk, & Brauer, 2008; Shankardass, et al., 2009). My group examined the synergistic effects of growing up in a community with higher levels of traffic-related air pollution and community violence on childhood asthma risk in an urban Boston birth cohort study (Clougherty, et al., 2007). We developed models to estimate traffic-related pollution (nitrogen dioxide) for 413 children and ascertained lifetime community violence exposure based on parental report. In analyses adjusted for maternal education, race/ethnicity, maternal history of allergy, child's gender, and tobacco smoke exposure, we found an elevated risk of asthma for those in high-pollution areas only among children who also lived in communities with above-median exposure to violence levels (OR = 1.6, 95% CI = 1.1–2.3).

Summary

Taken together, these data support a link between violence exposure and childhood asthma expression. While the research summarized herein addresses specific components of the conceptual model depicted in figure 8-1, future studies should take a more integrated approach that tests the pathways more comprehensively. This will require larger samples. The likelihood of multiple mechanistic pathways with complex interdependencies must be considered when examining the independent influence of traumatic stress, as well as the interaction of violence and physical environmental toxins, on asthma and allergy. Because social adversity (e.g., violence) and physical environmental hazards tend to cluster in the most socially disadvantaged, this line of research might better inform the etiology of growing health disparities. The design of future epidemiologic studies and effective intervention programs will need to address social stressors including violence and physical environmental toxins jointly in order to more effectively impact outcomes on a public health scale.

Disclosure Statement

During the preparation of this manuscript, the author was supported by Grant Nos. R01 HL080674-06, R01 HL095606-01, and R01 MD006086-01.

References

Aardal-Eriksson, E., Eriksson, T., & Thorell, L. H. (2001). Salivary cortisol, posttraumatic stress symptoms, and general health in the acute phase and during 9-month follow-up. *Biological Psychiatry, 50*, 986–993.

Alkon, A., Lippert, S., Vujan, N., Rodriguez, M. E., Boyce, W. T., & Eskenazi, B. (2006). The ontogeny of autonomic measures in 6- and 12-month-old infants. *Developmental Psychobiology, 48*(3), 197–208.

Alpern, L., & Lyons-Ruth, K. (1993). Preschool children at social risk: Chronicity and timing of maternal depressive symptoms and child behavior at school and at home. *Development and Psychopathology, 5*, 371–387.

Anisman, H., Zaharia, M. D., Meaney, M. J., & Merali, Z. (1998). Do early-life events permanently alter behavioral and hormonal responses to stressors? *International Journal of Developmental Neuroscience, 16*(3–4), 149–164.

Arck, P. C., Knackstedt, M. K., & Blois, S. M. (2006). Current insights and future perspectives on neuro-endocrine-immune circuitry challenging pregnancy maintenance and fetal health. *Journal Reproduktionsmed Endokrinol, 3*(2), 98–102.

Arnow, B. A. (2004). Relationships between childhood maltreatment, adult health and psychiatric outcomes and medical utilization. *Journal of Clinical Psychiatry, 65*(Suppl 12), 10–15.

Beijers, R., Jansen, J., Riksen-Walraven, M., & de Weerth, C. (2010). Maternal prenatal anxiety and stress predict infant illnesses and health complaints. *Pediatrics, 126*, e401–e409.

Belsky, J. (1984). The determinants of parenting: A process model. *Child Development, 55*, 83–96.

Benoit, D., & Parker, K. C. H. (1994). Stability and transmission of attachment across 3 generations. *Child Development, 65*, 1444–1456.

Berz, J. B., Carter, A. S., Wagmiller, R. L., Horwitz, S. M., Murdock, K. K., & Briggs-Gowan, M. (2007). Prevalence and correlates of early onset asthma and wheezing in a healthy birth cohort of 2- to 3-year olds. *Journal of Pediatric Psychology, 32*(2), 154–166.

Bienenstock, J., Goetzl, E. J., & Blennerhassett, M.G. (Eds.). (2003). *The autonomic nervous system, Volume 15: Autonomic neuroimmunology.* New York: Taylor & Francis.

Bjerg, A., Hedman, L., Perzanowski, M. S., Platts-Mills, T., Lundback, B., & Ronmark, R. (2007). Family history of asthma and atopy: In-depth analyses of the impact on asthma and wheeze in 7- to 8-year-old children. *Pediatrics, 120*(4), 741–748.

Bogat, G. A., DeJonghe, E., Levendosky, A. A., Davidson, W.S., & von Eye, A. (2006). Trauma symptoms among infants exposed to intimate partner violence. *Child Abuse & Neglect, 30*, 109–125.

Bogat, G. A., Leahy, K., von Eye, A., Maxwell, C., Levendosky, A. A., & Davidson, W. W. (2005). The influence of community violence on the functioning of women experiencing domestic violence. *American Journal of Community Psychology, 36*, 123–132.

Boynton-Jarrett, R., Rich-Edwards, J. W., Jun, H. J., Hibert, E. N., & Wright, R. J. (2011). Abuse in childhood and risk of uterine leiomyoma: The role of emotional support in biologic resilience. *Epidemiology, 22,* 6–14.

Bradshaw, C. P., & Garbarino, J. (2004). Social cognition as a mediator of the influence of family and community violence on adolescent development. *Annals of the New York Academy of Sciences, 1036,* 85–105.

Braveman, P., & Barclay, C. (2009). Health disparities beginning in childhood: A life-course perspective. *Pediatrics, 124,* S163–S175.

Braveman, P., Marchi, K., Egerter, S., Kim, S., Metzler, M., Stancil, T., et al. (2010). Poverty, near-poverty, and hardship around the time of pregnancy. *Maternal and Child Health Journal, 14,* 20–35.

Bremner, J. D. (2003). Long-term effects of childhood abuse on brain and neurobiology. *Child & Adolescent Psychiatric Clinics of North America, 12,* 271–292.

Briggs-Gowan, M. J., Ford, J. D., Fraleigh, L., McCarthy, K, & Carter, A. S. (2010). Prevalence of exposure to potentially traumatic events in a healthy birth cohort of very young children in the northeastern United States. *Journal of Traumatic Stress, 23,* 725–733.

Brown, J. R., Hill, H. M., et al. (2005). Traumatic stress symptoms in women exposed to community and partner violence. *Journal of Interpersonal Violence, 20,* 1478–1494.

Butler, R., Braff, D., et al. (1990). Physiological evidence of exaggerated startle response in a subgroup of Vietnam veterans with combat-related PTSD. *American Journal of Psychiatry, 147,* 1308–1312.

Cacioppo, J. T., Berntson, C. G., Malarkey, W. B., Kiecolt-Glaser, J. K., Sheridan, J. F., Poehlmann, K. M., et al. (1998). Autonomic, neuroendocrine, and immune responses to psychological stress: The reactivity hypothesis. *Annals of the New York Academy of Sciences, 840,* 664–673.

Caldji, C., Diorio, J., & Meaney, M. J. (2000). Variations in maternal care in infancy regulate the development of stress reactivity. *Biological Psychiatry, 48,* 1164–1174.

Campos, J. J., Frankel, C. B., Camras L. (2004). On the nature of emotion regulation. *Child Development, 75,* 377–394.

Card, J. P., Levitt, P, Gluhovsky, M., & Rinaman, L. (2005). Early experience modifies the postnatal assembly of autonomic emotional motor circuits in rats. *Journal of Neuroscience, 25*(40), 9102–9111.

Carlson, V., Cicchetti, D., et al. (1989). Finding order in disorganization: Lessons from research on maltreated infants' attachments to their caregivers. In D. Cicchetti and V. Carlson (Eds.), *Child maltreatment: Theory and research on the causes and consequences of child abuse and neglect* (pp. 494–528). New York: Cambridge University Press.

Carrion, V. G., Weems, C. F., Ray, R. D., Glaser, B., Hessl, D., & Reiss, A. L. (2002). Diurnal salivary cortisol in pediatric posttraumatic stress disorder. *Biological Psychiatry, 51,* 575–582.

Charney, D. S., Deutch, A. Y., Krystal, J. H., Southwick, S. M., & Davis, M. (1993). Psychobiologic mechanisms of posttraumatic stress disorder. *Archives of General Psychiatry, 50*(4), 295–305.

Chen, E., Fisher, E. B., Bacharier, L. B., & Strunk, R. C. (2003). Socioeconomic status, stress, and immune markers in adolescents with asthma. *Psychosomatic Medicine, 65*(6), 984–992.

Chen, E., Schreier, H. M., Strunk, R. C., & Brauer, M. (2008). Chronic traffic-related air pollution and stress interact to predict biologic and clinical outcomes in asthma. *Environmental Health Perspectives, 116,* 970–975.

Cichetti, D., & Cohen, D. J. (2006). Perspectives on developmental psychopathology. In D. Cicchetti and D. J. Cohen (Eds.), *Developmental psychopathology: Volume 1: Theory and methods* (pp. 3–20). New York: John Wiley & Sons.

Cicchetti, D., & Rogosch, F. A. (2001). Diverse patterns of neuroendocrine activity in maltreated children. *Development and Psychopathology, 13,* 677–693.

Clark, C., Ryan, L., Kawachi, I., Canner M. J., Berkman, L., & Wright, R. J., (2007). Witnessing community violence in residential neighborhoods: A mental health hazard for urban women. *Journal of Urban Health, 85*(1), 22–38.

Cloitre, M., Stolbach, B. C., Herman, J. L., van der Kolk, B., Pynoos, R., Wang, J., et al. (2009). A developmental approach to Complex PTSD: Childhood and adult cumulative trauma as predictors of symptom complexity. *Journal of Traumatic Stress, 22,* 399–408.

Clougherty, J., Levy, J. I., Kubzansky, L. D., Ryan, P. B., Suglia, S. F., Canner, M. J., et al. (2007). Synergistic effects of traffic-related air pollution and exposure to violence on urban asthma etiology. *Environmental Health Perspectives, 115*(8), 1140–1146.

Cohen, S., & Herbert, T. (1996). Health psychology: Psychological factors and physical disease from the perspective of human psychoneuroimmunology. *Annual Review of Psychology, 47,* 113–142.

Cohen, S., Janicki-Deverts, D., & Miller, G. E. (2007). Psychological stress and disease. *Journal of the American Medical Association, 298*(14), 1685–1687.

Cooley-Quille, M., Boyd, R. C., Frantz, E., & Walsh, J. (2001). Emotional and behavioral impact of exposure to community violence in inner-city adolescents. *Journal of Clinical Child Psychology, 30,* 199–206.

Coplan, J., Andrews, M. W., Rosenblum, L. A., Owens, M. J., Friedman, S., Gorman, J. M., et al. (1996). Persistent elevations of cerebrospinal fluid concentrations of corti-cotropin-releasing factor in adult nonhuman primates exposed to early-life stressors: Implications for the pathophysiology of mood and anxiety disorders. *Proceedings of the National Academy of Sciences, 93,* 1619–1623.

Cox, J. L., Chapman, G., Murray, D., & Jones, P. (1996). Validation of the Edinburgh Postnatal Depression Scale (EPDS) in non-postnatal women. *Journal of Affective Disorders, 39*(3), 185–189.

Cummings, E. M., El-Sheikh, M., Kouros, C. D., & Buckhalt, J. A. (2009). Children and violence: The role of children's regulation in the marital aggression-child adjustment link. *Clinical Child and Family Psychological Review, 12,* 3–15.

Cummings, E. M., Goeke-Morey, M. C., Schermerhorn, A. C., Merrilees, C. E., & Cairns, E. (2009). Children and political violence from a social ecological perspective: Implications from research on children and families in Northern Ireland. *Clinical Child and Family Psychological Review, 12,* 16–38.

Dawson, G., Hessl, D., & Frey, K. (1994). Social influences on early developing biological and behavioral systems related to risk for affective disorder. *Development and Psychopathology, 6,* 759–779.

De Bellis, M. D., Baum, A. S., Birmaher, B., Keshavan, M. S., Eccard, C. H., Boring, A. M., et al. (1999). Developmental traumatology, Part 1: Biological stress systems. *Biological Psychiatry, 9,* 1259–1270.

Devereux, G., Barker, R. N., & Seaton, A. (2002). Antenatal determinants of neonatal immune responses to allergens. *Clinical and Experimental Allergy, 32*(1), 43–50.

Devereux, G., Seaton, A., & Barker, R. N. (2001). In utero priming of allergen-specific helper T cells. *Clinical and Experimental Allergy, 31*(11), 1686–1695.

de Weerth, C., & Buitelaar, J. K. (2005). Physiological stress reactivity in human pregnancy—A review. *Neuroscience & Biobehavioral Reviews, 29,* 295–312.

Elenkov, I. J., & Chrousos, G. P. (1999). Stress hormones, Th1/Th2 patterns, pro/anti-inflammatory cytokines and susceptibility to disease. *Trends in Endocrinology & Metabolism, 10*(9), 359–368.

Elenkov, I. J., Iezzoni, D. G., Daly, A., Harris, A. G., & Chrousos, G. P. (2005). Cytokine dysregulation, inflammation and well-being. *Neuroimmunomodulation, 12,* 255–269.

Eskandari, F., Webster, J. I., & Sternberg, E. M. (2003). Neural immune pathways and their connection to inflammatory diseases. *Arthritis Research & Therapy, 5,* 251–265.

Essex, M. J., Klein, M. H., Cho, E., & Kraemer, H. C. (2002). Maternal stress beginning in infancy may sensitize children to later stress exposure: Effects on cortisol and behavior. *Biological Psychiatry, 52*(8), 776–784.

Fainsilber Katz, L. (2007). Domestic violence and vagal reactivity to peer provocation. *Biological Psychology, 74,* 154–164.

Fairbank, J. A., & Fairbank, D. W. (2009). Epidemiology of child traumatic stress. *Current Psychiatry Reports, 11,* 289–295.

Feinberg, A. P. (2007). Phenotypic plasticity and the epigenetics of human disease. *Nature, 447*(7143), 433–440.

Feldt, K., Raikkonen, K., Eriksson, J. G., Andersson, S., Osmond, C., Barker, D.J., et al. (2007). Cardiovascular reactivity to psychological stressors in late adulthood is predicted by gestational age at birth. *Journal of Human Hypertension, 21*(5), 401–410.

Felitti, V. J. (2009). Adverse childhood experiences and adult health. *Academic Pediatrics, 9,* 131–132.

Field, T., & Diego, M. (2008). Vagal activity, early growth and emotional development. *Infant Behavior and Development, 31,* 361–373.

Field, T., Diego, M., Hernandez-Reif, M., Vera, Y., Gil, K., Schanberg, S., Kuhn, C., et al. (2004). Prenatal maternal biochemistry predicts neonatal biochemistry. *International Journal of Neuroscience, 114*(8), 933–945.

Field, T., Diego, M., & Hernandez-Reif, M. (2006). Prenatal depression effects on the fetus and newborn: A review. *Infant Behavior and Development, 29,* 445–455.

Field, T., Hernandez-Reif, M., Diego, M., Schanberg, S., & Kuhn, C. (2006). Stability of mood states and biochemistry across pregnancy. *Infant Behavior and Development, 29,* 262–267.

Ford, J. D., Fraleigh, L. A., Albert D.B., & Connor, D.F. (2010). Child abuse and autonomic nervous system hyporesponsivity among psychiatrically impaired children. *Child Abuse and Neglect, 34,* 507–515.

Francis, D. D., Caldji, C., Champagne, F., Plotsky, P. M., & Meaney, M. J. (1999). The role of corticotropin-releasing factor-norepinephrine systems in mediating the effects of early experience on the development of behavioral and endocrine responses to stress. *Biological Psychiatry, 46*(9), 1153–1166.

Gelfand, E. W. (2009). Pediatric asthma: A different disease. *Proceedings of the American Thoracic Society, 6,* 278–282.

Goland, R. S., Jozak, S., Warren, W. B., Conwell, I. M., Stark, R. I., & Tropper, P. J. (1993). Elevated levels of umbilical cord plasma corticotropin-releasing hormone in growth-related fetuses. *Journal of Clinical Endocrinology and Metabolism, 77,* 1174–1179.

Gold, D. R., & Wright, R. (2005). Population disparities in asthma. *Annual Review of Public Health, 26,* 89–113.

Goodman, S. H., & Gotlib, I. H. (1999). Risk for psychopathology in the children of depressed mothers: A developmental model for understanding mechanisms of transmission. *Psychological Review, 106,* 458–490.

Gotlib, I. H., & Goodman, S. H. (1999). Children of parents with depression. In W. K. Silverman and T. H. Ollendick (Eds.), *Developmental issues in the clinical treatment of children and adolescents* (pp. 415–432). Needham Heights, MA: Allyn & Bacon.

Gunnar, M. R., Bruce, J., Hickman, S.E. (2001). Salivary cortisol response to stress in children. *Advances in Psychosomatic Medicine, 22*, 52–60.

Hahn, E. L., & Bacharier, L. B. (2005). The atopic march: The pattern of allergic disease development in childhood. *Immunology & Allergy Clinics of North America, 25*(2), 231–246.

Halken, S. (2003). Early sensitisation and development of allergic airway disease—Risk factors and predictors. *Paediatric Respiratory Reviews, 4*(2), 128–134.

Heaton, T., Rowe, J., Turner, S., Aalberse, R. C., de Klerk, N., Surivaarachchi, D., et al. (2005). An immunoepidemiological approach to asthma: Identification of in-vitro T-cell response patterns associated with different wheezing phenotypes in children. *Lancet, 365*, 142–149.

Heim, C., Newport, D. J., Heit, S., Graham, Y. P., Wilcox, M., Bonsall, R., et al. (2000). Pituitary-adrenal and autonomic responses to stress in women after sexual and physical abuse in childhood. *Journal of the American Medical Association, 284*, 592–597.

Henning, K., Leitenberg, H., Coffey, P., Bennett, T., & Jankowski, M. K. (1997). Long-term psychological adjustment to witnessing interparental physical conflict during childhood. *Child Abuse and Neglect, 21*(6), 501–515.

Herlenius, E., & Lagercrantz, H. (2004). Development of neurotransmitter systems during critical periods. *Experimental Neurology, 190*(Suppl. 1), S8–S21.

Hertsgaard, L., Gunnar, M. R., Larson, M., Brodersen, L., & Lehman, H. (1995). Adrenocortical responses to the strange situation in infants with disorganized/disoriented attachment relationships. *Child Development, 66*, 1100–1106.

Hessl, D., Dawson, G., Frey, K., Panagiotides, H., Self, J., Yamada, E., et al. (1998). A longitudinal study of children of depressed mothers: Psychobiological findings related to stress. In D. M. Hann, L. C. Huffman, K. K. Lederhendler, & D. Minecke (Eds.), *Advancing research on developmental plasticity: Integrating the behavioral sciences and the neurosciences of mental health* (p. 256). Bethesda, MD: National Institutes of Mental Health.

Hien, D., & Bukszpan, C. (1999). Interpersonal violence in a "normal" low-income control group. *Women Health, 29*(4), 1–16.

Hien, D., Cohen, L., Campbell, A. (2005). Is traumatic stress a vulnerability factor for women with substance use disorders? *Clinical Psychology Review, 25*(6), 813–823.

Holberg, C. J., Morgan, W. J., Wright, A. L., & Martinez, F. D. (1998). Differences in familial segregation of FEV1 between asthmatic and nonasthmatic families: Role of maternal component. *American Journal of Respiratory and Critical Care Medicine, 158*, 162–169.

Holman, E. A., Silver, R. C., & Waitzkin, H. (2000). Traumatic life events in primary care patients: A sutdy in an ethnically diverse sample. *Archive of Family Medicine, 9*(9), 802–810.

Holt, S., Buckley, H., & Whelan, S. (2008). The impact of exposure to domestic violence on children and young people: A review of the literature. *Child Abuse and Neglect, 32*, 797–810.

Igosheva, N., Klimova, O., Anischenko, T., & Glover, V. (2004). Prenatal stress alters cardiovascular responses in adult rats. *Journal of Physiology, 557*(Pt 1), 273–285.

Illi, S., von Mutius, E., Lau, S., Nickel, R., Niggemann, B., Sommerfeld, C., et al. (2001). The pattern of atopic sensitization is associated with the development of asthma in childhood. *Journal of Allergy and Clinical Immunology, 108*(5), 709–714.

Johnke, H., Norberg, L. A., Vach, W., Host, A., & Andersen, K. E. (2006). Patterns of sensitization in infants and its relation to atopic dermatitis. *Pediatric Allergy & Immunology, 17*, 591–600.

Jolley, S. N., Elmore, S., Barnard, K. E., & Carr, D. B. (2007). Dysregulation of the hypo-thalamic-pituitary-adrenal axis in postpartum depression. *Biological Research for Nursing, 8*, 210–222.

Jones, N. A., Field, T., Fox, N. A., Davalos, M., Lundy, B, & Hart, S. (1998). Newborns of mothers with depressive symptoms are physiologically less developed. *Infant Behavior and Development, 21*, 537–541.

Jun, H. J., Corliss, H. L., Boynton-Jarrett, R., Spiegelman, D., Austin, S. B., & Wright, R. J. (2011). Growing up in a domestic violence environment: Relationship with devel-opmental trajectories of BMI during adolescence into young adulthood. *Journal of Epidemiology and Community Health* [Epub ahead of print]. Retrieved from http://jech. bmj.com.ezp-prod1.hul.harvard.edu/content/early/2011/01/31/jech.2010.110932. long on January 23, 2012.

Kaufman, J., Birmaher, B., Perel, J., Dahl, R.E., Moreci, P., Nelson, B., et al. (1997). The corticotropin-releasing hormone challenge in depressed abused, depressed nonab-used, and normal control children. *Biological Psychiatry, 42*(8), 669–679.

Keenan, K, Grace, D., Gunthorpe, D. (2003). Examining stress reactivity in neonates: Relations between cortisol and behavior. *Child Development, 74*, 1930–1942.

Kessler, R. C., Sonnega, A., Bromet, E., Hughes, M., & Nelson, C. B. (1995). Posttraumatic stress disorder in the National Comorbidity Survey. *Archives of General Psychiatry, 52*, 1048–1060.

King, J. A., Mandansky, D., King, S., Fletcher, K. E., & Brewer, J. (2001). Early sexual abuse and low cortisol. *Psychiatry and Clinical Neurosciences, 55*, 71–74.

Kliewer, W. (2006). Violence exposure and cortisol responses in urban youth. *International Journal of Behavioral Medicine, 13*(2), 109–120.

Kumar, A., & Ghosh, B. (2009). Genetics of asthma: A molecular biologist perspective. *Clinical and Molecular Allergy, 7*, 7.

Kumari, M., Chandola, T., Brunner, E., & Kivimaki, M. (2010). A nonlinear relationship of generalized and central obesity with diurnal cortisol secretion in the Whitehall II study. *Journal of Clinical Endocrinology & Metabolism, 95*, 4415–4423.

Larsson, C. A., Gullberg, B., Rastam, L., Linblad, U. (2009). Salivary cortisol differs with age and sex and sows inverse associations with WHR in Swedish women: A cross-sectional study. *BMC Endocrine Disorders, 9*, 16.

Liao, S. Y., Liao, T. N., Chiang, B. L., Huang, M. S., Chen, C. C., Chou, C. C., et al. (1996). Decreased production of IFN gamma and increased production of IL-6 by cord blood mononuclear cells of newborns with a high risk of allergy. *Clinical and Experimental Allergy, 26*, 397–405.

Lipschitz, D. S., Rasmusson, A. M., & Southwick, S.M. (1998). Childhood posttraumatic stress disorder: A review of neurobiologic sequelae. *Psychiatric Annals, 28*, 452–457.

Litonjua, A. A., Carey, V. J., Burge, H. A., Weiss, S.T., & Gold, D. R. (1998). Parental his-tory and the risk for childhood asthma. Does mother confer more risk than father? *American Journal of Respiratory and Critical Care Medicine, 158*(1), 176–181.

Liu, D., Diorio, J., Tannenbaum, B., Caldji, C., Francis, D., Freedman, A., et al. (1997). Maternal care, hippocampal glucocorticoid receptors, and hypothalamic-pituitary-adrenal response to stress. *Science, 277*, 1659–1662.

Lupien, S. J., King, S., Meaney, M. J., & McEwen, B. S. (2000). Child's stress hormone levels correlate with mother's socioeconomic status and depressive state. *Biological Psychiatry, 48*, 976–980.

Lyons-Ruth, K., & Block, D. E. (1996). The disturbed caregiving system: Relations among childhood trauma, maternal caregiving, and infant affect and attachment. *Infant Mental Health Journal, 17*, 257–275.

Margolin, G., & Gordis, E. B. (2000). The effects of family and community violence on children. *Annual Review of Psychology, 51,* 445–479.

Martinez, F. D., Wright, A. L., Taussig, L. M., Holberg, C. J., Halonen, M., & Morgan, W. J. (1995). Asthma and wheezing in the first six years of life. *New England Journal of Medicine, 332,* 133–138.

Mason, J. W., Kosten, T. R., Southwick, S. M., & Giller, E. L., Jr. (1990). The use of psychoendocrine strategies in post-traumatic stress disorder. *Journal of Applied Social Psychology, 20,* 1822–1846.

McCrory, E., De Brito, S. A., & Viding, E. (2010). Research review: The neurobiology and genetics of maltreatment and adversity. *Journal of Child Psychology and Psychiatry, 51,* 1079–1095.

McEwen, B. S. (2002). Protective and damaging effects of stress mediators: The good and bad sides of the response to stress. *Metabolism: Clinical & Experimental, 51*(6 Suppl 1), 2–4.

Miles, E. A., Warner, J. A., Jones, A. C., Colwell, B. M., Bryant, T. N., & Warner, J. O. (1996). Peripheral blood mononuclear cell proliferative responses in the first year of life in babies born to allergic parents. *Clinical and Experimental Allergy, 26,* 780–788.

Monk, C., Sloan, R. P., et al. (2004). Fetal heart rate reactivity differs by women's psychiatric status: An early marker for developmental risk? *Journal of the American Academy of Child & Adolescent Psychiatry, 43,* 283–290.

Mossman, T. R., & Coffman, R. L. (1989). Th1 and Th2 cells: Different patterns of lymphokine secretion lead to different functional properties. *Annual Review of Immunology, 7,* 145–173.

Mossman, T. R., & Sad, S. (1996). The expanding universe of T-cell subsets: Th1, Th2 and more. *Immunology Today, 17,* 138–146.

Mrazek, D. A., Klinnert, M., Mrazek, P. J., Brower, A., McCormick, D., Rubin, B., et al. (1999). Prediction of early-onset asthma in genetically at-risk children. *Pediatric Pulmonology, 27*(2), 85–94.

Myers, H. F. (2009). Ethnicity- and socio-economic status-related stresses in context: An integrative review and conceptual model. *Journal of Behavioral Medicine, 32,* 9–19.

Neigh, G. N., Gillespie, C. F., & Nemeroff, C. B., (2009). The neurobiological toll of child abuse and neglect. *Trauma, Violence & Abuse, 10,* 389–410.

Nierop, A., Bartsikas, A., Zimmermann, R., & Ehlert, U. (2006). Are stress-induced cortisol changes during pregnancy associated with postpartum depressive symptoms? *Psychosomatic Medicine, 68,* 931–937.

Odelram, H., Bjorksten, B., Leander, E., & Kjellman, N. I. (1995). Predictors of atopy in newborn babies. *Allergy, 50*(7), 585–592.

Ogawa, J. R., Sroufe, L. A., Weinfield, N. S., Carlson, E. A., & Egeland, B. (1997). Development and the fragmented self: Longitudinal study of dissociative symptomatology in a nonclinical sample. *Development and Psychopathology, 9,* 855–879.

Oosterman, M., De Schipper, J. C., Fisher, P., Dozier, M., & Schuengel, C., (2010). Autonomic reactivity in relation to attachment and early adversity among foster children. *Development and Psychopathology, 22,* 109–118.

Orr, S., Lasko, N., Shalev, A. Y., & Pitman, R. K. (1995). Physiologic responses to loud tones in Vietnam veterans with posttraumatic stress disorder. *Journal of Abnormal Psychology, 104,* 75–82.

Paige, S., Reid, G., Allen, M. G., & Newton, J. E. (1990). Psychophysiological correlates of posttraumatic stress disorder in Vietnam veterans. *Biological Psychiatry, 27,* 419–430.

Panettieri, R. A., Covar, R., Grant, E., Hillyer, E. B., & Bacharier, L. (2008). Natural history of asthma: Persistence versus progression—Does the beginning predict the end? *Journal of Allergy and Clinical Immunology, 121,* 607–613.

Peden, D. B. (2000). Development of atopy and asthma: Candidate environmental influences and important periods of exposure. *Environmental Health Perspectives, 108*(Suppl 3), 475–482.

Perry, B. D., Pollard, R. A., Blakley, T. L., Baker, W. L., & Vigilante, D. (1995). Childhood trauma, the neurobiology of adaptation, and use-dependent development of the brain: How "states" become "traits". *Infant Mental Health Journal, 16*, 271–291.

Prescott, S. L., Macaubas, C., Holt, B. J., Smallacombe, T. B., Loh, R., Sly, P. D., et al. (1998). Transplacental priming of the human immune system to environmental allergens: Universal skewing of initial T cell responses toward the Th2 cytokine profile. *Journal of Immunology, 160*, 4730–4737.

Pryce, C. R., Ruedi-Bettschen, D., Dettling, A. C., & Feldon, J. (2002). Early life stress: Long-term physiological impact in rodents and primates. *News Physiological Science, 17*, 150–155.

Raison, C. L., & Miller, A. H. (2003). When not enough is too much: The role of insufficient glucocorticoid signaling in the pathophysiology of stress-related disorders. *American Journal of Psychiatry, 260*, 1554–1565.

Reinisch, J. M., Simon, N. G., Karow, W. G., Gandelman, R., et al. (1978). Prenatal exposure to prednisone in humans and animals retards intra-uterine growth. *Science, 202*, 436–438.

Rich-Edwards, J., Mohllajee, A. P., Kleinman, K., Hacker, M. R., Majzoub, J., Wright, R. J., et al. (2008). Elevated mid-pregnancy corticotrophin-releasing hormone is associated with prenatal, but not postpartum, maternal depression. *Journal of Clinical Endocrinology and Metabolism, 93*(5), 1946–1951.

Rich-Edwards, J. W., James-Todd, T., Mohlajee, A., Kleinman, K., Burke, A., Gillman, M. W., et al. (2010). Lifetime maternal experiences of abuse and risk of pre-natal depression in two demographically distinct populations in Boston. *International Journal Epidemiology, 40*, 375–384.

Rich-Edwards, J. W., Spiegelman, D., Livdoti Hibert, E. N., Jun, H. J., Todd, T. J., Kawachi, I., et al. (2010). Abuse in childhood and adolescence as a predictor of type 2 diabetes in adult women. *American Journal of Preventative Medicine, 39*, 529–536.

Rigterink, T., Fainsilber Katz, L., & Hessler, D. M. (2010). Domestic violence and longitudinal associations with children's physiological regulation abilities. *Journal of Interpersonal Violence, 25*, 1669–1683.

Riley, E. H., Wright, R. J., Jun, H. J., Hibert, E. N., & Rich-Edwards, J. W. (2010). Hypertension in adult survivors of child abuse: Observations from the Nurses' Health Study II. *Journal of Epidemiology and Community Health, 64*, 413–418.

Robinson, D. S., Hamid, Q., Ying, S., Tsicopoulos, A., Barkans, J., Bentley, A. M., et al. (1992). Predominant Th2 like bronchoalveolar T-lymphocyte population in atopic asthma. *New England Journal of Medicine, 326*, 298–304.

Robinson, J. L., & Acevedo, M. C. (2001). Infant reactivity and reliance on mother during emotion challenges: Predictors of cognition and language skills in a low-income sample. *Child Development, 72*, 402–415.

Saglani, S., & Bush, A. (2007). The early-life origins of asthma. *Current Opinions in Allergy and Clinical Immunology, 7*(1), 83–90.

Saltzman, K. M., Holden, G. W., & Holahan, C. J. (2005). The psychobiology of children exposed to marital violence. *Journal of Clinical Child and Adolescent Psychology, 34*(1), 129–139.

Schechter, D. S. (2004). How post-traumatic stress affects mothers' perceptions of their babies: A brief video feedback intervention makes a difference. *Zero to Three, 24*, 43–49.

Schmidt, L. A., Fox, N. A., Rubin K. H., Sternberg, E. M., Gold, P. W., Smith, C. C., et al. (1997). Behavioral and neuroendocrine responses in shy children. *Developmental Psychobiology, 30,* 127–140.

Schuder, M. R., & Lyons-Ruth, K. (2004). "Hidden trauma" in infancy: Attachment, fearful arousal, and early dysfunction of the stress response system. In J. D. Osofsky (Ed.), *Young children and trauma: Intervention and treatment* (pp. 69–104). New York: Guilford Press.

Seckl, J. R. (1997). Glucocorticoids, feto-placental 11-beta-hydroxysteroid dehydrogenase type 2, and the early life origins of adult disease. *Steroids, 62,* 89–94.

Seckl, J. R. (2001). Glucocorticoid programming of the fetus: Adult phenotypes and molecular mechanisms. *Molecular and Cellular Endocrinology, 185*(1–2), 61–71.

Seng, J. S., Low, L. K., Ben-Ami, D., & Liberzon, I. (2005). Cortisol level and perinatal outcome in pregnant women with posttraumatic stress disorder: A pilot study. *Journal of Midwifery and Women's Health, 50,* 392–398.

Shankardass, K., McConnell, R., Jerrett, M., Milam, J., Richardson, J., & Berhane, K. (2009). Parental stress increases the effect of traffic-related air pollution on childhood asthma incidence. *Proceedings of the National Academy of Sciences, 106,* 12406–12411.

Shenk, C. E., Noll, J. G., Putnam, F. W., & Trickett, P. K. (2010). A prospective examination of the role of childhood sexual abuse and physiological asymmetry in the development of psychopathology. *Child Abuse and Neglect, 34,* 752–761.

Sheridan, M., & Nelson, C. A. (2009). Neurobiology of fetal and infant development: Implications for infant mental health. In C. H. Zeanah (Ed.), *Handbook of infant mental health* (pp. 37–59). New York: Guilford.

Shimomitsu, T., & Odagiri, Y. (2001). Endocrinological assessment of extreme stress. *Advances in Psychosomatic Medicine, 22,* 35–51.

Springer, K. W. (2009). Childhood physical abuse and midlife physical health: Testing a multi-pathway life course model. *Social Science & Medicine, 69,* 138–146.

Sternthal, M. J., Bosquet Enlow, M., Cohen, S., Canner M. J., Staudenmayer, J., Tsang, K., et al. (2009). Maternal interpersonal trauma and cord blood IgE levels in an inner-city cohort: A life-course perspective. *Journal of Allergy and Clinical Immunology, 124,* 954–960.

Sternthal, M. J., Jun, H. J., Earls, F., & Wright, R .J. (2010). Community violence and urban childhood asthma: A multilevel analysis. *European Respiratory Journal, 36,* 1400–1409.

Straus, M. A. (1996). The revised Conflict Tactics Scales (CTS2): Development and preliminary psychometric data. *Journal of Family Issues, 17,* 283–316.

Suglia, S. F., Staudenmayer, J., Cohen, S., Bosquet Enlow, M., Rich-Edwards, J. W., & Wright, R. J. (2010a). Cumulative stress and cortisol disruption among Black and Hispanic pregnant women in an urban cohort. *Psychological Trauma: Theory Research Practice and Policy, 2*(4), 326–334.

Suglia, S., Staudenmayer, J. Cohen, S., & Wright, R. J. (2010b). Posttraumatic stress symptoms related to community violence and children's diurnal cortisol response in an urban community-dwelling sample. *International Journal of Behavioral Medicine, 17,* 43–50.

Swahn, M. H.& Bossarte, R. M. (2006). The associations between victimization, reeling unsafe, and asthma episodes among US high-school students. *American Journal of Public health, 96,* 802–804.

Tariq, S. M., Arshad, S. H., Matthews, S. M., & Hakim, E. A. (1999). Elevated cord serum IgE increases the risk of aeroallergen sensitization without increasing respiratory allergic symptoms in early childhood. *Clinical and Experimental Allergy, 29*(8), 1042–1048.

Tout, K., de Haan, M., Campbell, E. K., & Gunnar, M. R. (1998). Social behavior correlates of cortisol activity in child care: Gender differences and time-of-day effects. *Child Development, 69,* 1247–1262.

Trickett, P. K., Duran, L., & Horn, J. L. (2003). Community violence as it affects child development: Issues of definition. *Clinical Child and Family Psychology Review, 6*(4), 223–236.

True, M., Pisani, L., & Oumar, F. (2001). Infant-mother attachment among the Dogon in Mali. *Child Development, 75,* 1451–1466.

Undem, B. J., Kajekar, R., Hunter, D. D., & Myers, A. C. (2000). Neural integration and allergic disease. *Journal of Allergy and Clinical Immunology, 106*(5 Suppl), S213–S220.

Undem, B. J., & Weinreich, D. (2003). Neuroimmune interactions in the lung. In J. Bienenstock, E. J. Goetzle, and M. G. Blennerhassett (Eds.), *The autonomic nervous system, Volume 15: Autonomic neuroimmunology* (pp. 280–295). New York: Taylor & Francis.

Vallee, M., Mayo, W., Dellu, F., Le Moal, M., Simon, H., & Maccari, S. (1997). Prenatal stress induces high anxiety and postnatal handling induces low anxiety in adult offspring: Correlation with stress-induced corticosterone secretion. *Journal of Neuroscience, 17*(7), 2626–2636.

van Ijzendoorn, M. H., Schuengel, C., & Bakermans-Kranenburg, M. J. (1999). Attachment and loss: Frightening maternal behavior linking unresolved loss and disorganized infant attachment. *Journal of Consulting & Clinical Psychology, 67,* 54–63.

von Hertzen, L. C. (2002). Maternal stress and T-cell differentiation of the developing immune system: Possible implications for the development of asthma and atopy. *Journal of Allergy and Clinical Immunology, 109*(6), 923–928.

Ward, A. M., Moore, V. M., Steptoe, A., Cockington, R. A., Robinson, J. S., & Phillips, D. I. (2004). Size at birth and cardiovascular responses to psychological stressors: Evidence for prenatal programming in women. *Journal of Hypertension, 22*(12), 2295–2301.

Ward, M. J., & Carlson, E. A. (1995). The predictive validity of the Adult Attachment Interview for adolescent mothers. *Child Development, 66,* 69–79.

Wegman, H. L., & Stetler, C. (2009). A meta-analytic review of the effects of childhood abuse on medical outcomes in adulthood. *Psychosomatic Medicine, 71*(8), 805–812.

Whitelaw, N. C., & Whitelaw, E. (2009). Transgenerational epigenetic inheritance in health and disease. *Current Opinion in Genetics & Development, 18,* 273–279.

Williams, H. E., & Flohr, C. (2006). How epidemiology has challenged 3 prevailing concepts about atopic dermatitis. *Journal of Allergy and Clinical Immunology, 118*(1), 209–213.

Williams, R. (2007). The psychosocial consequences for children of mass violence, terrorism and disasters. *International Review of Psychiatry, 19,* 263–277.

Wonnacott, K. M., & Bonneau, R. H. (2002). The effects of stress on memory cytotoxic T lymphocyte-mediated protection against herpes simplex virus infection at mucosal sites. *Brain Behavior and Immunity, 16,* 104–117.

Wright, R., & Bosquet Enlow, M. (2008). Maternal stress and perinatal programming in the expression of atopy. *Expert Reviews in Clinical Immunology, 4,* 535–538.

Wright, R. J. (2006). Health effects of socially toxic neighborhoods: the violence and urban asthma paradigm. *Clinics in Chest Medicine, 27,* 413–421.

Wright, R. J. (2007). Prenatal maternal stress and early caregiving experiences: Implications for childhood asthma risk. *Pediatric and Perinatal Epidemiology, 21,* 8–14.

Wright, R. J. (2009). Moving towards making social toxins mainstream in children's environmental health. *Current Opinion in Pediatrics, 21*(2), 222–229.

Wright, R. J. (2010). Perinatal stress and early life programming of lung structure and function. *Biological Psychology, 84,* 46–56.

Wright, R. J., Cohen, R. T., & Cohen, S. (2005). The impact of stress on the development and expression of atopy. *Current Opinions in Allergy and Clinical Immunology, 5*(1), 23–29.

Wright, R. J., Cohen, S., Carey, V., Weiss, S. T., & Gold, D.R. (2002). Parental stress as a predictor of wheezing in infancy: A prospective birth-cohort study. *American Journal of Respiratory & Critical Care Medicine, 165,* 358–365.

Wright, R. J., Finn, P., Contreras, J. P., Cohen, S., Wright, R. O., Wand, M., et al. (2004). Chronic caregiver stress and IgE expression, allergen-induced proliferation and cytokine profiles in a birth cohort predisposed to atopy. *Journal of Allergy and Clinical Immunology, 113,* 1051–1057.

Wright, R. J., Fisher, K., Chiu, Y. H-M., Cohen, S., & Coull, B. (2011). Disruption of maternal diurnal cortisol in pregnancy and prenatal body mass index (BMI) are associated with repeated wheeze up to age 2 years in urban children: Project ACCESS. *American Journal of Respiratory and Critical Care Medicine, 183,* A3799.

Wright, R .J., Mitchell, H., Visness, C. M., Cohen, S., Stout, J., Evans, R., et al. (2004). Community violence and asthma morbidity: The Inner-City Asthma Study. *American Journal of Public health, 94*(4), 625–632.

Wright, R. J., Rodriguez, M., & Cohen, S. (1998). Review of psychosocial stress and asthma: An integrated biopsychosocial approach. *Thorax, 53,* 1066–1074.

Wright, R. J., & Subramanian, S. V. (2007). Advancing a multilevel framework for epidemiological research on asthma disparities. *Chest, 132,* 757S–769S.

Yehuda, R. (2001). Biology of posttraumatic stress disorder. *Journal of Clinical Psychiatry, 62,* 41–46.

Yehuda, R., & Bierer, L. M. (2008). Transgenerational transmission of cortisol and PTSD risk. *Progress in Brain Research, 167,* 121–134.

Yehuda, R., Engel, S. M., Brand, S. R., Seckl, J., Marcus, S. M., & Berkowitz, G. S. (2005). Transgenerational effects of posttraumatic stress disorder in babies of mothers exposed to the World Trade Center attacks during pregnancy. *Journal of Clinical Endocrinology and Metabolism, 90*(7), 4115–4118.

Yehuda, R., Teicher, M. H., Seckl, J. R., Grossman, R. A., Morris, A., & Bierer, L. M. (2007). Parental posttraumatic stress disorder as a vulnerability factor for low cortisol trait in offspring of Holocaust survivors. *Archives of General Psychiatry, 64,* 1040–1048.

PART V

Responses to Disasters and Terrorism

9

An Exploration of Causality in the Development
and Timing of Disaster-Related PTSD

CAROL S. NORTH

Untangling the causes of psychopathology is a daunting endeavor for scientific research. Attempts to explain the mental health problems that follow traumatic events. particularly disasters, are destined to encounter unique complexities. To begin with, the unpredictability of disasters inserts practical challenges into attempts to conduct research on mental health outcomes. Norris (1992) (p. 416) noted, "Establishing cause and effect is exceedingly difficult in traumatic stress research where prospective designs are rarely feasible." In general, the determination of causality is most directly and readily accomplished through experimental designs such as randomized controlled trials, which are not possible in studies examining the effects of disasters. (Institutional human studies review boards do not look kindly upon research designs that call for the random assignment of major trauma to research participants.) Additional difficulties in studying the etiology of trauma-related psychopathology are inherent in established definitions of trauma-related syndromes. Yet other complexities arise from the confounding of preexisting risk factors for trauma with post-trauma outcomes.

Post-traumatic stress disorder (PTSD) is an uncharacteristic psychiatric diagnosis in the current diagnostic nomenclature, which defines most psychiatric disorders atheoretically and agnostically with regard to etiology. Unlike most other psychiatric disorders, PTSD is defined in relation to a potentially etiologic source: exposure to a traumatic event. The diagnostic construct of PTSD is thus caught in a "Catch-22" situation, because the traumatic event is needed to anchor the symptoms of the disorder so as to define a coherent syndrome, yet assumptions of traumatic causation conflict with the current approach in psychiatric nosology, which is atheoretical and agnostic regarding etiology (North, 2011; North et al., 2009). Including assumptions about etiology within the diagnostic criteria for a disorder will serve to inhibit scientific investigation into the causes that are already "known" (North, 2011; North, Surís, Davis, & Smith, 2009). A potential solution to this apparent quandary is to continue to require the temporal and contextual association of post-traumatic symptoms with exposure to a qualifying traumatic event while refraining from defining PTSD in terms of a causal process (North, 2011; North et al., 2009). This agnostic approach provides a coherent syndrome that permits research into the etiology of the disorder.

Research on the mental health effects of trauma is complicated by preexisting individual risk factors for trauma exposure that might be confounded with risk factors for mental health outcomes following trauma exposure, making it virtually impossible to untangle causal relationships between trauma exposure and psychopathology (North, 2011). The study of the mental health effects of disasters, however, provides opportunities to avoid much of the confounding that has plagued research on mental health problems associated with other types of trauma (Hasin, Keyes, Hatzenbuehler, Aharonovich, & Alderson, 2007). Not all disasters are equal-opportunity events (e.g., Hurricane Katrina, which disproportionately affected those with the least resources and an overrepresentation of predisaster socioeconomic, health, and mental health vulnerabilities) (Greenough et al., 2008; North, King, et al., 2008). Many disasters, however, such as the Oklahoma City bombing, strike more randomly, thereby avoiding many of the selection biases associated with other kinds of trauma such as motorcycle accidents.

Disasters create a ready environment for the development of PTSD, a well-established outcome among disaster survivors (Norris et al., 2002). Most people who are exposed to disasters, however, do not develop PTSD or, for that matter, any psychiatric illness (Breslau et al., 1998; North, 2007; North, Hong, & Pfefferbaum, 2008). PTSD by definition cannot occur in the absence of exposure to trauma such as disaster. Therefore, exposure to the disaster is necessary for the development of PTSD, but it is not a "necessary and sufficient" explanation for the development of PTSD. Disaster trauma must certainly be a contributor, however, because people who are exposed to a disaster can develop a psychiatric disorder (i.e., PTSD) that they never would have had otherwise. If not everyone who is exposed to a disaster develops PTSD, then there must be other contributory factors that help determine who among the exposed individuals will or will not develop PTSD.

This chapter first reviews predictors of PTSD and its course that are described in the existing literature. This is followed by an examination of illustrative data from an epidemiologic study of the Oklahoma City bombing. It can be seen through these considerations that efforts to sort out causal associations within these relationships are stymied by unusual features embedded within current definitions pertaining to PTSD, its onset, and its remission that create confusion for research investigation.

Predictors of the Development and Timing of PTSD
in Prior Disaster Studies

Previous research has identified a number of predictors of PTSD in disaster-exposed populations. A comprehensive review of disaster mental health research by Norris and colleagues (2002) found that among the most consistent predictors of PTSD was female gender, with 49 of 50 articles reporting significant gender differences and a female predominance of PTSD. This review also found preexisting psychopathology to be one of the best predictors of postdisaster psychiatric problems. Preexisting personality in relation to PTSD following disasters has received less study, yet personality has also been found to be strongly predictive of PTSD (Norris et al., 2002). Because PTSD is conceptualized in relation to a traumatic exposure, it is intuitive that trauma exposure (including indicators of the trauma severity and the dose of the exposure) would predict the development of PTSD. Indeed, the level of exposure (estimated via proxy variables such as injury severity and perceived threat to life) has been found by a number of studies to predict the likelihood of developing PTSD (Norris et al., 2002). Other predictors of PTSD identified by the Norris et al. (2002) review are age (among adults; youth is protective, with greater risk found among older and especially middle-aged adults), membership in an ethnic minority and/or socioeconomically disadvantaged group, marital status (marriage being a protective factor for men and a risk factor for women), other life stressors, and lack of social support.

The factors that determine the timing and course of PTSD might differ from those that determine the likelihood of developing PTSD (Schnurr, Lunney, & Sengupta, 2004). Despite the abundance of predictors of PTSD that have been discovered, relatively few predictors have been identified for the occurrence of delayed-onset PTSD compared to acute-onset PTSD and PTSD remission, and the evidence has often been conflicting. Delayed-onset PTSD is apparently a more prevalent finding among military veterans, and it has been found to be associated with psychiatric comorbidity (Andrews, Brewin, Philpott, & Stewart, 2007; Andrews, Brewin, Stewart, Philpott, & Hejdenberg, 2009; Gray, Bolton, & Litz, 2004; Prigerson, Maciejewski, & Rosenheck, 2001). A variable that has repeatedly been found to be associated with the timing of PTSD onset is the occurrence of intervening life stressors, although studies are inconsistent regarding whether the association is positive (Andrews et al., 2009; Buckley, Blanchard, & Hickling, 1996) or negative (Horesh, Solomon, Zerach, & Elin-Dor, 2010).

Many people with PTSD eventually recover from it, but some do not, suggesting that there should be some potentially identifiable factors that might determine who will and who will not recover from PTSD. Numerous studies have identified predictors of *chronic PTSD*, but very few prospective studies have examined predictors of *remission from PTSD*, which is a fundamentally different concept. Traumatized populations examined in the studies of PTSD remission have included military veterans, motor vehicle accident survivors, primary care patients, and community populations (Blanchard et al., 1997; Koren, Arnon, & Klein, 2001; Perkonigg et al., 2005; Schnurr et al., 2004; Zlotnick et al., 2004). Predictors of PTSD remission identified by more than one of these studies are early post-trauma responses (PTSD symptom severity, avoidance symptoms, and psychosocial functioning), other traumatic and stressful events during the follow-up period, and postincident psychiatric comorbidity. Additional predictors of PTSD remission identified by single studies in this list are the severity of physical injury sustained during the traumatic event, the degree of physical recovery, trauma suffered by a close family member during the follow-up period, fewer years of education, being married, and a self-competence rating indicating an ability to cope with trauma.

Evidence from the Oklahoma City Bombing Study

A sample of 182 directly exposed survivors of the Oklahoma City bombing randomly selected from the Oklahoma State Department of Health's public registry of survivors was assessed at index approximately six months after the disaster, with a 71% participation rate. This was a highly exposed sample, as evidenced by the fact that 87% had a disaster-related injury and 77% required medical attention for injuries. The sample had nearly equal gender representation but was 89% Caucasian, with a mean age of 43 years and an average education level of two years of college; nearly two-thirds were married. A follow-up study was conducted nearly seven years after the disaster, with a 62% follow-up rate (n = 113). Study attrition from index to follow-up was associated with demographic variables of divorced/separated marital status (with study attrition in 35% of divorced/separated versus 15% of others, p = 0.002) and fewer years of education (13.7 versus 14.8, p < 0.001) but was not associated with any other demographic variables, injuries sustained in the bombing, or psychiatric disorders. Detailed descriptions of the methods used in these studies are available in previous publications (North et al., 1999; North, Pfefferbaum, Kawasaki, Lee, & Spitznagel, 2010).

The Diagnostic Interview Schedule (DIS-IV) (Robins et al., 2000) was used to assess full *Diagnostic and Statistical Manual of Mental Disorders* (4th ed., text revision) (*DSM-IV-TR*) (American Psychiatric Association, 2000) diagnostic criteria for psychiatric disorders at index and follow-up. The Disaster Supplement provided information on disaster exposure variables and other relevant experiences, including the number of other lifetime traumatic events and the number of other stressful events after the disaster. The most prevalent postdisaster disorder was PTSD (34%), and the second most prevalent postdisaster diagnosis was major depression (23%). Less than one-half (45%) had one or more postdisaster psychiatric disorders at index (North et al., 1999). The Temperament and Character Inventory (Cloninger, 1987; Svrakic, Whitehead, Przybeck, & Cloninger, 1993), a self-administered dimensional measure of personality traits, was administered in order to assess personality at index, with an 83% completion rate (n = 151). Low levels of both cooperativeness and self-directedness occurring together were considered to indicate an unhealthy personality structure with underdeveloped executive functions, which is considered a core feature of personality disorders (Svrakic et al., 1993).

Predictors of PTSD

In the Oklahoma City bombing study, group C (avoidance/numbing) symptoms were strongly predictive of PTSD: 94% of those meeting group C criteria at index were diagnosed with PTSD at index (North et al., 1999). Symptom group C was associated with a number of other indicators of psychiatric illness (predisaster psychopathology, postdisaster psychiatric comorbidity, receiving mental health treatment, taking psychotropic medication, coping by drinking alcohol, and problems functioning). Symptom groups B (intrusion) and D (hyperarousal) were highly prevalent (about 80% each), and in the absence of group C they did not show these associations. These findings suggest that with the current construction of the diagnostic criteria for PTSD, avoidance and numbing represent the core of the psychopathology, and intrusion and hyperarousal are normative responses that by themselves do not indicate psychiatric illness (North et al., 1999).

Variables not associated with PTSD in bivariate analyses were age, marital status, and lifetime history of other traumatic events (p > 0.05 in all comparisons). Those with PTSD sustained nearly twice as many injuries in the bombing (2.7 in those with PTSD versus 1.5 in others; df = 86.45, t = 4.58, p < 0.001). PTSD was also associated with the number of adverse life events after the disaster (5.1 among those with PTSD versus 3.1 among others; df = 82.48, t = −3.47, p < 0.001). This finding is consistent with conclusions about trauma exposure drawn by Norris (1992, p. 416): "With regard to overall levels of perceived stress, these events appear to be only one of many sources of stress in people's lives." Among other predictors of PTSD in Oklahoma City bombing survivors, women were approximately twice as likely as men to develop PTSD after the bombing (45% versus 23%; χ^2 = 9.75, p = 0.002). One's level of education was protective, with PTSD occurring in only 20% of those with and 39% of those without a college degree (χ^2 = 5.27, p = 0.022). However, in a multiple logistic regression model predicting PTSD (dependent variable) based on the independent covariates of female sex and college education (entered simultaneously into the model), only female sex was significantly predictive (β = 0.96, SE = 0.34, df = 1, Wald χ^2 = 8.01, p = 0.005), and college education was not (β = −0.21, SE = 0.37, df = 1, Wald χ^2 = 0.33, p = 0.567). Coupled with the finding of a significant association of female sex and education (45% of men and 20% of women having a college degree; χ^2 = 13.22, p < 0.001) and no interaction of female sex and education in the prediction of PTSD, this suggests that the association of no college education with PTSD is confounded with female sex, which might serve as a moderator for the association between education and PTSD.

Bombing-related PTSD was also more than twice as prevalent among those with a predisaster psychiatric disorder (45% versus 26%; χ^2 = 7.21, p = 0.007), among those with a personality constellation of combined low cooperativeness and low self-directedness (50% versus 23%; χ^2 = 10.76, p = 0.001), and among those with both a predisaster psychiatric disorder and a personality constellation of low cooperativeness/low self-directedness (64% versus 25%; χ^2 = 14.34, p < 0.001). The personality constellation was insignificantly associated with having a predisaster diagnosis, however (52% versus 37%; χ^2 = 3.11, p = 0.078). In a limited multiple logistic regression model predicting PTSD (dependent variable) based on the independent covariates of predisaster psychiatric disorder and personality constellation of low cooperativeness/low self-directedness (simultaneously entered into the model), only the personality measure was significantly associated with PTSD (β = 1.12, SE = 0.38, Wald ^{2} = 8.87, p = 0.003); predisaster psychiatric disorder was not associated (β = 0.63, SE = 0.37, Wald χ^2 = 2.93, p = 0.087). A term characterizing the interaction of the personality measure and predisaster psychiatric diagnosis that was added as an independent variable was not significantly associated with PTSD. These analyses are consistent with the possibility that the contribution of predisaster psychiatric illness to PTSD after the bombing was largely mediated through personality characteristics. It is noteworthy also that 33% of those with PTSD did not have these vulnerabilities, and 24% of bombing survivors without either of these vulnerabilities developed PTSD.

A multiple regression model was constructed to predict PTSD based on the list of variables significantly associated with PTSD in the above bivariate analyses (not including education, because it was confounded with female sex), which were entered simultaneously into the model (see Fig. 9.1). In this model, female gender and number of injuries remained strongly associated with PTSD. Predisaster psychiatric diagnosis, however, was not predictive of PTSD, whereas the personality constellation of low cooperativeness/low self-directedness was predictive. It appears that the association of preexisting psychopathology with PTSD after the bombing might have been largely a function of the effects of personality. A majority of variance in the occurrence of PTSD was unexplained by this model: a generalization of R^2 computed using the method of Nagelkerke (1991) was 0.38 (indicating that the model explained only 38% of the variance). Therefore, most of what might predict PTSD was not determined by this study.

Independent variables	df	β	SE	Wald χ^2	p	OR	95% CL	
Female sex	1	1.26	0.44	8.18	**0.004**	3.54	1.49	8.42
Predisaster psychiatric disorder	1	0.75	0.44	2.93	0.087	2.13	0.90	5.05
Personality combination of low cooperativeness and low self-directedness	1	0.93	0.45	4.32	**0.038**	2.54	1.06	6.11
Number of injuries*	1	0.29	0.10	7.91	**0.005**	1.34	1.09	1.65
Number of postdisaster life events*	1	0.50	0.18	6.69	**0.010**	1.60	1.12	2.28

*(Number of injuries truncated at 7; number of life events truncated at 4)

Figure 9.1 Multivariate model of variables predicting PTSD related to the Oklahoma City bombing.

The Course of PTSD and Post-traumatic Symptoms

A prospective seven-year follow-up study identified no incident (new) cases of PTSD (defined as new onset of disaster-related symptoms leading to PTSD beginning more than six months after the bombing, consistent with the *DSM-IV-TR* definition of delayed-onset PTSD as "onset of symptoms is at least 6 months after the stressor") (American Psychiatric Association, 2000, p. 468).

Nine survivors not fulfilling criteria for bombing-related PTSD at index were identified as having developed bombing-related PTSD at some time during the interval before follow-up. At index, all nine met group B (intrusion) and group D (hyperarousal) symptom group criteria, but six lacked just one group C (avoidance/numbing) symptom, and three lacked two group C symptoms. When these nine Oklahoma City bombing cases of PTSD first diagnosed after six months were compared with the 36 cases of PTSD diagnosed at the six-month assessment, none of the significant predictors of PTSD described earlier predicted a first diagnosis of PTSD after six months. Thus, of PTSD cases not identified until the seven-year follow-up assessment, at six months, all were already close to the diagnostic threshold in terms of symptom levels (lacking only one or at most two group C symptoms) for a diagnosis of PTSD. This progression of symptoms indicates a development of PTSD that was well underway and nearly complete by six months, not delayed onset until after six symptom-free months. This finding is confirmed by data from a prospectively conducted follow-up study of survivors of a mass shooting episode in Killeen, Texas, demonstrating the same pattern of near-threshold symptoms in cases not meeting symptom criteria at index but meeting full criteria by three years, with avoidance/numbing symptoms similarly playing a pivotal role in an individual's crossing over the diagnostic threshold (North, McCutcheon, Spitznagel, & Smith, 2002).

The postdisaster prevalence of disaster-related PTSD in the follow-up sample of Oklahoma City bombing survivors, including both cases diagnosed at index and those identified at follow-up, was 41% (n = 46). At follow-up, 26% of the sample had active bombing-related PTSD in the current month. Only 37% of those with PTSD related to the bombing were in full remission, defined by *DSM-IV-TR* as a state in which "[t]here are no longer any symptoms or signs of the disorder" (American Psychiatric Association, 2000, p. 2); 63% were still symptomatic. (Because the DIS obtains a lifetime symptom count for PTSD—and, in the case of disaster-specific PTSD, a postdisaster symptom count—but not a current symptom count, the determination of partial remission could not be provided.) Among those who did not develop PTSD, 36% acknowledged active post-traumatic symptoms at seven years.

Remission from PTSD was not predicted by any of the demographic, exposure, predisaster diagnosis, personality, or psychiatric comorbidity variables found to predict the development of PTSD in this sample. However, the number of other postdisaster adverse life events reported at seven years was negatively associated with PTSD remission (2.1 events among those who remitted compared to 4.0 among those not remitted; t = 3.28, df = 44, p = 0.002).

Problems with Definitions of PTSD Onset and Recency

At least some of the discrepancies in reported findings might be definitional in origin (Andrews et al., 2007; Prigerson et al., 2001; Smid, Mooren, van der Mast, Gersons, & Kleber, 2009). Nonuniform definitions of onset and recency that have been used in trauma research have plagued efforts to identify consistent predictors of the course of PTSD.

The *DSM-IV-TR* definitions of onset and remission of PTSD are imprecise and leave much room for interpretation. Delayed onset of PTSD as defined by *DSM-IV-TR* occurs when "at least 6 months have passed between the traumatic event and the onset of the symptoms" (American Psychiatric Association, 2000, p. 465). This definition might be interpreted to mean that the disorder begins when the symptoms begin (akin to schizophrenia, which one would say began when the person started hearing voices, even if full criteria were not met for another six months), but not all researchers have followed this interpretation. Andrews and colleagues (2007, p. 1319) noted, "There is no clarification of whether 'the onset of the symptoms' refers to *any* symptoms that might eventually lead to the disorder or only to full-blown PTSD itself." These authors identified two different interpretations of the criteria for delayed-onset PTSD used in research studies. "Definition 1" considers delayed-onset PTSD as occurring when diagnostic criteria are not fulfilled by six months after a disaster but are later met. This is a diagnostic-threshold-based definition of onset. "Definition 2" considers delayed-onset PTSD as occurring when full criteria for PTSD are met after a six-month period during which no PTSD symptoms were present. This is a symptom-based definition of onset.

The proposed *DSM-5* criteria for delayed onset of PTSD diverge substantially from the symptom-based definition in *DSM-IV-TR* with the adoption of a threshold-based definition: "diagnostic threshold is not exceeded until 6 months or more after the event(s) (although onset of some symptoms may occur sooner than this)" (*DSM-5* Task Force, 2010). This proposed change represents a major departure from historical definitions of onset of disorders in prior versions of the diagnostic criteria and will disrupt the comparability of onset data in future studies with onset data from the large body of previous work. Regardless of the definition of PTSD onset, however, Andrews and coworkers (2009) observed the development of delayed-onset PTSD in military personnel to begin with hyperarousal symptoms early in the course of deployment, followed by a gradual but steady process of symptom accumulation that ultimately led to the full complement of PTSD symptoms.

In the Oklahoma City bombing study, all cases of PTSD not identified at six months but meeting full criteria later had not just some symptoms but almost enough symptoms to otherwise fulfill the diagnostic criteria at six months. However, the high prevalence of post-traumatic symptoms (96%) in the overall sample within the first six months virtually precluded any potential for delayed-onset PTSD using the symptom-based definition of onset. Alternatively, problems are evident with the diagnostic-threshold-based definition of onset of PTSD (based on meeting full diagnostic criteria), because the examination of symptoms in cases identified according to this definition demonstrated that PTSD is well underway and nearing the diagnostic threshold at six months, only to cross the diagnostic threshold with the subsequent development of one or two symptoms in group C. This scenario does not paint a clear picture of commencement of the disorder after six months.

The definition of PTSD remission has similar problems. Although remission is not specifically defined for PTSD in *DSM-IV-TR*, the manual's definition of remission for psychiatric disorders in general is a state in which "[t]here are no longer any symptoms or signs of the disorder" (American Psychiatric Association, 2000, p. 2). The disappearance of all symptoms as a requirement for remission is a far more stringent criterion than having dropped below the symptom threshold required for diagnosis, as reflected in the relatively low seven-year remission rates (37%) for established PTSD cases among Oklahoma City bombing survivors. Dropping below the symptom threshold is consistent with the *DSM-IV-TR* definition of *partial remission*: "The full criteria for the disorder were previously met, but currently only some of the symptoms or signs of the disorder remain"

(American Psychiatric Association, 2000, p. 2). (Of note, all the prospective studies
of the course of PTSD reviewed in an earlier section of this chapter used criteria
for remission corresponding to the *DSM-IV-TR* definition of partial remission.)

A literal interpretation of *DSM-IV-TR* suggests, therefore, that its definitions
of both onset and remission of PTSD hinge on the presence or absence of *any*
post-traumatic symptoms (i.e., *onset* of PTSD as beginning with the first symptoms, and *remission* as commencing with the disappearance of all PTSD symptoms). Determining the start and end of PTSD based on the presence of any
symptoms is problematic for definitions of both onset and remission. For onset,
early post-traumatic symptoms are so common that there is little room for people
with no symptoms to go on to develop full PTSD later. In order to achieve remission, survivors of the Oklahoma City bombing with PTSD had to have fewer current
symptoms than the 36% of people without PTSD who reported current symptoms
at follow-up. Determining the start and end of PTSD based on a diagnostic symptom threshold for definitions of onset and remission is also problematic; the
Oklahoma City bombing survivors who crossed over the diagnostic symptom
threshold for PTSD after six months were apparently already highly symptomatic
before six months, and those who cross back under the diagnostic symptom threshold might also still be quite symptomatic and impaired.

Ultimately, the most useful definitions of timing of onset and remission will
likely require the determination of an allowable level of symptoms to be used both
as a normative, nonpathological baseline from which individuals might later
develop full PTSD and as a nonpathological symptom platform reached by individuals who have effectively returned to a semblance of their baseline mental
health status. Because the group C symptoms appear to represent the core of psychopathology in PTSD and have been shown to be the critical symptoms in crossing the diagnostic threshold, with group B and D criteria not performing in these
ways (North et al., 1999, 2002), a potentially useful paradigm might be to define
onset and remission based on the presence or absence of group C symptoms,
which have been found by Andrews's group (2009) to begin later than hyperarousal symptoms. The development of better paradigms for defining onset and
remission, and the testing of their validity, will be important for the success of
future research into the determinants of delayed onset and remission of PTSD.

Conclusions

Available data indicate that disaster exposure by itself does not account for all
of the PTSD that develops in relation to it. Preexisting personal psychological vulnerabilities appear to play a significant role in the development of PTSD
after disaster exposure. Two-thirds of the PTSD in Oklahoma City bombing survivors could potentially be explained by preexisting psychopathology in terms of

predisaster psychiatric disorders and personality characteristics (presuming, of course, that personality was consistent over time and that the measure actually provided a measure of preexisting personality in this sample). Although these predisaster psychological vulnerabilities appear to play an important role in the development of subsequent PTSD, even their contribution appears to be limited, based on the substantial proportions of those with PTSD who did not have these vulnerabilities (33%) and of bombing survivors without these vulnerabilities who developed PTSD (24%). Explanations for PTSD in the group without vulnerabilities, as well as for the apparent resilience among those with vulnerabilities but not PTSD, are needed. The multiple regression analysis presented in the Oklahoma City bombing survivors study suggests that disaster exposure severity as measured by physical injuries, other postdisaster stressors, and female sex are also significant contributors to PTSD, independent of the effects of preexisting psychopathology and personality characteristics. These other variables provide further potential explanations for the development of PTSD in survivors without personal psychiatric vulnerabilities and the resilience among survivors without these vulnerabilities.

Causality is not necessarily implied even in the face of strong statistical associations such as many of those found in association with disaster-related PTSD. Of course, where there is no association, causality cannot be found. For the significant associations found, however, an important question is how much causality can be attributed to them. The scientific validation of causal inference from epidemiologically demonstrated associations requires that one account for confounding variables; assess criteria for causality (examining strength, consistency, and specificity of the association), temporality (i.e., whether the causal factor occurred before the outcome), dose-response relationship, and biological plausibility; and consider alternative explanations (See, 2000). Multiple regression models examined in the Oklahoma City bombing study found education to be sex-mediated and predisaster psychiatric disorders to be personality-mediated in the prediction of PTSD. In these models, female sex, severity of disaster exposure (measured by the number of injuries as a proxy variable), number of intervening postdisaster stressful life events, and personality characteristics all yielded independent, significant prediction of PTSD, providing the causal inference elements of strength and specificity of these associations with PTSD. Findings from other trauma and disaster studies support the causal inference element of consistency for the association of PTSD with female sex, disaster exposure severity (injuries), and other stressful life events. The temporality criterion is met when the PTSD outcome occurs after the occurrence of these other variables. The dose-response relationship is met via the association of disaster exposure severity (number of injuries) with PTSD independent of the other variables. Thus, a great deal of evidence points to the independent direct contributions of female sex, disaster exposure, other stressful life events, and personality characteristics in the development of PTSD following exposure to disaster.

Despite the considerable potential explanation of PTSD provided by the collection of these independent variables, there remains a great deal of unexplained variance outside of the collection of these variables in the explanation of PTSD following disasters. There are a number of other variables not included in this model that might influence the course of psychiatric stability after disaster exposure, and many of these have been examined in previous research, such as other aspects of the exposure experience beyond what has been measured—for example, the amount of injury, the amount of life disruption caused by the disaster, community recovery, the receipt of mental health treatment, personal social support, coping skills, and cognitive processing of the experience. The causal effects of many of these variables are difficult to study because of extensive confounding with preexisting personal characteristics. In order to explain the frequent occurrence of failure to develop PTSD after disaster despite preexisting psychological vulnerabilities, an additional factor of personal resilience might be invoked. Although the concept of resilience is the subject of an extensive literature, this topic is beyond the scope of this chapter.

Untangling the causalities of delayed-onset forms of PTSD and of remission from PTSD includes considerations separate from those related to the development of PTSD after disaster. The definition of PTSD and the examination of its predictors are complicated enough by the unusual characteristics of the diagnosis delineated in this chapter, and defining onset and remission of PTSD and its predictors is further complicated by unresolved definitional issues that are destined to shape the predictors of these characteristics of PTSD in future determinations of criteria for these aspects of PTSD.

Disclosure Statement

C.S.N. wishes to disclose research funding from NIAAA, NIDDK, VA, the American Psychiatric Association, and the American Orthopaedic Association; speaker's fees from the Texas Department of State Health Services; and consultant fees from the University of Oklahoma Health Sciences Center and Tarrant County Public Health (Texas). Points of view in this document are those of the author(s) and do not necessarily represent the official position of the Department of Veterans Affairs or the United States Government.

References

American Psychiatric Association. (2000). *Diagnostic and Statistical Manual of Mental Disorders* (4th ed., text revision). Washington, DC.

Andrews, B., Brewin, C. R., Philpott, R., & Stewart, L. (2007). Delayed-onset posttraumatic stress disorder: A systematic review of the evidence. *American Journal of Psychiatry, 164,* 1319–1326.

Andrews, B., Brewin, C. R., Stewart, L., Philpott, R., & Hejdenberg, J. (2009). Comparison of immediate-onset and delayed-onset posttraumatic stress disorder in military veterans. *Journal of Abnormal Psychology, 118,* 767–777.

Blanchard, E. B., Hickling, E. J., Forneris, C. A., Taylor, A. E., Buckley, T. C., Loos, W. R., et al. (1997). Prediction of remission of acute posttraumatic stress disorder in motor vehicle accident victims. *Journal of Traumatic Stress, 10,* 215–234.

Breslau, N., Kessler, R. C., Chilcoat, H. D., Schultz, L. R., Davis, G. C., & Andreski, P. (1998). Trauma and posttraumatic stress disorder in the community: The 1996 Detroit area survey of trauma. *Archives of General Psychiatry, 55,* 626–632.

Buckley, T. C., Blanchard, E. B., & Hickling, E. J. (1996). A prospective examination of delayed onset PTSD secondary to motor vehicle accidents. *Journal of Abnormal Psychology, 105,* 617–625.

Cloninger, C. R. (1987). A systematic method for clinical description and classification of personality variants. A proposal. *Archives of General Psychiatry, 44,* 573–588.

DSM-5 Task Force. (2010). *DSM-5 development: 309.81 posttraumatic stress disorder.* American Psychiatric Association. Retrieved January 26, 2011, from http://www.dsm5.org/ProposedRevisions/Pages/proposedrevision.aspx?rid = 165

Gray, M. J., Bolton, E. E., & Litz, B. T. (2004). A longitudinal analysis of PTSD symptom course: Delayed-onset PTSD in Somalia peacekeepers. *Journal of Consulting and Clinical Psychology, 72,* 909–913.

Greenough, P. G., Lappi, M. D., Hsu, E. B., Fink, S., Hsieh, Y. H., Vu, A., et al. (2008). Burden of disease and health status among Hurricane Katrina-displaced persons in shelters: A population-based cluster sample. *Annals of Emergency Medicine, 51,* 426–432.

Hasin, D. S., Keyes, K. M., Hatzenbuehler, M. L., Aharonovich, E. A., & Alderson, D. (2007). Alcohol consumption and posttraumatic stress after exposure to terrorism: Effects of proximity, loss, and psychiatric history. *American Journal of Public Health, 97,* 2268–2275.

Horesh, D., Solomon, Z., Zerach, G., & Ein-Dor, T. (2010). Delayed-onset PTSD among war veterans: The role of life events throughout the life cycle. *Social Psychiatry and Psychiatric Epidemiology, 46,* 863–870.

Koren, D., Arnon, I., & Klein, E. (2001). Long term course of chronic posttraumatic stress disorder in traffic accident victims: A three-year prospective follow-up study. *Behavior Research and Therapy, 39,* 1449–1458.

Nagelkerke, N. J. D. (1991). A note on a general definition of the coefficient of determination. *Biometrika, 78,* 691–692.

Norris, F. H. (1992). Epidemiology of trauma: Frequency and impact of different potentially traumatic events on different demographic groups. *Journal of Consulting and Clinical Psychology, 60,* 409–418.

Norris, F. H., Friedman, M. J., Watson, P. J., Byrne, C. M., Diaz, E., & Kaniasty, K. (2002). 60,000 disaster victims speak: Part I. An empirical review of the empirical literature, 1981–2001. *Psychiatry, 65,* 207–239.

North, C. S. (2007). Epidemiology of disaster mental health response. In R. J. Ursano, C. S. Fullerton, L. Weisæth, & B. Raphael (Eds.), *Textbook of disaster psychiatry* (pp. 29–47). New York: Cambridge University Press.

North, C. S. (2011). Assessing the link between disaster exposure and mental illness. In L. B. Cottler (Ed.) *Mental health in public health* (pp. 104–117). New York: Oxford University Press.

North, C. S., Hong, B. A., & Pfefferbaum, B. (2008). P-FLASH: Development of an empirically-based post-9/11 disaster mental health training program. *Missouri Medicine, 105,* 62–66.

North, C. S., King, R. V., Fowler, R. L., Polatin, P., Smith, R. P., LaGrone, A., et al. (2008). Psychiatric disorders among transported hurricane evacuees: Acute-phase findings in a large receiving shelter site. *Psychiatric Annals, 38,* 104–113.

North, C. S., McCutcheon, V., Spitznagel, E. L., & Smith, E. M. (2002). Three-year follow-up of survivors of a mass shooting episode. *Journal of Urban Health, 79,* 383–391.

North, C. S., Nixon, S. J., Shariat, S., Mallonee, S., McMillen, J. C., Spitznagel, E. L., et al. (1999). Psychiatric disorders among survivors of the Oklahoma City bombing. *Journal of the American Medical Association, 282,* 755–762.

North, C. S., Pfefferbaum, B., Kawasaki, A., Lee, S., & Spitznagel, E. L. (2011). Psychosocial adjustment of directly exposed survivors 7 years after the Oklahoma City bombing. *Comprehensive Psychiatry, 52,* 1–8.

North, C. S., Surís, A. M., Davis, M., & Smith, R. P. (2009). Toward validation of the diagnosis of posttraumatic stress disorder. *American Journal of Psychiatry, 166,* 1–8.

Perkonigg, A., Pfister, H., Stein, M. B., Hofler, M., Lieb, R., Maercker, A., et al. (2005). Longitudinal course of posttraumatic stress disorder and posttraumatic stress disorder symptoms in a community sample of adolescents and young adults. *American Journal of Psychiatry, 162,* 1320–1327.

Prigerson, H. G., Maciejewski, P. K., & Rosenheck, R. A. (2001). Combat trauma: Trauma with highest risk of delayed onset and unresolved posttraumatic stress disorder symptoms, unemployment, and abuse among men. *Journal of Nervous and Mental Disease, 189,* 99–108.

Robins, L. N., Cottler, L. B., Compton, W. M., Bucholz, K., North, C. S., & Rourke, K. M. (2000). Diagnostic Interview Schedule for the DSM-IV (DIS-IV). St. Louis, MO: Washington University.

Schnurr, P. P., Lunney, C. A., & Sengupta, A. (2004). Risk factors for the development versus maintenance of posttraumatic stress disorder. *Journal of Traumatic Stress, 17,* 85–95.

See, A. (2000). Use of human epidemiology studies in proving causation. *Defense Counsel Journal, 4,* 478–487.

Smid, G. E., Mooren, T. T., van der Mast, R. C., Gersons, B. P., & Kleber, R. J. (2009). Delayed posttraumatic stress disorder: Systematic review, meta-analysis, and meta-regression analysis of prospective studies. *Journal of Clinical Psychiatry, 70,* 1572–1582.

Svrakic, D. M., Whitehead, C., Przybeck, T. R., & Cloninger, C. R. (1993). Differential diagnosis of personality disorders by the seven-factor model of temperament and character. *Archives of General Psychiatry, 50,* 991–999.

Zlotnick, C., Rodriguez, B. F., Weisberg, R. B., Bruce, S. E., Spencer, M. A., Culpepper, L., et al. (2004). Chronicity in posttraumatic stress disorder and predictors of the course of posttraumatic stress disorder among primary care patients. *Journal of Nervous and Mental Disease, 192,* 153–159.

10

Causal Thinking and Complex Systems Approaches for Understanding the Consequences of Trauma

MELISSA TRACY, MAGDALENA CERDÁ,
AND SANDRO GALEA

Despite recent advances in methods for causal inference and a large body of research on trauma victims, much remains to be understood about the causes and consequences of trauma. Existing epidemiologic approaches to causal inference are insufficient to capture the effects of complex relations between trauma and psychopathology, which affect each other and are affected by the situation of individuals in social networks and larger environments (Galea, Riddle, & Kaplan, 2010).

In this chapter, we describe the potential advantages of complex systems approaches for studying the consequences of trauma. We review the evidence demonstrating the need for such an approach, including the dynamic relations governing trauma and its consequences, the influence of connections between individuals on exposure and reactions to trauma, and the particular challenges of studying mass traumatic events. We also illustrate a complex systems approach to the study of trauma, using an agent-based model to examine the course of psychopathology under differing mass traumatic event conditions and to assess the influence of one's social network on risk for and consequences of traumatic event exposure.

Causal Inference in the Study of Trauma and its Consequences

Although exposure to some traumatic events is unpredictable and unavoidable, certain characteristics might predispose individuals to traumatic experiences (Breslau, Davis, & Andreski, 1995). In addition, reactions to trauma depend not only on the nature of the traumatic experience but on personal characteristics, the presence of support networks, the environment in which affected individuals reside, and numerous other factors (Brewin, Andrews, & Valentine, 2000). Understanding the consequences of trauma, then, requires careful consideration of the causes of both trauma exposure and reactions to trauma, including psychopathology such as post-traumatic stress disorder (PTSD).

Advances in methods for causal inference and analysis have enabled insight into potential causes of various health conditions. These advances include sufficient-component cause models for considering multiple causation, multilevel models for considering the influence of conditions beyond the individual on individual health, and counterfactual thinking and marginal structural models that allow one to better address potential confounding and time-varying relations between exposures and confounders. Although these methods have the potential to further our understanding of the causes and consequences of trauma, their limitations are likely to leave many challenging questions unanswered.

Multiple Causation and Sufficient-Component Cause Models

One challenge complicating the isolation of causes is the fact that a variety of causes work in conjunction to produce most disease. These multiple causes might originate at different levels (i.e., individual and community levels), and multiple combinations of causes might lead to the same outcome. In the case of psychopathology, a common consequence of exposure to trauma, causal candidates range from genetic factors to early life experiences to recent life events to residence in disadvantaged neighborhoods (Galea, Ahern, et al., 2007; Kendler, Karkowski, & Prescott, 1999; Shrout, 1998).

Sufficient-component cause models aim to delineate the various causal mechanisms sufficient to produce a particular disease, thereby identifying necessary causes (without which disease could never occur) and clarifying relations between component causes (Greenland & Brumback, 2002; Rothman, Greenland, Poole, & Lash, 2008). However, it is difficult to distinguish causal mechanisms without detailed data on intermediate factors operating between exposures and disease, which are often not available from typical epidemiologic studies (Greenland & Brumback, 2002). Furthermore, sufficient-component cause models are unable to adequately account for dynamic processes that influence disease, including interactions between individuals (Koopman & Lynch, 1999). Such processes, reflecting changes in individual behaviors and characteristics based on past experiences, as well as interactions with others, are critical for understanding exposure and reactions to trauma. Thus, sufficient-component cause models have limited utility for investigating the complex processes that underlie the relation between the causes and consequences of trauma.

Multilevel Determinants and Hierarchical Models

Factors operating beyond the individual level, including conditions in areas where individuals reside or otherwise spend their time, might have important influences on individual health. In the case of trauma, conditions of family and social networks and the neighborhoods in which individuals live can shape the response individuals have to the experience of trauma. For example, several studies have found that the risk of mental health problems associated with a history of victimization is stronger for residents of less violent and more affluent neighborhoods (Latzman & Swisher, 2005; Molnar, Browne, Cerdá, & Buka, 2005; Mrug & Windle, 2010). Although multilevel models (Diez Roux, 2000) have allowed the consideration of the effects of these kinds of group-level exposures on individual outcomes, they cannot be used to consider dynamic relations between individuals and the networks in which they exist (Auchincloss & Diez Roux, 2008; Galea et al., 2010). Such a gap is critical given that interpersonal relations and networks might affect the likelihood of exposure to primary and secondary sources of trauma, as well as the capacity of individuals to recover from such trauma. Furthermore, macro-level factors, such as municipal policies, also influence one's capacity to recover from trauma (particularly in the case of mass trauma), but the role of such factors is difficult to study with traditional analytic approaches, which would require data from multiple sites with varying policies and exposures.

Counterfactual Thinking and Marginal Structural Models

Formalization of the concept of counterfactuals, or potential outcomes models, for use in epidemiology (Maldonado & Greenland, 2002) has provided a useful platform for causal inference using observational data. Counterfactual measures compare two conditions, at least one of which is contrary to fact (Greenland & Brumback, 2002; Greenland et al., 2005; Maldonado & Greenland, 2002). For example, a counterfactual, or causal, contrast could measure the difference in PTSD prevalence between a population exposed to a mass traumatic event and the same population during the same time period had they not been exposed to that trauma. Because at least one of these conditions is contrary to fact (i.e., the population was either exposed or unexposed during a given time period), an estimate of the PTSD prevalence from a different population or from the same population at a different time must be substituted for the counterfactual condition in order to estimate the causal effect of exposure to the mass traumatic event on PTSD prevalence. The extent to which these substitute conditions match what would have occurred in the population of interest under the counterfactual scenario reflects the presence or absence of confounding (Maldonado & Greenland, 2002).

Randomized trials are often used to minimize potential confounding by assigning the exposure or treatment condition at random; however, certain exposures, including traumatic events, cannot be ethically studied in this way. Marginal structural models and propensity score matching attempt to replicate randomized trials using observational data, and marginal structural models in particular have the additional advantage of allowing some dynamic relations between exposures and potential confounders (Hernán et al., 2005; Robins, Hernán, & Brumback, 2000). However, these models are also unable to incorporate changing relations between individuals, which might play a crucial role in some processes, including trauma exposure and the development of psychopathology.

Causal inference in epidemiology, then, has been hampered by a lack of methods sufficient to adequately and simultaneously consider dynamic relations between multiple causes that originate across multiple levels and that are affected by dynamic connections between individuals. These complicated elements are characteristic of many health problems, but they are particularly salient for understanding trauma and psychopathology. The use of complex systems approaches is one possible way forward.

Advantages of Complex Systems Approaches

Complex systems approaches have several advantages over traditional regression-based models for the study of trauma and its consequences. Complex systems approaches are computational approaches that use computer-based algorithms to model dynamic interactions between individuals and between individuals and their environment (Galea, Hall, & Kaplan, 2009; Galea et al., 2010).

In this discussion, we focus on agent-based models (ABMs), one type of complex systems model, in which agents with a defined set of features interact with each other and their environment according to initial preset rules, with the possibility of adapting their behavior to changes in their environment, as well as based on their past history of experiences and interactions with other agents (Bonabeau, 2002; Gilbert, 2006). Emerging population-level patterns can then be compared under different behavioral rules and in agent populations with differing characteristics (Epstein, 1999; Epstein & Axtell, 1996). These models have been popular in fields outside the health sciences for decades and are frequently used in ecology, economics, political science, and sociology. A classic example of an ABM is Schelling's segregation model, which demonstrated that population-level patterns of residential segregation can emerge even when individual-level preferences do not favor segregation (Bruch & Mare, 2006; Schelling, 1978).

Features of Complex Systems Models

ABMs are characterized by agent heterogeneity and autonomy and by the incorporation of networks, dynamics, adaptation, and other forms of feedback. Agent heterogeneity allows agents to differ from each other on a range of characteristics, and agent autonomy allows each agent to operate independently of all other agents. Stochasticity can be incorporated when designating agent characteristics and behaviors (Auchincloss & Diez Roux, 2008), thereby moving beyond deterministic processes. These features enable the replication of real-world populations and their actions, including the generation of health states.

Interactions between individuals are explicitly part of ABMs, as are interactions between individuals and their environment. Embedding agents in social networks, neighborhoods, and other types of nonrandom relationships acknowledges multiple levels of influence on exposures and outcomes, including trauma and psychopathology.

The ability to incorporate adaptation and feedback, which is critical in many processes, is another key advantage of ABMs. Agent experiences and behaviors are influenced by past experiences and changes in the environment, allowing reciprocal relations between exposures and outcomes to be explicitly modeled rather than merely referred to under the specter of possible reverse causality.

Applying Complex Systems Approaches to Trauma and Psychopathology

These features of ABMs hold particular advantages for studying the consequences of trauma. For example, agent heterogeneity and autonomy reflect the reality of how individuals with different characteristics have differential risks of being exposed to certain types of traumatic experiences, and how they demonstrate variability in their reactions to the same traumatic event.

Adaptation and feedback in ABMs can also accommodate complex situations that mirror the complex realities of trauma exposure and psychopathology. For example, trauma and psychopathology are often thought to influence each other, and having a past history of psychopathology is a strong predictor of future psychopathology. Furthermore, exposure to a traumatic event might begin a cascade of circumstances that impact an individual's long-term health. These types of complex situations, with bidirectional relations and varying timing of different exposures, overwhelm the limits of regression-based methods but can be successfully investigated using ABMs.

Finally, the embedding of agents in social and community networks, with changes in those networks as time progresses, allows the consideration of the dynamic relations between network membership and trauma. For example, agents might react to a violent assault in their neighborhood by moving to a new location, disrupting their existing social networks but forming new social bonds in their new area, which might further change their exposure to traumatic events. Agent movement can also eventually change the character of the neighborhoods being both vacated and favored for relocation, altering the probability of exposure to violence among residents of those areas.

Counterfactual Thinking and Complex Systems Models

The population-level patterns emerging from the initial rules that govern agent reactions and interactions under varying circumstances might provide crucial insight into the processes that underlie the production of population health. Using a counterfactual approach, "experiments" can be run with ABMs in order to compare population patterns of disease under different conditions, including potential interventions and macro-level policies to mitigate the persistence or spread of disease or health behaviors (e.g., Halloran, Longini, Nizam, & Yang, 2002; Levy, Nikolayev, & Mumford, 2005). This approach allows the comparison of conditions in a more satisfying way than is typically possible with other types of causal models that consider counterfactuals because using ABMs, each condition could actually be observed in the same agent population, and complex relations could be explicitly included in the models (Auchincloss & Diez Roux, 2008; Galea et al., 2010). Thus, the true effects of the conditions or interventions might be more readily apparent with ABMs than when using other methods subject to confounding and other limitations.

Complex Relations in Exposure to and Consequences of Trauma

Research into trauma and its consequences, like research on psychopathology, is particularly suited to a complex systems approach because of the reciprocal relations between trauma and psychopathology, the influence of others on trauma risk and psychopathology risk, and the challenges of studying the long-term effects of mass traumatic events. The literature summarized here will be used to inform the development of an ABM that can extend our understanding of the consequences of trauma beyond what can be accomplished using traditional analytic approaches.

Dynamic Relations between Trauma and Psychopathology

Complex associations between trauma and psychopathology have challenged past research efforts. These complexities include reciprocal relations between trauma and psychopathology, multiple psychological consequences of traumatic events, and multiple stressors arising from traumatic experiences, all of which might influence psychopathology.

Reciprocal Relations between Trauma and Psychopathology

Studies of the consequences of trauma have long been plagued by the inability of researchers to adequately distinguish the directionality of trauma and psychopathology. Except for a limited number of studies with exceptionally detailed timing of events and symptoms (e.g., Grant, Yager, Sweetwood, & Olshen, 1982; Kendler, Karkowski, & Prescott, 1998), most work in this area relies on retrospective reports of stressful life events, including traumatic experiences, by individuals who might or might not exhibit psychological symptoms at the time of reporting (Kessler et al., 1997). These studies generally show support for the role of traumatic events in the onset and persistence of psychopathology, but they also provide evidence that psychopathology results in increased exposure to future life events, including trauma (Billings & Moos, 1982; Breslau, Davis, Peterson, & Schultz, 1997; Grant et al., 1982; Orcutt, Erickson, & Wolfe, 2002; Patton, Coffey, Posterino, Carlin, & Bowes, 2003).

Past experience of traumatic events also increases one's risk for subsequent traumas, independent of sociodemographic and personality characteristics that might influence trauma exposure (Breslau et al., 1995). Furthermore, past experience of psychopathology is a strong predictor of future psychopathology (e.g., Breslau, Peterson, & Schultz, 2008; Brewin et al., 2000; Grant, Patterson, Olshen, & Yager, 1987; Norris et al., 2002). Therefore, there are reciprocal relations between trauma and psychopathology, as well as strong feedback between past and future experiences of trauma and of psychopathology, that are difficult to incorporate using traditional analytic approaches. These cyclic, repeated patterns raise questions about the etiologic periods for trauma (i.e., how does the timing of exposure matter?), the directionality of the association between trauma and mental illness, and the effects of accumulated instances of trauma versus single exposures on psychopathology.

Multiple Psychological Reactions to Traumatic Experiences

Understanding relations between the different kinds of psychopathology that might arise after traumatic events has also proven to be quite challenging. For example, several competing hypotheses have been offered to explain the frequent co-occurrence of PTSD and depression after trauma: (1) one disorder leads to the other, (2) PTSD and depression are distinct consequences of exposure to trauma, or (3) co-occurrence is due to a common vulnerability to both PTSD and depression that arises from a set of factors that also increase vulnerability to traumatic exposures (Breslau, Davis, Peterson, & Schultz, 2000; Shalev et al., 1998). Similar questions arise about multiple other types of comorbid psychiatric disorders, including substance use disorders, conduct disorders, and forms of anxiety other than PTSD (de Graaf, Bijl, ten Have, Beekman, & Vollebergh, 2004a, 2004b; Fergusson, Goodwin, & Horwood, 2003; Hayatbakhsk et al., 2007; Hettema, Kuhn, Prescott, & Kendler, 2006; Moffitt et al., 2007; Windle and Davies, 1999). Complex systems approaches, which can test multiple hypotheses about the relation and sequencing of post-trauma psychopathology for consistency with observed patterns, might have an advantage over other studies attempting to distinguish between possible explanations for patterns of comorbidity.

Multiple Stressors Arising from Traumatic Experiences

Traumatic experiences include and trigger a wide variety of stressors that might elevate risk for mental health problems (Norris et al., 2002). These stressors range from experiences during the traumatic event—including perceived life threat, physical injury, and the witnessing of horrific scenes—to personal and financial loss resulting from traumatic events and ongoing health and financial problems and other hardships in the aftermath of traumatic events. Many studies combine these diverse stressors into measures of trauma exposure severity (e.g., Hardin, Weinrich, Weinrich, Hardin, & Garrison, 1994), which obscures the distinct effects of various experiences during and after traumatic events. Although it is difficult to assess these related stressors independently using traditional analytic techniques, particularly given their role as potential mediators between trauma exposure and psychopathology, there is increasing evidence that post-trauma stressors are critical in both the development and the persistence of psychopathology after trauma, over and above the influence of direct trauma experiences (Galea, Brewin, et al., 2007; Galea, Tracy, Norris, & Coffey, 2008; Nandi, Tracy, Beard, Vlahov, & Galea, 2009). Using complex systems approaches to overcome the limitations of traditional analyses investigating the mental health effects of the cascade of stressors triggered by traumatic events could inform appropriate post-trauma interventions.

An examination of the diverse stressors and consequences arising from traumatic experiences, and the dynamic relations between them, would be an important step forward in the field. Additional exploration of how these complex relations are affected by the links between individuals would be an even greater contribution.

The Influence of Social Networks on Exposure to and Consequences of Trauma

Consideration of the connections between individuals is critical to understanding the occurrence of certain behaviors and health conditions in populations.

In the classic case of infectious disease transmission, patterns of contact between individuals determine whether and how widely infections, such as sexually transmitted infections, are spread in a given population (e.g., Jolly, Muth, Wylie, & Potterat, 2001; Morris & Kretzschmar, 1997). Recent studies have also demonstrated the important role of social networks in transmitting noninfectious health conditions such as obesity (Christakis & Fowler, 2007).

It is increasingly clear that social networks also influence mental health (Greenblatt, Becerra, & Serafetinides, 1982; Kawachi & Berkman, 2001), with dynamic relations existing between social networks and corresponding social support, exposure to trauma, and psychopathology. In this discussion, the term "social network" primarily refers to an individual's close friends and family members who would be leaned on for support in times of need and whose life circumstances are of concern to the individual.

The Influence of Social Networks on Exposure to Trauma

At the most basic level, one's social network might promote certain behaviors, such as alcohol abuse or criminal activities, that put one at risk for serious accidents or violent encounters (e.g., Beck & Treiman, 1996; Fleisher & Krienert, 2004). One's personal social network is also embedded within larger networks that determine area levels of social cohesion and social capital (Kawachi & Berkman, 2001), which are thought to influence area levels of violence (Kennedy, Kawachi, Prothrow-Stith, Lochner, & Gupta, 1998; Sampson, Raudenbush, & Earls, 1997). Residing in an area with high levels of violence increases one's likelihood of being exposed to violence (Curry, Latkin, & Davey-Rothwell, 2008).

TRAUMATIC LOSS Social networks might also influence exposure to trauma through the sudden, unexpected death of a close friend or relative, which is listed among potential criterion stressors for PTSD in the *Diagnostic and Statistical Manual of Mental Disorders* (4th ed.) (*DSM-IV*) (American Psychiatric Association, 1994). Studies of traumatic bereavement have long highlighted the mental health consequences of unexpected deaths for surviving family members and friends, often focusing on deaths characterized by violence (i.e., accidents, suicides, homicides) and reactions including depression, complicated grief, and PTSD (Amick-McMullan, Kilpatrick, & Resnick, 1991; Kaltman & Bonnano, 2003; Murphy et al., 1999; Zisook, Chentsova-Dutton, & Shuchter, 1998). These traumatic loss experiences are quite common, with about one-quarter of most adult samples reporting at least one such experience in their lifetime (Frans, Rimmö, Åberg, & Fredrikson, 2005; Freedy et al., 2010; Norris, 1992). They also have significant mental health consequences. For example, about 14% of Detroit residents reporting a tragic loss in their lifetime met criteria for PTSD; this is lower than the risk of PTSD associated with assaultive violence events like being mugged, shot, or stabbed (21%) but higher than the risk of PTSD associated with other types of injuries or shocking events such as being in a serious car accident or witnessing a violent death or serious injury (6%) (Breslau et al., 1998; Breslau, Peterson, Poisson, Schultz, & Lucia, 2004).

SECONDARY TRAUMATIZATION The traumatic events experienced by members of one's social network might also increase risk for the development of psychopathology. Numerous studies have described the mental health effects of exposure to traumatic events experienced by others, alternatively termed "vicarious traumatization," "secondary traumatization," and "compassion fatigue." Most of these studies have focused on professionals exposed to details of the traumatic experiences of others through their work with trauma victims (e.g., mental health professionals, social workers) or those exposed to the immediate aftermath of a mass traumatic event (e.g., emergency services personnel and other rescue workers, journalists). This work clearly shows that traumatic deaths and injuries, as well as descriptions of traumatic experiences, can have long-term mental health consequences—including post-traumatic stress, anxiety, and depressive symptoms, as well as increased substance use and a disrupted sense of security—for individuals who are not related to the trauma victims other than through their professional or volunteer efforts (Figley, 1995; Lerias & Byrne, 2003; Palm, Polusny, & Follette, 2004; Perrin et al., 2007; Ursano, Fullerton, Kao, & Bhartiya, 1995).

Other studies have demonstrated the mental health impacts of traumatic events among family members, with a significant body of work focusing on psychological symptoms among the partners of soldiers traumatized by their combat experiences (e.g., Dirkzwager, Bramsen, Ader, & van der Ploeg, 2005; Solomon et al., 1992). The expansion of potentially traumatic events in *DSM-IV* criteria for PTSD (American Psychiatric Association, 1994) to include learning of traumatic events experienced by a close friend or relative has spurred further research into the prevalence of this type of trauma and its consequences. Estimates of the proportion of adults who report learning of a traumatic event to a close friend or relative in their lifetime have ranged from about 12% in a national U.S. sample (Kessler, Sonnega, Bromet, Hughes, & Nelson, 1995) to about 60% among Detroit residents aged 18 to 45 years (Breslau et al., 1998). Although these traumas are rarely rated as the "worst" or most distressing events by individuals who have experienced multiple traumas in their lifetime, they result in a nonnegligible burden of PTSD, with the conditional risk of PTSD related to learning of traumas to others ranging from about 3% (Breslau, 2009; Breslau et al., 1998, 2004) to about 10% among women (Kessler et al., 1995). This is consistent with prior work suggesting that vicarious traumatization usually results in less severe psychological reactions than direct traumatic experiences do (McCann & Pearlman, 1990; Motta, Joseph, Rose, Suozzi, & Leiderman, 1997).

The Influence of Trauma on Social Networks

Traumatic events might also influence social networks. An obvious example is the disruption of existing personal networks that occurs when a close friend or family member dies in an unexpected or violent manner (Kawachi & Berkman, 2001). Social networks might also deteriorate in the aftermath of mass traumatic events, particularly those requiring relocation or affecting communities as a whole, as networks are physically disrupted or simply overwhelmed by simultaneous needs (Bland et al., 1997; Kaniasty & Norris, 1993; Norris, Baker, Murphy, & Kaniasty, 2005). Violence in communities also has the potential to erode social cohesion in an area (Galea, Karpati, & Kennedy, 2002; Kawachi, 1999), which reflects the collapse of larger social networks in the area. Therefore, exposure to trauma can influence and be influenced by social networks. This is a particularly important issue if we are to understand how to best promote individual and community capacity for post-trauma recovery.

The Influence of Social Networks on Psychopathology

There is also a large body of evidence supporting the substantial direct effects of social networks, and primarily the various types of social support derived from those networks, on psychopathology (e.g., Greenblatt et al., 1982; Kessler & McLeod, 2002). Briefly, the influence of members of one's social network might encourage or discourage behaviors (e.g., physical activity) that promote psychological health; inclusion in a supportive network or, conversely, social isolation might also directly influence mental wellbeing (Kawachi & Berkman, 2001; Oxman, Berkman, Kasl, Freeman, & Barrett, 1992).

Of course, being embedded in a large social network does not guarantee mental health benefits. Network membership might actually be detrimental, for example, when one is faced with the demands of being in a caregiver role or otherwise obligated to one's network (Kawachi & Berkman, 2001) or when experiencing negative reactions from network members (e.g., blame, avoidance) or other failures on their part to provide assistance during times of need (Brown, Andrews, Harris, Adler, & Bridge, 1986; Guay, Billette, & Marchand, 2006; Kaniasty & Norris, 1993; Ullman & Filipas, 2001).

Numerous studies have investigated the effect of social networks and social support specifically during times of trauma and other stress, in line with theories that characterize social support as a stress-buffering factor, important only during such stressful times (Brown et al., 1986; Kawachi & Berkman,

2001). Although most of these studies are not longitudinal, these studies have generally found that individuals reporting greater social support or larger social network connections have a lower likelihood of psychopathology when exposed to traumatic experiences than individuals reporting lower levels of social support or fewer social network connections (e.g., Kaspersen, Matthiesen, & Götestam, 2003; Paykel, 1994). Recent meta-analyses of risk factors for PTSD have also identified social support as a strong predictor of PTSD among adults exposed to trauma (Brewin et al., 2000; Ozer, Best, Lipsey, & Weiss, 2003).

The Influence of Psychopathology on Social Networks

In yet another example of bidirectional relations, PTSD and other post-trauma psychopathology can affect social networks, as evidenced by numerous studies reporting a decrease in received and perceived social support over time among individuals with PTSD (Guay et al., 2006; Kaspersen et al., 2003). Psychological symptoms such as withdrawal and avoidance might directly reduce the frequency of social contacts; these and other symptoms might also strain existing relationships, further deteriorating support networks (Dirkzwager et al., 2005; Guay et al., 2006; Kaniasty & Norris, 1993; Kaspersen et al., 2003).

In summary, complicated and multidirectional relations exist among social networks, traumatic events, and post-trauma psychopathology. Existing approach-es, which generally treat social support as an unchanging characteristic of individuals (Galea et al., 2010) and aim to estimate the main effects of social support on mental health or consider social support as a mediator or moderator of relations between trauma and mental health, are clearly unable to adequately address and understand these complex relations. Complex systems approaches, with their ability to realistically model social networks, thus have great potential to further our understanding of how connections between individuals influence and are influenced by reactions to both individual and mass traumatic events.

Particular Challenges of Studying Mass Traumatic Events

Several reviews of post-disaster psychopathology have highlighted the particular challenges associated with studying the consequences of mass traumatic events (e.g., Galea, Nandi, & Vlahov, 2005; Norris et al., 2002). These challenges range from difficulty identifying incident cases of psychopathology to trouble synthesizing risk factors for psychopathology across differing mass traumatic events. Complex systems approaches could address some of these challenges while also shedding light on the utility of various post-disaster interventions for improving population mental health.

Lack of Information on Predisaster Psychological Functioning

Because of the unpredictable nature of mass traumatic events, information on the psychological health and preexisting risk factors of those exposed to such events is generally not available, except in a few instances in which existing samples were afflicted by disasters or other instances of mass violence (e.g., Cerdá, Tracy, & Galea, in press; Littleton, Grills-Taquechel, & Axsom, 2009; Norris & Murrell, 1988). Because PTSD is linked to specific events, cases of PTSD related to a mass traumatic event can technically be considered incident cases even among those with a prior history of PTSD resulting from other traumatic experiences. However, this ignores the potential role of prior PTSD or other dimensions of pretrauma functioning in determining responses to subsequent trauma, as well as the potential of current PTSD and other psychopathology to influence retrospective reports of past trauma, history of prior mental health problems, and other risk factors (Brewin et al., 2000; Galea et al., 2005). By utilizing a simulated population with known levels of predisaster psychopathology, ABMs could facilitate the direct assessment of changes in psychopathology after mass traumatic events.

Lack of Comparability across Mass Traumatic Events

Heterogeneity across mass traumatic events and the populations they affect make comparisons across such events challenging, further hindering the synthesis of information about risk factors for mental health consequences of these types of events. As noted by Galea et al. (2005), even ostensibly similar types of mass violence (i.e., bombings) might not be comparable in their effects, because they might occur in radically different settings, with different witnesses, victims, and shades of terror. Similarly, in areas that have experienced ongoing terrorism and mass violence (e.g., the Middle East), traumatic experiences themselves begin to fade as predictors of psychopathology. For example, in a study of Israeli residents exposed to ongoing terrorism, salient predictors of depressive symptoms were household income, social support, and economic loss resulting from terrorism, rather than direct exposure to or threat of traumatic experiences, which were commonplace among the individuals surveyed (Tracy, Hobfoll, Canetti-Nisim, & Galea, 2008). A single bus bombing taking place in an area unaccustomed to such violence would likely have a very different impact on the mental health of area residents than one taking place in a setting afflicted with ongoing terrorism. The characteristics of those affected by mass traumatic events, including their personal and community resources, influence their responses to and recovery from mass traumatic events, further complicating efforts to estimate the effects of these events. The ability of complex systems models to simulate alternate mass traumatic event scenarios in the same population followed over time could potentially address some of these challenges.

Difficulty Assessing Post-trauma Interventions

Finally, complex systems models can allow a comparison of the development and course of PTSD and other post-trauma psychopathology when different post-trauma interventions are employed in the population, similar to the use of these models to simulate the effects of different containment strategies for outbreaks of infectious diseases such as smallpox (Halloran et al., 2002) and different policy effects on smoking prevalence (Levy et al., 2005). In the case of mass disasters, individual- and community-level interventions could be compared, including crisis counseling, psychological first aid, and screening for symptoms during routine primary care visits (Everly, Phillips, Kane, & Feldman, 2006; Gibson et al., 2006; Ursano, Fullerton, & Norwood, 2003), using data from existing studies of the effects of these approaches. These models can offer valuable insight into the best intervention strategies under different mass traumatic event scenarios, depending on the extent of the destruction, the characteristics of those affected, and the recovery environment.

Illustrating a Complex Systems Approach to Understanding Trauma and Psychopathology

In order to further illustrate the potential of complex systems approaches for the study of trauma and psychopathology, we developed an ABM incorporating dynamic relations between individual and mass traumatic experiences and psychopathology, as well as multiple levels of influence, including social networks and neighborhoods. We use this model to (1) compare the longitudinal course of psychopathology in populations experiencing different mass traumatic event conditions and (2) explore how connections between individuals simultaneously influence both risk of traumatic experiences and consequences of those experiences.

Developing an Agent-Based Model of Trauma and Psychopathology

In describing our ABM, we aim to demonstrate how the literature summarized above, as well as existing data collected for other purposes, can be used to inform decisions about agent experiences and behaviors and dynamic relations between different levels of the model. This ABM includes only a small subset of the potential relations between agent, network, and neighborhood characteristics; trauma; and post-trauma psychopathology and thus addresses only a fraction of the questions that could be asked about trauma, psychopathology, and the influence of multiple levels. Although narrow in scope, this model clearly moves beyond the capabilities of traditional regression-based approaches, and its simplicity allows clear insights to emerge regarding the factors driving population mental health after mass traumatic events.

Agents, Households, Networks, and Neighborhoods

We first created a population of 2,000 adult agents (i.e., individuals) with the following characteristics: age, sex, race/ethnicity, educational attainment, marital status, household size, and household income. The ABM was developed using Recursive Porous Agent Simulation Toolkit software, which utilizes Java programming language. Baseline values were assigned so that the distribution of these characteristics in the agent population would match that in the U.S. population according to the 2000 U.S. Census (Bureau of the Census, 2000).

Agents were grouped into "households" ranging from one to seven members, with a household size of one reflecting an unmarried agent living alone. Agents were grouped via the following procedure: (1) Agents with a marital status of "married" were paired with another "married" agent who was within 10 years of the first agent's age; of the opposite sex; and of the same race/ethnicity, household size, and household income. (2) Additional "unmarried" agents were added to these married pairs in order to achieve the specified household size for each agent (these additional household members were matched based on their race/ethnicity, household size, and household income). (3) Remaining agents were joined to households, relaxing the race/ethnicity and household income criteria in order to satisfy household size criteria. Each agent household was then randomly assigned to a location within one of 16 neighborhoods of equal size on a 200 × 200 square grid. In this model, then, an agent's "neighbors" were all agents residing in the same neighborhood, rather than the more restricted range of agents occupying adjacent cells or cells within a certain radius on the grid, as in many ABMs (e.g., Bruch & Mare, 2006). The average household income in each neighborhood was calculated from the agent households residing in that neighborhood. The overall median household income for the 16 neighborhoods was identified; neighborhoods at or above this level were considered "high income," whereas those below the median were considered "low income." This is an example of how neighborhood characteristics can arise from the characteristics of neighborhood residents, although other area-level features without individual-level analogues (e.g., collective efficacy, presence of certain types of businesses or places for recreation, municipal policies) can also be considered in ABMs. Although agent households were randomly assigned to neighborhoods in this model, it is also possible to sort agents into neighborhoods based on their income or other characteristics.

Agents were assigned a particular number of close friends, ranging from zero to six or more, with the distribution as reported in the national 2004 General Social Survey (McPherson, Lovin-Smith, & Brashears, 2006). Close friends were matched to each agent based on geographic proximity (i.e., the probability of two agents residing a short distance apart being matched as close friends was considerably higher than the probability of two agents on opposite ends of the grid being joined in friendship). The size of each agent's social network was calculated as the sum of his or her household members and close friends. Agents with a greater than average number of family and friends were considered to have a high level of social ties, whereas those with social networks of below-average size were considered to have a low level of social ties.

The model so far thus consists of several levels of influence, with agents joined in friendship networks and nested in households that, in turn, are nested in neighborhoods, as depicted in Figure 10.1. This structure allows agents to be influenced by and to exert influence over each of these levels as the model progresses through time.

Agent Experiences during the Model

Each step of the ABM roughly represents one year in time. At each time step, then, agents aged by one year. Additionally, some agents died, based on all-cause mortality probabilities according to age, race/ethnicity, and sex for the 2000 U.S.

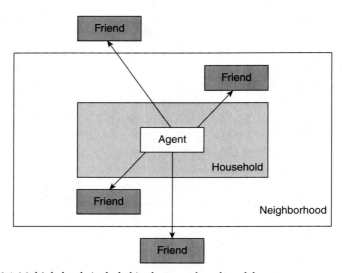

Figure 10.1 Multiple levels included in the agent-based model.

population (Miniño, Arias, Kochanek, Murphy, & Smith, 2002); these agents were "reborn" at the next time step as an unmarried 18-year-old agent with otherwise the same characteristics as the deceased agent. This allowed the agent population size to remain constant throughout the model run, although agent deaths disrupted social networks in a realistic manner and had other effects as described below.

INDIVIDUAL TRAUMATIC EXPERIENCES Besides aging and dying, agents experienced traumatic events and psychopathology during this illustrative model. At each time step, each agent had a certain probability of directly experiencing each of eight traumatic events: (1) natural disaster, (2) serious accident, (3) assault with a weapon, (4) assault without a weapon, (5) unwanted sexual contact, (6) serious illness or injury, (7) witnessing the serious injury or death of someone else, and (8) another extraordinarily stressful event. These are a subset of criterion A traumatic events potentially related to PTSD (American Psychiatric Association, 1994). The probability of experiencing each event was estimated from a population-based cohort study among residents of the New York City metropolitan area (Galea, Ahern, et al., 2008), so that an agent's probability of experiencing each event could be selected from a probability distribution specific to the agent's age, sex, race/ethnicity, marital status, education level, household income, and neighborhood income. The New York City metropolitan area cohort study used to estimate trauma probabilities included four interviews over a period of about three years (Galea, Ahern, et al., 2008). At each follow-up interview, participants were asked to report whether each of the eight traumatic events of interest had occurred since the last interview (about one year earlier). Three probabilities were calculated for each traumatic event based on the study participant's age, sex, race/ethnicity, (1) marital status, (2) education level, and (3) household income. These probabilities were used to rescale a β probability distribution with shape parameters $\alpha = 2$ and $\beta = 5$, also incorporating neighborhood income according to the following procedure: If an agent of a particular age, sex, and race/ethnicity resided in a "high income" neighborhood, his or her probability of trauma was selected from a $\beta(2,5)$ distribution rescaled to be bound by the lowest and highest of the three probabilities corresponding to the agent's marital status, education level, and household income. The $\beta(2,5)$ distribution is skewed to the right (i.e., the bulk of values lie to the left of the mean), thus favoring the selection of lower probabilities of trauma for residents of high-income neighborhoods. Conversely, if an agent resided in a "low income" neighborhood, the inverse of the $\beta(2,5)$ distribution was used so that probabilities in the higher end of the distribution would be favored. For example, black males ages 18–24 had a probability between 0 and 0.16 of witnessing a serious injury or violent death, and black females ages 25–34 had a probability between 0 and 0.04 of experiencing unwanted sexual contact. Estimated probabilities were consistent with previous studies finding younger age (Norris, 1992), less education, and black race (Breslau et al., 1995) to be associated with exposure to trauma. For simplification, the probabilities of exposure to trauma in this iteration of the model were not directly influenced by prior traumatic experiences or psychopathology, though additions described later allow for the indirect influence of prior trauma on future trauma and PTSD. Once an agent's probability of trauma was selected, a random number between 0 and 1 was selected. If this number was less than the agent's selected trauma probability, the agent experienced that traumatic event at that time step.

Two additional traumatic events were possible at each time step. If any member of the agent's social network (i.e., friends or household members) died, that agent experienced the trauma of the sudden death of a loved one at that time step. (We used all-cause mortality estimates as the basis for agent deaths in this model; these deaths would not necessarily be "sudden" in real life. Future iterations of the model could utilize rates of homicide, suicide, and accident mortality in order to more closely reflect tragic deaths.) Finally, if any member of the agent's social network experienced a traumatic event, the agent was designated as having experienced a secondary traumatic event, consistent with *DSM-IV* criteria, which includes learning of traumatic events to others as traumas in their own right (American Psychiatric Association, 1994). We distinguished secondary traumas from direct traumas because some studies suggest that learning of traumas to others is quite common in some populations (e.g., Breslau et al., 1998), and we aimed to track the prevalence of both direct and secondary trauma over time.

DEVELOPMENT AND RESOLUTION OF PTSD Agents who experienced traumatic events also had a certain probability of developing PTSD as a result of those events at any given time step. This probability was based on the type of traumatic event experienced and on the agent's age, sex, race/ethnicity, marital status, education level, household income, and prior history of PTSD (i.e., having had PTSD at any previous time step of the model). The probability of PTSD was calculated from a logistic regression equation developed using the same urban population-based study from which trauma probabilities were estimated. Information on the probability of PTSD given secondary trauma was not available from this study. In line with previous studies suggesting that secondary trauma is not associated with mental health consequences as severe as those resulting from direct trauma (Breslau et al., 1998; Kessler et al., 1995; McCann & Pearlman 1990), agents experiencing secondary trauma were assigned a probability of PTSD half that associated with experiencing any of the direct traumas in the model, again using a logistic regression equation including agent sociodemographic characteristics.

PTSD probabilities were further adjusted according to the agent's level of social ties, such that agents with low social ties had an increased probability of PTSD whereas those with high social ties had a decreased probability. Specifically, the probability of PTSD increased by 30% for an agent with low social ties (e.g., from 0.10 to 0.13) and decreased by 30% for an agent with high social ties (e.g., from 0.10 to 0.07). We are here expressly equating a large social network with a high level of positive social support, which is proven to have protective effects on mental health after trauma (Brewin et al., 2000; Ozer et al., 2003). Although this simplifying assumption ignores the possibility of small networks offering higher quality support than larger networks, as well as the potential for negative support from networks of any size, it allows social support to arise from connections between individuals, rather than be operationalized as a static characteristic of individuals. For traumatic events, a random number between 0 and 1 was selected; if this number was less than the agent's calculated probability of PTSD, the agent developed PTSD in that time step.

Resolution of PTSD was governed by an exponential decay function loosely based on patterns of symptom duration among untreated individuals with PTSD, as reported by Kessler et al. (1995). Resolution of PTSD among agents in the model was thus consistent with sharp declines in the first year after the development of symptoms, with more gradual declines thereafter (Breslau, 2009; Kessler et al., 1995).

SUMMARIZING AGENT EXPERIENCES An initial burn-in period of 10 time steps was run in order to develop a history of traumatic event experiences and psychopathology among agents; no other agent characteristics changed during this period. Following the burn-in period, the model was continued for 30 time steps in order to simulate the experiences of the agents during 30 years of life, thus providing a view of long-term population mental health in the context of traumatic experiences. At each time step, the following measures were calculated for the agent population: (1) the percentage of agents who directly experienced a traumatic event at that time step; (2) the percentage who experienced a secondary trauma; (3) the percentage who developed a new case of PTSD at that time step (these are considered incident cases even if agents had PTSD from another trauma earlier in the model run); (4) the total percentage with PTSD at that time step, combining both new and unresolved cases (i.e., PTSD prevalence); and (5) the percentage who had ever developed PTSD up to that time (i.e., cumulative incidence). We were thus able to graph the trajectory of trauma and PTSD over the course of each model run, as illustrated in Figure 10.2. Each model presented in this chapter was run 10 times, with results averaged across the 10 runs to ensure that results were not unduly influenced by any unusual pattern of results from a single model run.

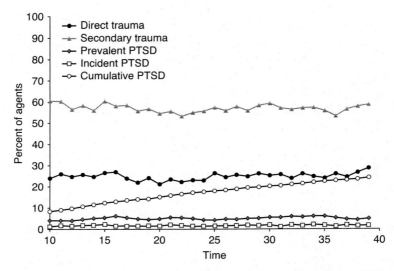

Figure 10.2 Trauma and PTSD prevalence, PTSD incidence, and cumulative PTSD incidence over one run of the agent-based model.

In this sample model run, the prevalence of direct and secondary trauma exposure in the population was around 25% and 55%, respectively. Annual PTSD incidence and prevalence were about 2% and 5%, respectively, and 24% of the population had developed PTSD at least once in their lifetime by the end of the model run. The average duration of PTSD was about 30 months. Although these numbers (particularly direct trauma exposure, PTSD prevalence, and duration of symptoms) are not without precedent (Breslau, 2009; Norris, 1992), they reflect the particular urban sample from which probabilities were calculated, as well as the assumptions governing PTSD occurrence and resolution in the model (e.g., all cases of PTSD resolve at the same rate). As we move on to demonstrate how this ABM can be used to address specific research questions, our focus is not on the absolute values observed in the model but rather on the prevalence of trauma and psychopathology in one model run relative to those observed in another model run, reflecting a comparison condition.

Model Summary

Relations among agent, network, and neighborhood characteristics and experiences are depicted in Figure 10.3. Summarizing the model thus far, heterogeneous agents are embedded in social networks consisting of the other members of their household and their close friends; the physical location in which they live

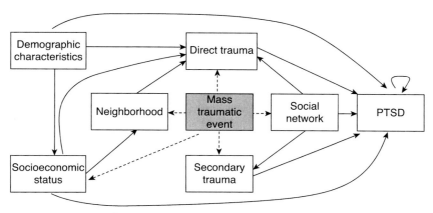

Figure 10.3 Diagram of relations in the agent-based model.

influences who their close friends are. The characteristics of their neighbors (i.e., income) influence their environment, which in turn affects their exposure to traumatic events. Agents' social networks also expose them to trauma through sudden deaths or their own traumatic events. PTSD risk varies according to the type of trauma experienced and the agent's characteristics; having many social ties decreases an agent's probability of developing PTSD. Once an agent has PTSD, he or she is more likely to develop PTSD when exposed to future traumatic events. We now add some additional features to the model in the interest of comparing the effects of different mass traumatic event conditions.

The Course of Psychopathology after Mass Traumatic Events

Our first research objective was to compare the patterns of PTSD across populations experiencing mass traumatic events of differing magnitude and severity. The use of our ABM, with its backdrop of typical individual traumatic experiences and corresponding psychopathology, will allow insights into how mass traumatic events change population levels of PTSD (by comparing PTSD rates in the same population before and after the mass trauma) and how different types of mass traumatic events influence the long-term burden of psychopathology in the affected populations. The "experiments" we describe here could not be replicated in real-world populations and thus overcome some of the central challenges facing disaster research, including the creation of a counterfactual to exposure to a mass traumatic event, accounting for pretrauma psychiatric conditions, and accounting for the interdependent effects of social networks on the likelihood of exposure to trauma and subsequent psychopathology. In the models that follow, we focus on mass traumatic events occurring at one point in time, reflecting a natural disaster or single act of terrorism, rather than situations of ongoing mass violence. Agents residing in the four neighborhoods in the center of the agent physical space (about 25% of the agent population) were directly exposed to the mass traumatic event. We also ran models with mass traumatic events affecting different proportions of the populations (25%, 50%, 75%) and (when agents were sorted into neighborhoods by income) affecting only low- or high-income areas. The substantive findings from these models were similar to those from models with mass traumatic events affecting the central four neighborhoods.

Mass Traumatic Event without Other Repercussions

First, we consider a mass traumatic event that occurs with no other tangible repercussions—it happens, agents are exposed to it, and there are no other direct consequences such as property damage or displacement. An example of this type of trauma would be a mass shooting (e.g., Littleton et al., 2009), which traumatizes survivors through the horrific scenes they witnessed but doesn't directly result in any financial or other tangible losses. The probability of developing PTSD from this mass traumatic event was based on the affected agents' sociodemographic characteristics and prior history of PTSD, using a logistic regression equation among participants in the aforementioned cohort study (Galea, Ahern, et al., 2008) who lived close to the site of the September 11 terrorist attacks.

Figure 10.4 shows the PTSD incidence at each time step for a population experiencing such a mass traumatic event at time 15 and one experiencing no mass traumatic event. In the population with no mass traumatic event, the PTSD incidence remained constant throughout the model run as agents experienced direct and secondary traumas at typical levels. In the population exposed to a mass traumatic event, there was a spike in new cases of PTSD at time 15 as those exposed to the mass traumatic event developed post-traumatic stress reactions to their experiences. This is not surprising, as many studies have documented an elevated incidence of PTSD after disasters (Galea et al., 2005; Galea, Tracy, et al., 2008). However, an examination of the "years" following the mass traumatic event indicates that the PTSD incidence remained elevated in the population for the remainder of the model run; that is, new cases of PTSD continued to arise at a higher-than-expected rate after the population was exposed to a mass traumatic event. Delayed-onset cases of PTSD (Andrews, Brewin, Philpott, & Stewart, 2007) are not supported by our model, which assumes that agents develop PTSD from a particular traumatic event in the same time step in which the event occurs. Therefore, these new cases of PTSD are related to traumas other than the mass traumatic event that occurred at time 15.

What could explain this elevated PTSD incidence? One explanation offered by the ABM, incorporating feedback, is that a history of PTSD, built up in the

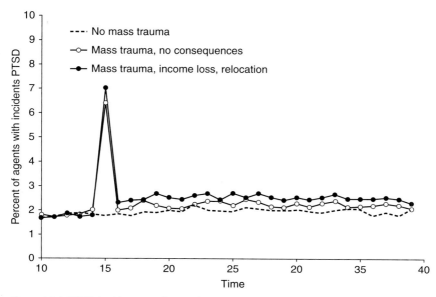

Figure 10.4 PTSD incidence under varying mass traumatic event scenarios.

population through the occurrence of the mass traumatic event, increases the likelihood that individuals will respond to future traumatic events with PTSD. This finding indicates that mass traumatic events are significant for population mental health, not only because of their direct influence on psychological symptoms but because of their ability to initiate a cycle of psychopathology. This can be further demonstrated by another addition to our model, in which we consider a mass traumatic event with tangible consequences for affected populations.

Mass Traumatic Event Leading to Other Stressors

In this second mass traumatic event scenario, agents who were exposed to the mass traumatic event also experienced a drop in their income level, reflecting the financial loss that frequently results from a disaster. Affected agents might also be displaced to a different neighborhood on the grid, with the probability of relocation dependent on their income level and the size of their social network. Although displaced agents moved together with their households, they lost their connections to close friends and were considered to have a low level of social ties for the remainder of the model. This type of mass traumatic event reflects a natural disaster like a hurricane, which might make some properties uninhabitable, leading to extended displacement, and might result in substantial property damage and job loss (e.g., Galea, Tracy, et al., 2008). This scenario is depicted in

Figure 10.3, in which a mass traumatic event not only comprises direct and secondary exposure to trauma in the population but influences socioeconomic status, neighborhood location and characteristics, and social network ties.

Figure 10.4 also shows the trajectory of PTSD incidence in the population experiencing this type of mass traumatic event at time 15. Again there was a spike in PTSD incidence at time 15, and again PTSD incidence remained elevated for the remainder of the model, but at even higher levels than when a mass traumatic event occurred without major repercussions. Similar patterns have been observed for the duration of symptoms after mass traumatic events, with health problems persisting at the highest levels among the subset of individuals who were forced to relocate after a mass traumatic event, but with nonrelocated victims also experiencing health problems at higher levels than a control group (Yzermans et al., 2005). However, as noted above, the patterns observed in the ABM reflect not prevalent cases of PTSD that are persisting over time but rather new cases of PTSD resulting from later traumatic experiences. In addition to the influence of one's past history of PTSD on risk for future PTSD, these results suggest that mass traumatic events might initiate a cascade of events that put affected individuals at increased risk for other traumatic experiences. In this example, experiencing a loss of income leads to an increased probability of trauma, as well as increased vulnerability to PTSD after exposure to trauma; agents might relocate to lower income neighborhoods, which also increases their exposure to trauma, and relocated agents experience a decline in social support, which increases their susceptibility to PTSD when exposed to future traumatic events. The combination of these forces results in an even greater susceptibility to PTSD in the face of future traumatic events in the population.

Several recent studies have highlighted the importance of postdisaster stressors, such as financial loss and displacement, for the development and maintenance of psychopathology after such events (Galea, Brewin, et al., 2007; Galea, Tracy, et al., 2008b). The use of an ABM has furthered this work by clarifying the substantial role of these posthurricane stressors as triggers of new traumas and new cases of psychopathology, related only indirectly to the original mass traumatic event. Future empirical studies focusing on the implications of posthurricane stressors for new cases of PTSD and other mental health problems in the aftermath of mass traumatic events might lend important insights into who should be targeted by postdisaster interventions in order to maximize long-term population mental health.

The Influence of Social Networks on Trauma and Psychopathology

Our second research objective was to examine the influence of social networks on trauma and psychopathology. A complex systems approach has the advantage of simultaneously accounting for the potentially competing effects of social networks on both trauma exposure and risk for PTSD following trauma exposure. We repeated the model outlined above, with about 25% of the population affected by a mass traumatic event in the four central neighborhoods at time 15, but varying the proportion of agents with a high level of social ties. We focus on results from three of these models for illustrative purposes.

In the first model, 50% of the agent population had a high level of social ties. This is the default condition in the model because agents with a social network that is at or above the average size are considered to have high social ties. In the second and third models, 90% and 10% of the agent population had a high level of social ties, respectively. Together, these three models allowed us to compare trajectories of trauma and PTSD in populations with low, medium, and high social ties and, in particular, to examine whether the protection offered by a high level of social ties outweighed the increased exposure to trauma that such close ties might entail.

As indicated in Table 10.1, populations with higher levels of social ties (i.e., models in which 50% and 90% of the population had a large social network) were exposed to more traumas, both directly (reflecting the influence of the deaths of network members) and indirectly (reflecting secondary traumas that occur when people learn of traumas to family members and close friends). However, the annual PTSD prevalence and incidence, as well as the cumulative PTSD incidence over the course of the model, remained lower in populations with higher levels of social ties, despite increased exposure to trauma in these populations. These results suggest that the benefits of a high level of social ties, in terms of protection against PTSD, outweigh the hazards associated with having a large social network. These results held true when considering mass traumatic events resulting in income loss and potential displacement, as well as in populations not affected by a mass traumatic event. Although in these models we did not address additional relations that might be of import (e.g., the possibility that chronic PTSD symptoms strain relationships, leading to a disruption

Table 10.1 Trauma and PTSD Prevalence, PTSD Incidence, and Cumulative PTSD Incidence in Agent Populations with Varying Levels of Social Ties

Level of social ties in the population	Percentage with high social ties	Average percentage directly exposed to trauma	Average percentage exposed to secondary trauma	Average PTSD prevalence	Average PTSD incidence	Cumulative PTSD incidence
Low	10	25.4	56.5	7.8	3.9	32.5
Medium	50	26.8	67.0	6.6	2.4	29.5
High	90	28.3	77.7	5.7	2.0	27.1

of social networks and the breakdown of social support), our results are a first step toward better understanding the delicate balance between social networks as a risk factor for trauma exposure and as a protective factor against psychopathology after trauma.

Taken together, explorations of these two research questions demonstrate the utility of complex systems approaches like ABMs for studying the potential consequences of mass traumatic events, including for comparing the long-term burden of psychopathology after events with differing circumstances and for considering the dynamic effects that connections between individuals can have on both exposure and reactions to trauma. Running models as counterfactual "experiments," varying one condition while leaving other characteristics constant, allows the extension of research on trauma and psychopathology beyond what is possible in real-world populations and settings. Besides demonstrating the importance of accounting for feedback and network connections, these illustrative models suggest further avenues for future empirical work.

Conclusions

In this chapter, we have summarized the challenges surrounding causal thinking in epidemiology, with particular application to trauma and psychopathology. We have described the potential advantages of complex systems approaches to dealing with these challenges, as well as the aspects of trauma and psychopathology that are particularly conducive to complex systems approaches. We illustrate the use of these methods with an ABM designed to shed light on the effect of different mass traumatic event conditions on PTSD over time, and on the complex role of social networks as risk and protective factors for PTSD. Our findings demonstrate the utility of complex systems approaches for understanding the causes and consequences of trauma, providing insight into avenues for future empirical research, as well as important targets for post-trauma interventions.

Disclosure Statement

The authors have no conflicts of interest to disclose.

References

American Psychiatric Association. (1994). *Diagnostic and statistical manual of mental disorders* (4th ed.). Washington, DC: Author.

Amick-McMullan, A., Kilpatrick, D. G., & Resnick, H. S. (1991). Homicide as a risk factor for PTSD among surviving family members. *Behavior Modification*, 15(4), 545–549.

Andrews, B., Brewin, C. R., Philpott, R., & Stewart, L. (2007). Delayed-onset posttraumatic stress disorder: A systematic review of the evidence. *American Journal of Psychiatry*, 164(9), 1319–1326.

Auchincloss, A. H., & Diez Roux, A. V. (2008). A new tool for epidemiology: The usefulness of dynamic-agent models in understanding place effects on health. *American Journal of Epidemiology*, 168(1), 1–8.

Beck, K. H., & Treiman, K. A. (1996). The relationship of social context of drinking, perceived social norms, and parental influence to various drinking patterns of adolescents. *Addictive Behavior*, 21(5), 633–644.

Billings, A. C., & Moos, R. H. (1982). Stressful life events and symptoms: A longitudinal model. *Health Psychology*, 1(2), 99–117.

Bland, S. H., O'Leary, E. S., Farinaro, E., Jossa, F., Krogh, V., Violanti, J., et al. (1997). Social network disturbances and psychological distress following earthquake evacuation. *Journal of Nervous and Mental Disease*, 185(3), 188–195.

Bonabeau, E. (2002). Agent-based modeling: Methods and techniques for simulating human systems. *Proceedings of the National Academy of Sciences of the United States of America*, 99(Suppl 3), 7280–7287.

Breslau, N. (2009). The epidemiology of trauma, PTSD, and other posttrauma disorders. *Trauma, Violence, & Abuse*, 10, 198–210.

Breslau, N., Davis, G. C., & Andreski, P. (1995). Risk factors for PTSD-related traumatic events: A prospective analysis. *American Journal of Psychiatry*, 152, 529–535.

Breslau, N., Davis, G. C., Peterson, E. L., & Schultz, L. R. (1997). Psychiatric sequelae of posttraumatic stress disorder in women. *Archives of General Psychiatry*, 54, 81–87.

Breslau, N., Davis, G. C., Peterson, E. L., & Schultz, L. R. (2000). A second look at comorbidity in victims of trauma: The posttraumatic stress disorder-major depression connection. *Biological Psychiatry*, 48, 902–909.

Breslau, N., Kessler, R. C., Chilcoat, H. D., Schultz, L. R., Davis, G. C., & Andreski, P. (1998). Trauma and posttraumatic stress disorder in the community: The 1996 Detroit Area Survey. *Archives of General Psychiatry*, 55, 626–632.

Breslau, N., Peterson, E. L., Poisson, L. M., Schultz, L. R., & Lucia, V. C. (2004). Estimating post-traumatic stress disorder in the community: Lifetime perspective and the impact of typical traumatic events. *Psychological Medicine*, 34, 889–898.

Breslau, N., Peterson, E. L., & Schultz, L. R. (2008). A second look at prior trauma and the posttraumatic stress disorder effects of subsequent trauma: A prospective epidemiological study. *Archives of General Psychiatry*, 65(4), 431–437.

Brewin, C. R., Andrews, B., & Valentine, J. D. (2000). Meta-analysis of risk factors for post-traumatic stress disorder in trauma-exposed adults. *Journal of Consulting and Clinical Psychology*, 68, 748–766.

Brown, G. W., Andrews, B., Harris, T., Adler, Z., & Bridge, L. (1986). Social support, self-esteem and depression. *Psychological Medicine*, 16(4), 813–831.

Bruch, E. E, & Mare, R. D. (2006). Neighborhood choice and neighborhood change. *American Journal of Sociology*, 112(3), 667–709.

Bureau of The Census (2000). STF3A FILES.

Cerdá, M., Tracy, M., & Galea, S. (in press). A prospective population based study of changes in alcohol use and binge drinking after a mass traumatic event. *Drug and Alcohol Dependence*.

Christakis, N. A., & Fowler, J. H. (2007). The spread of obesity in a large social network over 32 years. *New England Journal of Medicine*, 357, 370–379.

Curry, A., Latkin, C., & Davey-Rothwell, M. (2008). Pathways to depression: The impact of neighborhood violent crime on inner-city residents in Baltimore, Maryland, USA. *Social Science and Medicine*, 67(1), 23–30.

de Graaf, R., Bijl, R. B., ten Have, M., Beekman, A. T., & Vollebergh, W. A. (2004a). Pathways to comorbidity: The transition of pure mood, anxiety and substance use disorders into comorbid conditions in a longitudinal population-based study. *Journal of Affective Disorder*, 82(3), 461–467.

de Graaf, R., Bijl, R. B., ten Have, M., Beekman, A. T., & Vollebergh, W. A. (2004b). Rapid onset of comorbidity of common mental disorders: Findings from the Netherlands Mental Health Survey and Incidence Study (NEMESIS). *Acta Psychiatrica Scandinavica*, 109(1), 55–63.

Diez Roux, A. V. (2000). Multilevel analysis in public health research. *Annual Review of Public Health*, 21, 171–192.

Dirkzwager, A. J. E., Bramsen, I., Ader, H., & van der Ploeg, H. M. (2005). Secondary traumatization in partners and parents of Dutch peacekeeping soldiers. *Journal of Family Psychology*, 19(2), 217–226.

Epstein, J. M. (1999). Agent-based computational models and generative social science. *Complexity*, 4(5), 41–60.

Epstein, J. M., & Axtell, R. (1996). *Growing artificial societies: Social science from the bottom up.* Washington, DC: Brookings Institution Press.

Everly, G. S., Jr., Phillips, S. B., Kane, D., & Feldman, D. (2006). Introduction to and overview of group psychological first aid. *Brief Treatment and Crisis Intervention*, 6(2), 130–136.

Fergusson, D. M., Goodwin, R. D., & Horwood, L. J. (2003). Major depression and cigarette smoking: Results of a 21-year longitudinal study. *Psychological Medicine*, 33(8), 1357–1367.

Figley, C. R. (1995). *Compassion fatigue: Coping with secondary traumatic stress disorder in those who treat the traumatized.* New York: Brunner-Routledge.

Fleisher, M. S., & Krienert, J. L. (2004). Life-course events, social networks, and the emergence of violence among female gang members. *Psychological Medicine*, 32(5), 607–622.

Frans, Ö., Rimmö, P.-A., Åberg, L., & Fredrikson, M. (2005). Trauma exposure and post-traumatic stress disorder in the general population. *Acta Psychiatrica Scandinavica*, 111, 291–299.

Freedy, J. R., Magruder, K. M., Zoller, J. S., Hueston, W. J., Carek, P. J., & Brock, C. D. (2010). Traumatic events and mental health in civilian primary care: Implications for training and practice. *Family Medicine Journal*, 42(3), 185–192.

Galea, S., Ahern, J., Nandi, A., Tracy, M., Beard, J., & Vlahov, D. (2007). Urban neighborhood poverty and the incidence of depression in a population-based cohort study. *Annals of Epidemiology*, 17(3), 171–179.

Galea, S., Ahern, J., Tracy, M., Hubbard, A., Cerdá, M., Goldmann, E., et al. (2008) Longitudinal determinants of post-traumatic stress in a population-based cohort study. *Epidemiology*, 19, 47–54.

Galea, S., Brewin, C. R., Gruber, M., Jones, R. T., King, D. W., King, L. A., et al. (2007). Exposure to hurricane-related stressors and mental illness after Hurricane Katrina. *Archives of General Psychiatry*, 64(12), 1427–1434.

Galea, S., Hall, C., & Kaplan, G. A. (2009). Social epidemiology and complex system dynamic modeling as applied to health behaviour and drug use research. *International Journal of Drug Policy*, 20, 209–216.

Galea, S., Karpati, A., & Kennedy, B. (2002). Social capital and violence in the United States, 1974–1993. *Social Science and Medicine,* 55, 1373–1383.

Galea, S., Nandi, A., & Vlahov, D. (2005). The epidemiology of post-traumatic stress disorder after disasters. *Epidemiologic Reviews,* 27, 78–91.

Galea, S., Riddle, M., & Kaplan, G. A. (2010). Causal thinking and complex system approaches in epidemiology. *International Journal of Epidemiology,* 39(1), 97–106.

Galea, S., Tracy, M., Norris, F., & Coffey, S. F. (2008). Financial and social circumstances and the incidence and course of PTSD in Mississippi during the first two years after Hurricane Katrina. *Journal of Traumatic Stress,* 21(4), 357–368.

Gibson, L. E., Ruzek, J. I., Naturale, A. J., Watson, P. J., Bryant, R. A., Rynearson, T., et al. (2006). Interventions for individuals after mass violence and disaster: Recommendations from the roundtable on screening and assessment, outreach, and intervention for mental health and substance abuse needs following disasters and mass violence. *Journal of Trauma Practice,* 5(4), 1–28.

Gilbert, N. (2006). *Agent-based models.* Thousand Oaks, CA: Sage.

Grant, I., Patterson, T., Olshen, R., & Yager, J. (1987). Life events do not predict symptoms: Symptoms predict symptoms. *Journal of Behavioral Medicine,* 10(3), 231–240.

Grant, I., Yager, J., Sweetwood, H. L., & Olshen, R. (1982). Life events and symptoms: Fourier analysis of time series from a three-year prospective inquiry. *Archives of General Psychiatry,* 39, 598–605.

Greenblatt, M., Becerra, R. M., & Serafetinides, E. A. (1982). Social networks and mental health: An overview. *American Journal of Psychiatry,* 139, 977–984.

Greenland, S. (2005). Epidemiologic measures and policy formulation: Lessons from potential outcomes. *Emerging Themes in Epidemiology,* 2, 5.

Greenland, S., & Brumback, B. (2002). An overview of relations among causal modeling methods. *International Journal of Epidemiology,* 31(5), 1030–1037.

Guay, S., Billette, V., & Marchand, A. (2006). Exploring the links between posttraumatic stress disorder and social support: Processes and potential research avenues. *Journal of Traumatic Stress,* 19(3), 327–338.

Halloran, M. E., Longini, I. M., Jr., Nizam, A., & Yang, Y. (2002). Containing bioterrorist smallpox. *Science,* 298(5597), 1428–1432.

Hardin, S., Weinrich, M., Weinrich, S., Hardin, T., & Garrison, C. (1994). Psychological distress of adolescents exposed to Hurricane Hugo. *Journal of Traumatic Stress,* 7, 427–440.

Hayatbakhsh, M. R., Najman, J. M., Jamrozik, K., Mamun, A. A., Alati, R., & Bor, W. (2007). Cannabis and anxiety and depression in young adults: A large prospective study. *Journal of the American Academy of Child and Adolescent Psychiatry,* 46(3), 408–417.

Hernán, M. A. (2005). Invited commentary: Hypothetical interventions to define causal effects—Afterthought or prerequisite? *American Journal of Epidemiology,* 162(7), 618–620.

Hettema, J. M., Kuhn, J. W., Prescott, C. A., & Kendler, K. S. (2006). The impact of generalized anxiety disorder and stressful life events on risk for major depressive episodes. *Psychological Medicine,* 36(6), 789–795.

Jolly, A. M., Muth, S. Q., Wylie, J. L., & Potterat, J. J. (2001). Sexual networks and sexually transmitted infections: A tale of two cities. *Journal of Urban Health,* 78(3), 433–445.

Kaltman, S., & Bonnano, G. A. (2003). Trauma and bereavement: Examining the impact of sudden and violent deaths. *Journal of Anxiety Disorders,* 17, 131–147.

Kaniasty, K., & Norris, F. H. (1993). A test of the social support deterioration model in the context of natural disaster. *Journal of Personality and Social Psychology,* 64, 395–408.

Kaspersen, M., Matthiesen, S. B., & Götestam, K. G. (2003). Social network as a moderator in the relation between trauma exposure and trauma reaction: A survey among UN soldiers and relief workers. *Scandinavian Journal of Psychology*, 44, 415–423.

Kawachi, I. (1999). Social capital and community effects on population and individual health. In N. E. Adler, M. Marmot, B. S. McEwen, & J. Stewart (Eds.), *Socioeconomic status and health in industrial nations: Social, psychological and biological pathways* (pp. 124–137). New York: New York Academy of Sciences.

Kawachi, I., & Berkman, L. F. (2001). Social ties and mental health. *Journal of Urban Health*, 78(3), 458–467.

Kendler, K. S., Karkowski, L. M., & Prescott, C. A. (1998). Stressful life events and major depression: Risk period, long-term contextual threat, and diagnostic specificity. *Journal of Nervous and Mental Disease*, 186(11), 661–669.

Kendler, K. S., Karkowski, L. M, & Prescott, C. A. (1999). Causal relationship between stressful life events and the onset of major depression. *American Journal of Psychiatry*, 156, 837–841.

Kennedy, B. P., Kawachi, I., Prothrow-Stith, D., Lochner, K., & Gupta, V. (1998). Social capital, income inequality and firearm violent crime. *Social Science and Medicine*, 47, 7–17.

Kessler, R. C. (1997). The effects of stressful life events on depression. *Annual Review of Psychology*, 48, 191–214.

Kessler, R. C., & McLeod, J. D. (2002). Social support and mental health in community samples. In S. Cohen & S. L. Syme (Eds.), *Social support and health*. New York: Academic Press.

Kessler, R. C., Sonnega, A., Bromet, E., Hughes, M., & Nelson, C. B. (1995). Posttraumatic stress disorder in the National Comorbidity Survey. *Archives of General Psychiatry*, 52, 1048–1060.

Koopman, J. S., & Lynch, J. W. (1999). Individual causal models and population system models in epidemiology. *American Journal of Public Health*, 89, 1170–1174.

Latzman, R., & Swisher, R. (2005). The interactive relationship among adolescent violence, street violence and depression. *Journal of Community Psychology*, 33, 355–371.

Lerias, D., & Byrne, M. K. (2003). Vicarious traumatization: Symptoms and predictors. *Stress and Health*, 19(3), 129–138.

Levy, D. T., Nikolayev, L., & Mumford, E. (2005). Recent trends in smoking and the role of public policies: Results from the SimSmoke tobacco control policy simulation model. *Addiction*, 100(10), 1526–1535.

Littleton, H., Grills-Taquechel, A., & Axsom, D. (2009). Resource loss as a predictor of posttrauma symptoms among college women following the mass shooting at Virginia Tech. *Violence and Victims*, 24(5), 669–686.

Maldonado, G., & Greenland, S. (2002). Estimating causal effects. *International Journal of Epidemiology*, 31, 422–429.

McCann, I. L., & Pearlman, A. (1990). Vicarious traumatization: A framework for understanding the psychological effects of working with victims. *Journal of Traumatic Stress*, 3, 131–149.

McPherson, M., Lovin-Smith, L., & Brashears, M. E. (2006). Social isolation in America: Changes in core discussion networks over two decades. *American Sociological Review*, 71, 353–375.

Miniño, A. M., Arias, E., Kochanek, K. D., Murphy, S. L., & Smith, B. L. (2002). Deaths: Final data for 2000. *National Vital Statistics Report*, 50(15), 1–119.

Moffitt, T. E., Caspi, A., Harrington, H., Milne, B. J., Melchior, M., Goldberg, D., et al. (2007). Generalized anxiety disorder and depression: Childhood risk factors in a birth cohort followed to age 32. *Psychological Medicine*, 37(3), 441–452.

Molnar, B. E., Browne, A., Cerdá, M., & Buka, S. L. (2005). Violent behavior by girls reporting violent victimization: A prospective study. *Archives of Pediatric Adolescent Medicine,* 159(8), 731–739.

Morris, M., & Kretzschmar, M. (1997). Concurrent partnerships and the spread of HIV. *AIDS,* 11(5), 641–648.

Motta, R., Joseph, J., Rose, R., Suozzi, J., & Leiderman, L. (1997). Secondary trauma: Assessing intergenerational transmission of war experiences with a modified Stroop procedure. *Journal of Clinical Psychology,* 53, 895–903.

Mrug, S., & Windle, M. (2010). Prospective effects of violence exposure across multiple contexts on early adolescents' internalizing and externalizing problems. *Journal of Child Psychology and Psychiatry,* 51(8), 953–961.

Murphy, S. A., Braun, T., Tillery, L., Cain, K. C., Johnson, L. C., & Beaton, R. D. (1999). PTSD among bereaved parents following the violent deaths of their 12- to 28-year-old children: A longitudinal prospective analysis. *Journal of Traumatic Stress,* 12, 273–291.

Nandi, A., Tracy, M., Beard, J. R., Vlahov, D., & Galea, S. (2009). Patterns and predictors of trajectories of depression after an urban disaster. *Annals of Epidemiology,* 19(11), 761–770.

Norris, F. H. (1992). Epidemiology of trauma: Frequency and impact of different potentially traumatic events on different demographic groups. *Journal of Consulting and Clinical Psychology,* 60(3), 409–418.

Norris, F. H., Baker, C. K., Murphy, A. D., & Kaniasty, K. (2005). Social support mobilization and deterioration after Mexico's 1999 flood: Effects of context, gender, and time. *American Journal of Community Psychology,* 36, 15–28.

Norris, F. H., Friedman, M. J., Watson, P. J., Byrne, C. M., Diaz, E., & Kaniasty, K. (2002). 60,000 disaster victims speak: Part I. An empirical review of the empirical literature, 1981–2001. *Psychiatry,* 65(3), 207–239.

Norris, F. H., & Murrell, S. A. (1988). Prior experience as a moderator of disaster impact on anxiety symptoms in older adults. *American Journal of Community Psychology,* 16(5), 665–683.

Orcutt, H. K., Erickson, D. J., & Wolfe, J. A. (2002). Prospective analysis of trauma exposure: The mediating role of PTSD symptomatology. *Journal of Traumatic Stress,* 15(3), 259–266.

Oxman, T. E., Berkman, L. F., Kasl, S., Freeman, D. H., Jr., & Barrett, J. (1992). Social support and depressive symptoms in the elderly. *American Journal of Epidemiology,* 135, 356–368.

Ozer, E. J., Best, S. R., Lipsey, T. L., & Weiss, D. S. (2003). Predictors of posttraumatic stress disorder and symptoms in adults: A meta-analysis. *Psychological Bulletin,* 129, 52–73.

Palm, K. M., Polusny, M. A., & Follette, V. M. (2004). Vicarious traumatization: Potential hazards and interventions for disaster and trauma workers. *Prehospital and Disaster Medicine,* 19(1), 73–78.

Patton, G. C., Coffey, C., Posterino, M., Carlin, J. B., & Bowes, G. (2003). Life events and early onset depression: Cause or consequence? *Psychological Medicine,* 33, 1203–1210.

Paykel, E. S. (1994). Life events, social support and depression. *Acta Psychiatrica Scandinavica,* 377, 50–58.

Perrin, M. A., DiGrande, L., Wheeler, K., Thorpe, L., Farfel, M., & Brackbill, R. (2007). Differences in PTSD prevalence and associated risk factors among World Trade Center disaster rescue and recovery workers. *American Journal of Psychiatry,* 164, 1385–1394.

Robins, J. M., Hernán, M. A., & Brumback, B. (2000). Marginal structural models and causal inference in epidemiology. *Epidemiology,* 11(5), 550–560.

Rothman, K. J., Greenland, S., Poole, C., & Lash, T. L. (2008). Causation and causal inference. In K. J. Rothman, S. Greenland, & T. L. Lash (Eds.), *Modern epidemiology* (pp. 5–31, 3rd ed.). Philadelphia: Lippincott Williams & Wilkins.

Sampson, R. J., Raudenbush, S. W., & Earls, F. (1997). Neighborhoods and violent crime: A multilevel study of collective efficacy. *Science, 277,* 918–924.

Schelling, T. C. (1978). *Micromotives and macrobehavior.* New York: W. W. Norton & Company.

Shalev, A. Y., Freedman, S., Peri, T., Brandes, D., Sahar, T., Orr, S. P., et al. (1998). Prospective study of posttraumatic stress disorder and depression following trauma. *American Journal of Psychiatry, 155,* 630–637.

Shrout, P. E. (1998). Causal modeling of epidemiological data on psychiatric disorders. *Social Psychiatry and Psychiatric Epidemiology, 33,* 400–404.

Solomon, Z., Waysman, M., Levy, G., Fried, B., Mikulincer, M., Benbenishty, R., et al. (1992). From front line to home front: A study of secondary traumatization. *Family Process, 31*(3), 289–302.

Tracy, M., Hobfoll, S. E., Canetti-Nisim, D., & Galea, S. (2008). Predictors of depressive symptoms among Israeli Jews and Arabs during the Al Aqsa Intifada: A population-based cohort study. *Annals of Epidemiology, 18*(6), 447–457.

Ullman, S. E., & Filipas, H. H. (2001). Predictors of PTSD symptom severity and social reactions in sexual assault victims. *Journal of Traumatic Stress, 14,* 369–389.

Ursano, R. J., Fullerton, C. S., Kao, T.-C., & Bhartiya, V. R. (1995). Longitudinal assessment of posttraumatic stress disorder and depression after exposure to traumatic death. *Journal of Nervous and Mental Disease, 183*(1), 36–42.

Ursano, R. J., Fullerton, C. S., & Norwood, A. E. (Eds.). (2003). *Terrorism and disaster: Individual and community mental health interventions.* Cambridge, UK: Cambridge University Press.

Windle, M., & Davies, P. T. (1999). Depression and heavy alcohol use among adolescents: Concurrent and prospective relations. *Development and Psychopathology, 11*(4), 823–844.

Yzermans, C. J., Donker, G. A., Kerssens, J. J., Dirkzwager, A. J. E., Soeteman, R. J. H., & ten Veen, P. M. H. (2005). Health problems of victims before and after disaster: A longitudinal study in general practice. *International Journal of Epidemiology, 34*(4), 820–826.

Zisook, S., Chentsova-Dutton, Y., & Shuchter, S. R. (1998). PTSD following bereavement. *Annals of Clinical Psychiatry, 10*(4), 157–163.

PART VI

Examining Trauma, Psychopathology, and Violence in the Military

11

Trauma, Psychopathology, and Violence in Recent Combat Veterans

DEIRDRE MACMANUS AND SIMON WESSELY

Nations have historically been apprehensive about their returning warriors (Leventman, 1978; Waller, 1944), with their anxiety centered on concern about the prospects of the soldiers' adaptive reintegration into civilian society. After the First World War, these fears often took the form of concerns about veterans becoming the focus for radical political action, but by the Second World War there was also increased concern about domestic upheaval, problems with reintegration, and what we would now call social exclusion (Allport, 2009).

In the present, Great Britain and the United States have, for the first time since the Second World War, once again been engaged in combat in two theaters of combat operation—Iraq and Afghanistan—although on nothing like the scale of prior wars. Nevertheless, since the commencement of the Iraq war, followed by the Afghanistan conflict, over 100,000 UK reserve and regular service personnel and nearly 2 million U.S. personnel have been deployed (Polusny et al., 2011). There is considerable interest in the adverse consequences for the physical and mental health of military personnel involved in these operations. Media accounts highlight some of the challenges facing troops in their transition back to civilian life. One area that has been a particular focus of interest has been that of violent behavior (Caesar, 2010). The media increasingly make claims that recent military deployments are particularly associated with subsequent increased rates of aggression, violent offending, and incarceration. Here is an abstract from a January 2009 article in the *New York Times*:

FORT CARSON, Colo. - For the past several years, as this Army installation in the foothills of the Rocky Mountains became a busy way station for soldiers cycling in and out of Iraq, the number of servicemen implicated in violent crimes has raised alarm. Nine current or former members of Fort Carson's Fourth Brigade Combat Team have killed someone or were charged with killings in the last three years after returning from Iraq.

Five of the slayings took place last year alone. In addition, charges of domestic violence, rape and sexual assault have risen sharply. (Alvarey and Frosch, 2009).

At the same time, there have been claims of an increase in the number of veterans being processed through the criminal justice systems in both the United States and the United Kingdom.

Most of the research in this area has come from the United States, with an inevitable focus on veterans of the Vietnam conflict. As the United Kingdom was not involved in that war, it is only recently that similar work has been started there, stimulated entirely by concerns about the social outcomes of those who served in Iraq and/or Afghanistan.[1] The outcomes of Vietnam veterans have not been of particular interest in the United Kingdom, other than the stimulus that they gave to the introduction of the diagnosis of post-traumatic stress disorder (PTSD) into the psychiatric lexicon. But also, on either side of the Atlantic, it should not be assumed that the Vietnam experience provides a blueprint for the current generation. For example, the U.S. military during the Vietnam War was a mixture of a conscript and volunteer forces; now it (and that in the United Kingdom) is all volunteer. Personnel policy on tour length and numbers of tours has changed. Today, military personnel are more likely to have served multiple tours in Iraq and/or Afghanistan, compared to the typical single tour that troops would have served during the Vietnam War. The political context of the wars is different, as is the nature of the military conflict. Attitudes are different—toward the armed forces in general and toward psychiatric disorders in particular—as is the general economic situation (Wessely & Jones, 2004). The conclusion is that, as ever, it is a mistake to assume that history will repeat itself; each conflict has its own particular characteristics and, thus, consequences.

Although research examining the impact of war on psychological functioning has mainly focused on clinical outcomes, such as PTSD, anxiety, and depression (Fear et al., 2007, 2010; Hotopf et al., 2006; Jones et al., 2002; Jordan et al., 1991; Kang, Natelson, Mahan, Lee, & Murphy, 2003; Pizarro, Silver, & Prause, 2006; Unwin et al., 1999), combat exposure might also increase service members'

---

1 A word on terminology: "Veterans" is used in the United States to describe anyone who has served in the armed forces but no longer does, as well as anyone who has served in any given conflict and who might or might not still be serving. In the United Kingdom, "veterans" is a term that is more ambiguous and which in the mind of both the public and members of the armed forces tends to conjure up images of elderly "veterans" of conflicts such as the Second World War or the Korean War. The preferred term in most quarters is "ex–service personnel," so there is frequent reference to the "ex-services community," for example. However, the second U.S. usage of "veterans," to refer to anyone who served in a particular named conflict, is also now getting wider currency, as in "Gulf" or "Iraq" veterans, although again in the United Kingdom this will almost invariably refer only to those who have left the armed forces (Dandeker, Wessely, Iversen, & Ross, 2006).

risk for engaging in "externalizing" behaviors such as antisocial behavior, aggression, and criminal behavior. It is suggested that military service and combat experience might affect individuals' propensities toward violence and criminal behavior through a variety of mechanisms. One possible mechanism is through training for combat, the aim of which is to reprogram prosocial aversion to violent acts and breed attitudes that enhance survival of both self and military colleagues (i.e., to break down barriers to committing violent acts) (Grossman & Siddle, 1999). But just how much does service life contribute to this, given that the armed forces in general, and the army in particular, actively recruit from those already at risk of subsequent offending behaviors, something that happens on both sides of the Atlantic? It is possible that aspects of military life actively improve the social trajectories of service personnel relative to what might have been if they had not been recruited. When viewed from a life course theory perspective, military service is a transition that can be a turning point in the lives of those that join. For those already on a path to antisocial behavior, it might be a positive turning point; however, for those who have no record of previous offending, it might increase their criminal propensity, whereas for others it might serve as simply a bridging environment in their criminal careers (Bouffard, 2005). None of these trajectories are mutually exclusive. Finally, another mechanism for an association between military service and violent behavior is the psychological and behavioral consequences of combat experiences, which are the main focus of this chapter.

In this chapter, we consider literature on the Vietnam War and subsequent conflicts. The majority of research discussed is from the United States. UK research groups have begun research in this area, as the extrapolation of results from the United States to the United Kingdom is limited due to differences in military combat strategies, criminal justice systems, and healthcare systems. Although literature from the United Kingdom is lacking, we make reference where possible to the British perspective on the problem. Most of the published literature found is limited to the research of violence among service men, most likely due to the limited number of women in combat situations.

Violent Crime among Veterans: The Prison Perspective

The numbers of veterans appearing in the criminal justice system has been a matter of concern in both the United Kingdom and the United States in recent years. There seems to be general acceptance that this is a reflection of their experiences during military service (Napo, 2009). However, it is important to try to clarify whether military service is indeed a specific risk factor, taking into consideration preservice vulnerability factors associated with both joining the armed forces and subsequent offending behaviors, as well as other factors such as mental health problems, substance misuse, and social problems. In many ways, veterans in the United States and the United Kingdom experience similar problems upon leaving the military and making the transition back to civilian life: housing, mental health, employment, relationship breakdown, and substance misuse are problems all too frequently encountered on either side of the Atlantic. Ten percent of State prisoners in the United States reported prior service in the U.S. Armed Forces (Bureau of Justice Statistics, 2004). An initial figure from the UK national probation union (Napo), which estimated that 9.1% of English and Welsh prisoners have served in the armed forces (Napo, 2009), seemed to represent a situation similar to that of the U.S. However, the UK government subsequently produced a lower estimate of 3.5% using a more robust method of record linkage between the prison census data and the personnel records kept by the Ministry of Defence (MoD), both of which are comprehensive data sources (Ministry of Defence, 2010). Napo's response was to ask the MoD to review their methodology, but one has to give more credence to the record linkage data than the estimates of individual probation officers made without any quality check against military records.

Prisons in both countries tell the same story of men who have offended after leaving service, often committing serious violent or sexual crimes. It is striking when comparing the most recent (2004) survey of the U.S. veteran prison population by the Bureau of Justice Statistics (2004) and the most recent analysis of the veteran prison population in English and Welsh prisons (Ministry of Defence, 2010) how similar these populations are. Both U.S. and UK veterans are less likely than the general population to offend but more likely to be in prison for violent and sexual offenses. Among State prisoners in the United States, 57% of veterans were categorized as "violent offenders," compared to 47% of nonveterans. In the United Kingdom, 33% of veterans are in prison for violence against a person, compared to 29% of the nonveteran prison population. These differences might not be large, but that is not the case when it comes to sexual offenses. Twenty-three percent of veterans were in U.S. prisons for sexual offenses, compared to 9% of civilian prisoners. In England and Wales, 25% of veterans are in prison for sexual offenses, compared to 11% of the civilian prison population.

However, the prison statistics tell a one-dimensional story. Those in prison are only a small proportion of those who offend, and the issues around offending behavior and ex-service personnel are not restricted to criminal convictions and incarceration; there is also violent and antisocial behavior that does not result in conviction. Such sparse data cannot tell us why these individuals are ending up in prison mostly for violent and sexual offenses. They do not examine the impact of sociodemographic, military, and premilitary factors. For this we need more comprehensive data that provide information on a range of variables and allow us to consider potential confounders of apparent associations between military experiences and violence/offending behavior.

Does Combat Trauma Lead to Subsequent Violent Behavior?

General Violence

Although research is emerging from the recent Iraq/Afghanistan conflicts, the majority of work in this area has utilized data from previous conflicts, mostly on Vietnam veterans. Yager, Laufer, and Gallops (1984), in a survey of 1,342 male veterans and nonveterans, found that, whereas deployment to Vietnam was not associated with increased rates of self-reported arrests/convictions, having been exposed to combat while on deployment was. Indeed, they found a correlation between the level of combat exposure and the frequency of violent offenses (Yager et al., 1984). This was a large study that considered a range of potential confounding factors in its analyses. The fact that they did not include veterans in prison in their sample suggests that they might even have underestimated the association. Calvert and colleagues examined a number of self-reported violent outcomes and their association with various Vietnam deployment experiences and found a significant association between increased combat exposure and the harming of others postdeployment by kicking, biting, or hitting (Calvert & Hutchinson, 1990). Regarding the 1991 Gulf War, a population-based survey of 3,695 U.S. military personnel that compared a group of combat veterans with a group of military personnel who had not been deployed found that, after adjustment for education, income, mental health characteristics, and previous antisocial behavior, combat experience was significantly associated with incarceration after the Gulf War (OR = 1.6; p = 0.039) (Black et al., 2005). Other studies have explored the importance of certain experiences whilst on deployment. Hiley-Young, Blake, Abueg, Rozynko, and Gusman (1995) examined premilitary, war zone, and postmilitary experiences in a small study of consecutive admissions (n = 177) to a U.S. Department of Veterans Affairs hospital unit and found that combat exposure alone did not predict postmilitary violent behavior. Rather, they found that of all the war zone experiences assessed, only participation in the killing of prisoners of war or civilians while on deployment was predictive of postmilitary violence (Hiley-Young et al., 1995).

A major problem inherent in many of these studies, however, is that they were carried out many years after the deployment in question, and, given that the studies often use self-report measures, this delay increases the potential problem of recall bias. They also frequently measure violence that is taking place many years after return from deployment/combat, and the association with deployment becomes increasingly blurred over time. An important point to highlight is that differing enlistment methods (the Vietnam War used draft enlistment, whereas military personnel have enrolled voluntarily for the conflicts in Iraq and Afghanistan) would suggest that the two cohorts are not entirely comparable with respect to predeployment demographic characteristics, possibly leading to variations in postdeployment adjustment problems (Elbogen et al., 2010).

Another more difficult issue is that combat is not random. Those in combat roles are invariably younger, for example. It is also possible, and indeed probable, that those in combat roles are more likely to be risk takers and perhaps have a greater propensity for violence. Educational levels might also differ. In the United Kingdom, regiments that are traditionally and for good reason associated with increased aggressiveness, such as the Parachute Regiment, and which are as a result more often deployed on dangerous combat missions are also more likely to recruit from areas of social disadvantage, where the recruits are likely to have lower educational attainment. Some confounders, such as age, can be dealt with statistically, but others, such as temperament, risk taking, and propensity to violence, are less amenable to analysis. The possibility that residual confounding accounts for the association between combat exposure and offending remains a real one.

In answer to the above problems, research into personnel returning from Iraq and Afghanistan is now turning its attention to violence and antisocial behavior. A population study surveyed over 80,000 U.S. troops immediately upon their return from deployment in Iraq and then again six months later (Milliken, Auchterlonie, & Hoge, 2007). The researchers found that 3.5% initially reported concerns/thoughts of interpersonal aggression, but this increased to 14% six months later (Milliken et al., 2007). In a study from the Walter Reid Institute of Army Research, 18,305 U.S. soldiers were surveyed 3 and 12 months following their return from deployment in Iraq (Thomas et al., 2010). They were asked how often in the past month they "got into a fight with someone and hit the person"; 18% reported fighting and hitting someone one or more times in the past month, with little change in this prevalence between 3 and 12 months postdeployment. Unfortunately these studies did not examine the factors associated with this postdeployment violence. However, Booth-Kewley and colleagues published a recent paper that aimed to examine factors associated with antisocial behavior in combat veterans using a sample of marines enlisted in the U.S. Armed Forces who had been deployed to Iraq or Afghanistan between 2002 and 2007 (Booth-Kewley, Larson, Highfill-McRoy, Garland, & Gaskin, 2010). They found that combat exposure was positively and significantly associated with antisocial behavior after adjustment for a range of potential confounders. Killgore and colleagues surveyed 1,252 Operation Iraqi Freedom veterans regarding different combat experiences immediately upon their return from deployment and again three months later (Killgore et al., 2008). They controlled for the confounding effects of age, sex, and other relevant sociodemographic factors. Although effect sizes were small, they found that specific combat experiences, such as exposure to violent combat, killing another person, and contact

with high levels of human trauma, were predictive of greater risk-taking propensity after homecoming. They also found that these combat experiences were
predictive of actual risk-related behaviors in the preceding month, including
greater alcohol use and increased verbal and physical aggression toward others.
This is consistent with the idea that some combatants might develop an "invincibility complex." Anecdotally, military personnel have come back from war
with feelings of invincibility. These might be evidenced through increased risk
taking, binge drinking, drug use, getting into fights, and other antisocial behaviors (Vaughan, 2006). However, more research is required in order to determine
whether this is a product of mainly their combat experiences or preexisting
characteristics of the individual.

There has been a distinct lack of discussion of the situation among British
combat veterans. Unfortunately, other than the aforementioned prison data,
research into violence in the military in the United Kingdom is only just underway for the first time in British military research. One piece of preliminary
research was published this year comparing a sample of postnational service
veterans with a comparable general population survey sample on a variety of
mental health and behavioral measures (Woodhead et al., 2010). The researchers found that male veterans reported more violent behaviors than nonveterans.
This association remained significant after adjustment for childhood adversity
(OR = 1.44, 95% CI = 1.01–2.06). Unfortunately the data set did not permit any
closer analysis of why this might be the case.

Important research in the United Kingdom is currently ongoing into the
impact of deployment to Iraq and Afghanistan on violence in UK military personnel. The relationship between deployment (and deployment-related experiences) and self-reported physical violence on homecoming is being explored in
a large cohort study of a representative sample of over 10,000 regular and reserve
UK Armed Forces personnel (information available from authors upon request).
This sample has been followed up since the beginning of UK Armed Forces
involvement in the Iraq war, in 2003, and two phases of data collection are now
completed. Preliminary results from baseline analyses show that the prevalence
of self-reported violence is approximately 13%. This was shown to
be strongly associated with premilitary antisocial behavior. However, even
after premilitary antisocial behavior and other sociodemographic and military
confounders were controlled for, violence on homecoming was shown to be
strongly associated with serving a combat role, and in particular with exposure
to multiple traumatic events during combat and having thoughts that one might
be killed. This research is part of an ongoing prospective study that will ultimately look at the role of premilitary, deployment, and postdeployment factors
in the etiology of postdeployment violence. The researchers also intend to link
their cohort data with official criminal records in order to provide them with an
objective measure of offending in addition to the self-report measure. This is

something that has not yet been done with such a rich cohort data set in either the United Kingdom or the United States.

Intimate Partner Violence

An area of great concern in society in both the United States and the United Kingdom is intimate partner violence (IPV). It has been recognized as a serious public health issue only since the 1970s, but interest in the difficulties faced by military families has increased in recent years, especially in the United States, due in part to the well-publicized domestic homicides, in 2002, at Fort Bragg, North Carolina, among U.S. Special Forces units who served in Afghanistan (Buncombe, 2002).

According to a 2005 systematic review, prevalence rates of IPV among active duty servicemen and veterans in the United States vary widely, with rates ranging from 13.5% to 58% (Marshall, Panuzio, & Taft, 2005). These rates of IPV perpetration among military samples are approximately one to three times higher than rates found in studies of IPV in the general population (Straus & Gelles, 1990).

In one study of IPV amongst U.S. Army servicemen within three months after their return from deployment to Bosnia, deployment was not shown to be associated with a rise in IPV perpetration (McCarroll et al., 2003). However, in a larger U.S. Army-wide study that examined self-reported violence in over 26,000 participants, after controlling for demographic variables, the probability of severe aggression was significantly greater for soldiers who had deployed in the past year than for soldiers who had not deployed (McCarroll et al., 2010).

More specific than deployment, combat exposure in the warzone is hypothesized to impact on the likelihood of the perpetration of IPV, for example, by exposing individuals to violence in such a manner that they come to view violence as an acceptable means of acting. Gimbel and Booth (1994) noted that although aggressive behaviors that are highly endorsed in the war zone are inappropriate in intimate relationships, these learned behaviors might be carried over and used for conflict resolution within intimate relationships—this putative link, for example, being part of the rationale for postdeployment interventions such as BATTLEMIND. This is a U.S.-developed psychoeducational process designed to help deployed military personnel psychologically readjust their mindset from that suited to a combat environment to one more appropriate for civilian life. Exposure to combat has been the most frequently examined correlate of IPV perpetration, and an association has been reported in some studies (Byrne & Riggs, 1996; Orcutt, King, & King, 2003; Prigerson, Macijewski, & Rosenheck, 2002), although this association was largely accounted for by PTSD symptoms. Interestingly, when Orcutt and colleagues (2003) used structural equation modeling on data from the National Vietnam Veterans Readjustment Study (NVVRS)

(Kulka et al., 1990) to examine the relationship between battlefield deployment and subsequent spousal aggression and violence, they found that perceived battlefield threat (not actual combat exposure), severity of PTSD symptoms, and a number of premilitary adverse experiences demonstrated direct associations with subsequent IPV. However, once PTSD symptomatology was accounted for, those who had engaged in higher levels of combat were significantly less likely to engage in partner violence. This suggested that battlefield exposures themselves might not contribute to interpersonal violence in the absence of the mediating effect of PTSD (Orcutt et al., 2003). However, certain war zone experiences (e.g., battlefield atrocities and killing) have been demonstrated to predict postdeployment spousal violence (Hiley-Young et al., 1995; Taft et al., 2005).

Again most of these studies examined Vietnam veterans several years after their deployment. Teten and colleagues (2010) examined partner aggression among male Afghanistan or Iraq veterans with PTSD and compared this aggression to that reported by Vietnam veterans with PTSD. Interestingly, no significant difference in aggression measures was found between the Operation Enduring Freedom (OEF)/Operation Iraqi Freedom (OIF) and Vietnam veteran groups.

Does Past Violence Predict Future Violence?

Findings that combat veterans are at increased risk for subsequent violent behavior have led to attempts to understand this relationship. Historical variables are important to consider in the etiology of postdeployment violence. Research from the general population has already shown that childhood disruptive behavior has potent effects on antisocial behavior and criminality, even into mid-adulthood (Simonoff et al., 2004). Premilitary antisocial behavior might reflect a predisposition for such behavior that might continue into adulthood irrespective of the impact of military service. Unfortunately, many studies neglect to include premilitary antisocial behavior as an important confounding factor in their analyses. When a sample of Vietnam veterans who had been incarcerated in Iowa State prisons were compared with a sample of Vietnam veterans from the community, a greater proportion of veteran inmates were found to have antisocial personality disorder with an onset prior to military service (Shaw, Churchill, Noyes, & Loeffelholz, 1987). Thirty-six percent met criteria for antisocial personality, compared to 7% of the control group. The findings indicated that although aggressive tendencies might result from combat exposure, the preexisting characteristics of the individual are an important consideration in the etiological pathway. Fontana and Rosenheck (2005) subsequently used structural equation modeling with an NVVRS sample of 1,198 Vietnam veterans and found that when a number of risk factors were included in the model, prewar antisocial behavior was a stronger predictor of Veteran violence than was combat exposure. This is the only study the authors are aware of that has modeled cross-sectional data in temporal sequence to try to draw an etiological model of postdeployment violence. This is still no substitute for a truly prospective study design. In another study, a history of past violence (not necessarily premilitary violence) surpassed other risk factors as a predictor of veteran violence in a sample of 630 U.S. combat veterans (Hartl, Rosen, Drescher, Lee, & Gusman, 2005). Other studies have also highlighted the roles played by childhood maltreatment, exposure to family violence, and prewar violent behavior in combat veterans' subsequent violent behavior (Begic & Jokic-Begic, 2001; Elbogen et al., 2010).

From Combat Trauma to Violence: What Role Does Psychopathology Play?

Post-traumatic Stress Disorder

Anger and aggressive behavior are particular concerns expressed by the families of veterans with PTSD (Biddle, Elliott, Creamer, Forbes, & Devilly, 2002; Calhoun et al., 2002; Jordan et al., 1992), and findings from the United States suggest high rates of postdeployment PTSD, with estimates of 10% to 20% of returning U.S. servicemen and service women experiencing symptoms (Hoge et al., 2004; Hoge, Terhakopian, Castro, Messer, & Engel, 2007; Vasterling et al., 2006). A recent meta-analysis revealed a strong relationship between PTSD and anger and hostility among trauma-exposed adults (Orth & Wieland, 2006), and combat exposure showed a stronger association with PTSD than did other traumatic events. It has been suggested that PTSD is the obvious choice as an important mediator in the association between combat (trauma) and antisocial behavior.

PTSD has been consistently shown to be significantly related to violence and aggressive acts in veterans (Beckham, Feldman, & Kirby, 1998; Beckham, Feldman, Kirby, Hertzberg, & Moore, 1997; Begic & Jokic-Begic, 2001; Hartl et al., 2005; Jakupcak et al., 2007; Kulka et al., 1990; Lasko, Gurvits, Kuhne, Orr, & Pitman, 1994; McFall, Fontana, Raskind, & Rosenheck, 1999; Taft, Kaloupek, et al., 2007). In one study, Vietnam combat veterans with PTSD reported an average of 20 acts of violence in the past year, compared to less than 1 act reported by combat veterans without PTSD (Beckham et al., 1997). In a study by McFall and colleagues (1999) comparing violence in Vietnam veteran inpatients with PTSD to that in veteran inpatients without PTSD, those with PTSD were approximately seven times more likely than those without to have engaged in one or more acts of violence during the four-month period prior to hospitalization (p < 0.001). They also reported that veterans with PTSD were more likely to destroy property and make violent threats with a weapon. In the study by Hiley-Young et al. (1995) described previously, the researchers found that the level of combat exposure predicted PTSD severity.

Similar results have been found in Iraq/Afghanistan veterans as well, with one study showing that a higher proportion of Iraq/Afghanistan veterans with PTSD (53.2%) and subthreshold PTSD (52.4%) reported at least one act of violence in the past four months than of the non-PTSD group (20.3%) (Jakupcak et al., 2007). Booth-Kewley and colleagues explored factors associated with antisocial behavior in a sample of 1,543 U.S. Marines who deployed to combat zones in support of conflicts in Iraq and Afghanistan during 2002–2007 (Booth-Kewley, Larson, et al., 2010). With all other variables controlled for, Marines who screened high on a standardized test for PTSD were over six times as likely to engage in antisocial behavior as those who did not.

A relatively large amount of research has also established that a relationship exists between PTSD and IPV perpetration among U.S. veterans. Higher rates of IPV perpetration have been found among Vietnam veterans with PTSD than among those without the disorder (Carroll, Rueger, Foy, & Donahoe, 1985; Jordan et al., 1992). In addition, positive associations have been reported between measures of PTSD symptom severity and IPV severity (Samper, Taft, King, & King, 2004), even when considered together with other IPV risk factors (Byrne and Riggs, 1996; Orcutt et al., 2003). As described previously, Orcutt and colleagues demonstrated in Vietnam veterans that PTSD acts as a mediator on the pathway from combat trauma to IPV. Teten and colleagues (2010), in a more recent study, examined partner aggression among male Afghanistan or Iraq veterans, with and without PTSD, who served during OEF and OIF. The sample groups were small, with only 27 and 31 participants in each, so it is unsurprising that only a few comparisons reached significance, but the odds ratios suggested that male OEF/OIF veterans with PTSD were two to three times more likely to perpetrate aggression toward their female partners.

So it appears that there is a relationship between PTSD and violence among military personnel. However, this link is not straightforward. The concept of PTSD is complex, and studies have found different aspects of the symptomatology to be specifically related to postdeployment violence, such as hyperarousal (McFall et al., 1999; Taft, Vogt, Marshall, Panuzio, & Niles, 2007), avoidance/numbing symptoms (McFall et al., 1999), or comorbid dysphoria (Taft, Vogt, et al., 2007). Elbogen et al. (2010) explored the correlates of anger and hostility in Iraq and Afghanistan war veterans. They found that aggressive impulses or urges, difficulty managing anger, and perceived problems controlling violent behavior were each significantly associated with PTSD hyperarousal symptoms. Other PTSD symptoms were less strongly and less consistently linked to anger and hostility (Elbogen et al., 2010). To add further complexity, Miller, Greif, and

Smith (2003) were interested in the different emotional and behavioral manifestations associated with PTSD amongst Vietnam combat veterans (Miller et al.,
2003; Miller, Kaloupek, Dillon, & Keane, 2004). They identified "internalizing"
and "externalizing" clusters of combat-related PTSD. Internalizers had high
prevalence rates of panic and depression and were more likely to experience
their distress internally through mood and thoughts. Externalizers, in contrast,
were more likely to express distress outwardly through behaviors and had high
rates of antisocial personality traits, alcohol-related behaviors, and histories of
delinquency (Miller et al., 2003, 2004). Rielage, Hoyt, and Renshaw (2010)
showed that this personality model of PTSD comorbidities can also be applied in
the Iraq and Afghanistan veteran population. Thus, the earlier studies showing
a link between PTSD and postdeployment violence might be overly simplistic.

Another as yet unaddressed question is the temporal nature of the relationship between PTSD and violence. The authors are unaware of any studies that
address the question of causality. In order to do this, a prospective study would
be required to establish the temporal sequence of the combat trauma, the development of PTSD, and subsequent violent behavior. As yet, all studies have collected data cross-sectionally and therefore cannot address this issue.

From a British perspective, even if one accepts that there is a link between
violence in combat veterans and PTSD, research to date in UK military personnel who have returned from Iraq and Afghanistan has not found the levels of
PTSD to be as high as in the United States. Several studies have shown this
(Grieger et al., 2006; Hoge et al., 2006; Hoge et al., 2007; Hotopf et al., 2006). A
large prospective study of a randomly selected representative sample of UK military personnel found the prevalence of PTSD to be 4% (Fear et al., 2010).
Deployment was not found to be significantly associated with a rise in PTSD, at
least not in Regulars, but there was an association between PTSD and being
employed in a combat role as opposed to a combat support role. With PTSD
rates predicted to be so much lower in the United Kingdom, the actual importance of this as a risk factor for violence might at first seem less important than
among U.S. military cohorts. However, in an important addition to the literature, Sundin and colleagues warn against the comparison of PTSD rates between
studies with different methodologies, never mind between studies carried out
in the United States and the United Kingdom. Even differences such as the use
of anonymous versus "on the record" surveys can result in significant differences (Sundin, Fear, Iversen, Rona, & Wessely, 2010).

Substance Misuse

Although PTSD is perhaps the most researched diagnosis when considering
violence in combat veterans, there is also literature suggesting that other
psychopathologies are linked with such violence. Substance abuse has been found

to be a strong factor in predicting aggressive behavior among combat veterans (Jakupcak et al., 2007; McFall et al., 1999). Importantly, it has also been found to elevate the risk of violence considerably in veterans with PTSD (McFall et al., 1999). PTSD with comorbid alcohol dependence might lead to greater violence than PTSD alone, hypothetically due to the effect on hyperarousal symptoms (Zoriic, Karlovic, Buljan, & Maruic, 2003). Similarly, positive direct relationships have been found between the frequency of IPV perpetration and alcohol abuse among NVVRS participants (Samper et al., 2004; Savarese, Suvak, King, & King, 2001), and alcohol consumption and PTSD hyperarousal symptoms jointly predicted IPV perpetration, such that alcohol consumption appeared to potentiate the impact of PTSD hyperarousal symptoms on IPV perpetration (Savarese et al., 2001).

Although the impact of problem drinking on postdeployment violence by UK military personnel has not yet been researched, we already know that alcohol misuse is a significant problem within the UK Armed Forces (Fear et al., 2007). Indeed, the most common disorders in the UK military are alcohol abuse (18.0%) and neurotic disorders (13.5%) (Iversen et al., 2009). Although no UK study has as yet linked these disorders to violence in the military, the main UK cohort study has observed that alcohol misuse increases following one's return from deployment to Iraq or Afghanistan (Fear et al., 2010). It is therefore reasonable to suspect, extrapolating from the U.S. research, that alcohol misuse is a potentially important risk factor for violence in UK combat veterans.

Depression and Other Diagnoses

A host of other psychiatric conditions have been associated with violence in U.S. veterans—for example, depression symptomatology, which Hartl and colleagues (2005) found to be a predictor of high-risk behaviors in Vietnam veterans. Also among NVVRS participants, diagnoses of a major depressive episode and drug abuse diagnoses were higher among partner-violent veterans with PTSD than among nonviolent veterans with the disorder, suggestive of an added risk associated with these comorbid diagnoses (Taft et al., 2005). Booth-Kewley, Highfill-McRoy, Larson, and Garland (2010) recently studied predictors of military discharge for bad conduct among male U.S. Marines following deployment to a combat zone in support of OEF or OIF and found that the strongest predictor of a discharge for bad conduct was a psychiatric diagnosis, especially if received subsequent to return from deployment.

Limitations of Research to Date

Methodological weaknesses inherent in much of the research reviewed in this chapter limit our interpretation of these findings. Although some studies have used data from recent deployments to Iraq and Afghanistan, the majority have utilized data from Vietnam veterans and have been conducted many years after the conflict ended. Such delay leads to a range of methodological problems, including recall bias and difficulties determining causal pathways between deployment-related hazards and later outcomes. The majority of studies to date also employed a cross-sectional design that limits the causal inferences that can be drawn. Many of these veteran studies are based on selected samples and are therefore not representative of all veterans and/or conflicts (Wessely & Jones, 2004). Measures of variables and outcomes vary greatly between studies, reducing comparability. Lastly, the lack of research using UK samples is a problem due to the limited generalizability of results from U.S. research to the United Kingdom. There are cultural, health service, and legal differences between the United States and the United Kingdom that do not permit easy extrapolation, nor should it be assumed that all deployments are similar. Furthermore, whereas some of the apparent differences in point prevalences of psychiatric disorders between U.S. and UK studies are partly explained by confounders such as combat exposure, age, proportion of reservists, tour length, and so on, it is less easy to explain the differences that are emerging on longitudinal follow-up, in which the scale of the increase in disorders over time since deployment does differ between the two countries, something that is hard to explain by simple confounding (Fear et al., 2010; Hotopf et al., 2006; Milliken et al., 2007; Sundin et al., 2010; Thomas et al., 2010). We cannot, therefore, assume that the prevalence and correlates of violent and offending behavior in combat veterans will be similar between the United States and the United Kingdom.

Conclusion

As both the United States and the United Kingdom face the long-term consequences of the past eight years of conflict in Iraq and Afghanistan, both are only too aware of the potential impact of combat trauma on their armed forces. However, before accepting the picture that sometimes can emerge from the media, which of course is much influenced by narratives and stories, it is the role of researchers to try to interpret evidence objectively.

There is evidence that veterans in both the United Kingdom and the United States have lower incarceration rates than nonveterans (although this needs further investigation) but that veterans in both countries are more likely than other prisoners to be serving time for a violent or sex offense. Does this mean veterans are committing more sexual and violent offenses than the general population, and if so, why? Examination of the literature on the impact of military service on the behavior of service personnel reveals a trend toward relating deployment experience, specifically combat trauma, to subsequent violence in U.S. military personnel, even after controlling for premilitary antisocial behavior. It also suggests an association between a range of psychopathologies—such as PTSD, substance misuse, and depression—and violence. Whether these psychopathologies are causal or a result of reverse causality (i.e. the violent behavior caused the mental health problems) can be addressed only by appropriately designed prospective studies, which should also adequately measure and account for premilitary antisocial behavior and a wide range of sociodemographic factors that might confound the association between combat trauma and subsequent violence in combat veterans. Similar research is urgently required in the United Kingdom also.

The impact on society of violence perpetrated by combat veterans as a result of their combat experiences depends on a number of factors. To try to ascertain the attributable risk fraction (i.e. the proportion of violence in the population that is attributable to combat veterans) would require that we know the prevalence of combat veterans who have behaved violently in the population and then assume causality between their combat experiences and subsequent violence. To do this would surely be to overlook the complexity of the multifactorial pathway to violence in combat veterans and also to ignore the potentially devastating impact of one act of violence on the lives of those servicemen or servicewomen, their families, and their potential victims.

The United States has a long-standing Department of Veterans Affairs that provides medical and psychiatric care to veterans, and they routinely screen for PTSD, depression, problem drinking, and military sexual trauma. Focused outreach work is done in the community and in prison to ensure that veterans receive support. By contrast, piecemeal services in the United Kingdom are provided by the veterans' charities in the voluntary sector, and provision can be patchy, and awareness poor. We know that overall the veterans' charities see only a very small fraction indeed of those with mental health problems; most continue to be seen, for better or worse, within the National Health System (Iversen, Dyson, et al., 2005; Iversen, Nikolaou, et al., 2005). For those veterans who fall through the net, veteran courts have been operating in the United States since 2008 and are now spreading across the country (Eligen, 2010). They offer tailored support for veterans who have committed offenses to help them get their lives back on track. The United Kingdom does not screen servicemen and women for postdeployment mental health problems (although we are now conducting, with the aid of U.S. funding, a randomized controlled trial of just such a program in the UK Armed Forces), and no such veteran court system is as yet in place in the United Kingdom.

Robust research findings to enlighten us as to the etiological pathway to violence in combat veterans are vital to those operating in the military, healthcare, and criminal justice systems in order to fully inform the need for and appropriate use of risk assessments and the implementation of strategies for the prevention of future violent behavior among active and ex-serving military personnel who have been involved in combat, as well as to inform the management of those already in the criminal justice system, in both the United Kingdom and the United States.

Acknowledgments

We would like to acknowledge the Medical Research Council, who provided the funding for Dr. MacManus's Clinical Research Fellowship, as well as King's Centre for Military Health Research and King's College London for providing a supportive research environment. Particular thanks are expressed to Dr. Nicola Fear, Reader in Military Epidemiology, for her supervisory role in Dr. MacManus's research. We would also like to acknowledge the work of Phillipa Hatton, Research Assistant at KCMHR, for her contribution to the background research for this chapter.

Disclosure Statement

D.M. has no potential conflicts of interest, financial or otherwise, to disclose.

S.W. is Honorary Consultant Advisor in Psychiatry to the British Army, a trustee of Combat Stress, and partially funded by the South London and Maudsley NHS Foundation Trust/Institute of Psychiatry/National Institute of Health Research Biomedical Research Centre. Professor Wessely has no potential conflicts of interest, financial or otherwise, to disclose.

References

Allport, A. (2009). *Demobbed: Coming home after the Second World War*. New Haven, CT: Yale University Press.

Alvarey, L., & Frosch, D. (2009, January 1). A focus on violence by returning GIs. *New York Times*. Retrieved January 3, 2011, from www.nytimes.com/2009/01/02/us/02veterans.html Beckham, J. C., Feldman, M. E., & Kirby, A. C. (1998). Atrocities exposure in Vietnam combat veterans with chronic posttraumatic stress disorder: Relationship to combat exposure, symptom severity, guilt, and interpersonal violence. *Journal of Traumatic Stress, 11,* 777–785.

Beckham, J. C., Feldman, M. E., Kirby, A. C., Hertzberg, M. A., & Moore, S. D. (1997). Interpersonal violence and its correlates in Vietnam veterans with chronic posttraumatic stress disorder. *Journal of Clinical Psychology, 53,* 859–869.

Begic, D., & Jokic-Begic, N. (2001). Aggressive behavior in combat veterans with posttraumatic stress disorder. *Military Medicine, 166,* 671–676.

Biddle, D., Elliott, P., Creamer, M., Forbes, D., & Devilly, G. J. (2002). Self-reported problems: A comparison between PTSD-diagnosed veterans, their spouses, and clinicians. *Behaviour Research and Therapy, 40,* 853–865.

Black, D. W., Carney, C. P., Peloso, P. M., Woolson, R. F., Letuchy, E., & Doebbeling, B. N. (2005). Incarceration and veterans of the first gulf war. *Military Medicine, 170,* 612–618.

Booth-Kewley, S., Highfill-McRoy, R. M., Larson, G. E., & Garland, C. F. (2010). Psychosocial predictors of military misconduct. *Journal of Nervous and Mental Disease, 198,* 91–98.

Booth-Kewley, S., Larson, G. E., Highfill-McRoy, R. M., Garland, C. F., & Gaskin, T. A. (2010). Factors associated with antisocial behavior in combat veterans. *Aggressive Behavior, 36,* 330–337.

Bouffard, L. A. (2005). The military as a bridging environment in criminal careers: Differential outcomes of the military experience. *Armed Forces & Society, 31,* 273–295.

Buncombe, A. (2002). US Army stunned by spate of murders at special forces base. *The Independent.* Retrieved January 3, 2011, from http://www.independent.co.uk/news/world/americas/us-army-stunned-by-spate-of-murders-at-special-forces-base-638547.html

Bureau of Justice Statistics. (2004). *Veterans in state and federal prison, 2004.* Washington. DC: Author.

Byrne, C. A., & Riggs, D. S. (1996). The cycle of trauma: Relationship aggression in male Vietnam veterans with symptoms of posttraumatic stress disorder. *Violence and Victims, 11,* 213–225.

Caesar, E. (2010). From hero to zero. *The Sunday Times.* Retrieved January 3, 2010, from www.timesonline.co.uk/tol/news/uk/article7084032.ece

Calhoun, P. S., Beckham, J. C., Feldman, M. E., Barefoot, J. C., Haney, T., & Bosworth, H. B. (2002). Partners' ratings of combat veterans' anger. *Journal of Traumatic Stress, 15,* 133–136.

Calvert, W. E., & Hutchinson, R. L. (1990). Vietnam veteran levels of combat: Related to later violence? *Journal of Traumatic Stress, 3,* 103–113.

Carroll, E. M., Rueger, D. B., Foy, D. W., & Donahoe, C. P., Jr. (1985). Vietnam combat veterans with posttraumatic stress disorder: Analysis of marital and cohabitating adjustment. *Journal of Abnormal Psychology, 94,* 329–337.

Dandeker, C., Wessely, S., Iversen, A., & Ross, J. (2006). What's in a name? Defining and caring for "veterans." *Armed Forces & Society, 32,* 161–177.

Elbogen, E. B., Wagner, H. R., Fuller, S. R., Calhoun, P. S., Kinneer, P. M., Mid-Atlantic Mental Illness Research Clinical Center Workgroup, et al. (2010). Correlates of anger and hostility in Iraq and Afghanistan war veterans. *American Journal of Psychiatry, 167,* 1051–1058.

Eligen, J. (2010, December 13). Queens court for veterans aims to help, not punish. *New York Times.* Retrieved January 3, 2010, from www.nytime.com/2010/12/14/nyregion/14vets.html

Fear, N., Iversen, A., Meltzer, H., Workman, L., Hull, L., Greenberg, N., et al. (2007). Patterns of drinking in the UK armed forces. *Addiction, 102,* 1749–1759.

Fear, N. T., Jones, M., Murphy, D., Hull, L., Iversen, A. C., Coker, B., et al. (2010). What are the consequences of deployment to Iraq and Afghanistan on the mental health of the UK armed forces? A cohort study. *Lancet, 375,* 1783–1797.

Fontana, A., & Rosenheck, R. (2005). The role of war-zone trauma and PTSD in the etiology of antisocial behavior. *Journal of Nervous and Mental Disease, 193,* 203–209.

Gimbel, C., & Booth, A. (1994). Why does military combat experience adversely affect marital relations? *Journal of Marriage and Family, 56,* 691–703.

Grieger, T. A., Cozza, S. J., Ursano, R. J., Hoge, C., Martinez, P. E., Engel, C. C., & Wain, H. J. (2006). Posttraumatic stress disorder and depression in battle-injured soldiers. *American Journal of Psychiatry, 163*(10), 1777–1783.

Grossman, D., & Siddle, B. (1999). Psychological effects of combat. In L. Curtis and J. Turpin (Eds.), *Encyclopedia of violence, peace, and conflict* (pp. 144–145). San Diego, CA: Academic Press.

Hartl, T. L., Rosen, C., Drescher, K., Lee, T. T., & Gusman, F. (2005). Predicting high-risk behaviors in veterans with posttraumatic stress disorder. *Journal of Nervous and Mental Disease, 193,* 464–472.

Hiley-Young, B., Blake, D. D., Abueg, F. R., Rozynko, V., & Gusman, F. D. (1995). Warzone violence in Vietnam: An examination of premilitary, military, and postmilitary factors in PTSD in-patients. *Journal of Traumatic Stress, 8,* 125–141.

Hoge, C., Castro, C., Messer, S., McGurk, D., Cotting, D., & Koffman, R. (2004). Combat duty in Iraq and Afghanistan, mental health problems, and barriers to care. *New England Journal of Medicine, 351,* 13–22.

Hoge, C., Auchterlonie, J., & Milliken, C. (2006). Mental health problems, use of mental health services, and attrition from military service after returning from deployment to Iraq or Afghanistan. *Journal of the American Medical Association, 295,* 1023–1032.

Hoge, C. W., Terhakopian, A., Castro, C. A., Messer, S. C., & Engel, C. C. (2007). Association of posttraumatic stress disorder with somatic symptoms, health care visits, and absenteeism among Iraq war veterans. *American Journal of Psychiatry, 164,* 150–153.

Hotopf, M., Hull, L., Fear, N., Browne, T., Horn, O., Iversen, A., et al. (2006). The health of UK military personnel who deployed to the 2003 Iraq war: A cohort study. *Lancet, 367,* 1731–1741.

Iversen, A., Dyson, C., Smith, N., Greenberg, N., Walwyn, R., Unwin, C., et al. (2005). "Goodbye and good luck": The mental health needs and treatment experiences of British ex-service personnel. *British Journal of Psychiatry, 186,* 480–486.

Iversen, A., Nikolaou, V., Greenberg, N., Unwin, C., Hull, L., Hotopf, M., et al. (2005). What happens to British veterans when they leave the armed forces? *European Journal of Public Health, 15,* 175–184.

Iversen, A., van Staden, L., Hughes, J., Browne, T., Hull, L., Hall, J., et al. (2009). The prevalence of common mental disorders and PTSD in the UK military: Using data from a clinical interview-based study. *BMC Psychiatry, 9,* 68.

Jakupcak, M., Conybeare, D., Phelps, L., Hunt, S., Holmes, H. A., Felker, B., et al. (2007). Anger, hostility, and aggression among Iraq and Afghanistan war veterans reporting PTSD and subthreshold PTSD. *Journal of Traumatic Stress, 20,* 945–954.

Jones, E., Hodgins-Vermaas, R., McCartney, H., Everitt, B., Beech, C., Poynter, D., et al. (2002). Post-combat syndromes from the Boer war to the Gulf war: A cluster analysis of their nature and attribution. *British Medical Journal, 324,* 321.

Jordan, B. K., Marmar, C. R., Fairbank, J. A., Schlenger, W. E., Kulka, R. A., Hough, R. L., et al. (1992). Problems in families of male Vietnam veterans with posttraumatic stress disorder. *Journal of Consulting and Clinical Psychology, 60,* 916–926.

Jordan, B. K., Schlenger, W. E., Hough, R., Kulka, R. A., Weiss, D., Fairbank, J. A., et al. (1991). Lifetime and current prevalence of specific psychiatric disorders among Vietnam veterans and controls. *Archives of General Psychiatry, 48,* 207–215.

Kang, H. K., Natelson, B. H., Mahan, C. M., Lee, K. Y., & Murphy, F. M. (2003). Posttraumatic stress disorder and chronic fatigue syndrome-like illness among gulf war veterans: A population-based survey of 30,000 veterans. *American Journal of Epidemiology, 157,* 141–148.

Killgore, W. D. S., Cotting, D. I., Thomas, J. L., Cox, A. L., McGurk, D., Vo, A. H., et al. (2008). Post-combat invincibility: Violent combat experiences are associated with increased risk-taking propensity following deployment. *Journal of Psychiatric Research, 42,* 1112–1121.

Kulka, R. A., Schlenger, W. E., Fairbank, J. A., Hough, R. L., Jordan, B. K., Marmar, C. R., et al. (Eds.). (1990). *The national Vietnam veterans readustment study: Tables of findings and technical appendices.* New York: Brunner/Mazel

Lasko, N. B., Gurvits, T. V., Kuhne, A. A., Orr, S. P., & Pitman, R. K. (1994). Aggression and its correlates in Vietnam veterans with and without chronic posttraumatic stress disorder. *Comprehensive Psychiatry, 35,* 373–381.

Leventman, S. (1978). Epilogue: Social and historical perspectives on the Vietnam veteran. In C. Figley (Ed.), *Stress disorders among Vietnam veterans* (pp. 291–295). New York: Brunner/Mazel.

Marshall, A. D., Panuzio, J., & Taft, C. T. (2005). Intimate partner violence among military veterans and active duty servicemen. *Clinical Psychology Review, 25,* 862–876.

McCarroll, J. E., Ursano, R. J., Liu, X., Thayer, L. E., Newby, J. H., Norwood, A. E., et al. (2010). Deployment and the probability of spousal aggression by U.S. army soldiers. *Military Medicine, 175,* 352–356.

McCarroll, J. E., Ursano, R. J., Newby, J. H., Liu, X., Fullerton, C. S., Norwood, A. E., et al. (2003). Domestic violence and deployment in US army soldiers. *Journal of Nervous and Mental Disease, 191,* 3–9.

McFall, M., Fontana, A., Raskind, M., & Rosenheck, R. (1999). Analysis of violent behavior in Vietnam combat veteran psychiatric inpatients with posttraumatic stress disorder. *Journal of Traumatic Stress, 12,* 501–517.

Miller, M. W., Greif, J. L., & Smith, A. A. (2003). Multidimensional personality questionnaire profiles of veterans with traumatic combat exposure: Externalizing and internalizing subtypes. *Psychological Assessment, 15,* 205–215.

Miller, M. W., Kaloupek, D. G., Dillon, A. L., & Keane, T. M. (2004). Externalizing and internalizing subtypes of combat-related PTSD: A replication and extension using the PSY-5 scales. *Journal of Abnormal Psychology, 113,* 636–645.

Milliken, C. S., Auchterlonie, J. L., & Hoge, C. W. (2007). Longitudinal assessment of mental health problems among active and reserve component soldiers returning from the Iraq war. *Journal of the American Medical Association, 298,* 2141–2148.

Ministry of Defence. (2010). *Data analytical services and advice: Estimating the proportion of prisoners in England and Wales who are ex-armed forces—Further analysis.* London: Author.

Napo. (2009). *Armed forces and the criminal justice system.* Napo the Trade Union and Professional Association for Family Court and Probation Staff: London.

Orcutt, H. K., King, L. A., & King, D. W. (2003). Male-perpetrated violence among Vietnam veteran couples: Relationships with veteran's early life characteristics, trauma history, and PTSD symptomatology. *Journal of Traumatic Stress, 16,* 381–390.

Orth, U., & Wieland, E. (2006). Anger, hostility, and posttraumatic stress disorder in trauma-exposed adults: A meta-analysis. *Journal of Consulting and Clinical Psychology, 74,* 698–706.

Pizarro, J., Silver, R. C., & Prause, J. (2006). Physical and mental health costs of traumatic war experiences among civil war veterans. *Archives of General Psychiatry, 63,* 193–200.

Polusny, M. A., Kehle, S. M., Nelson, N. W., Erbes, C. R., Arbisi, P. A., & Thuras, P. (2011). Longitudinal effects of mild traumatic brain injury and posttraumatic stress disorder comorbidity on postdeployment outcomes in national guard soldiers deployed to Iraq. *Archives of General Psychiatry, 68,* 79–89.

Prigerson, H. G., Maciejewski, P. K., & Rosenheck, R. A. (2002). Population attributable fractions of psychiatric disorders and behavioral outcomes associated with combat exposure among US men. *American Journal of Public Health, 92,* 59–63.

Rielage, J. K., Hoyt, T., & Renshaw, K. (2010). Internalizing and externalizing personality styles and psychopathology in OEF–OIF veterans. *Journal of Traumatic Stress, 23*, 350–357.

Samper, R. E., Taft, C. T., King, D. W., & King, L. A. (2004). Posttraumatic stress disorder symptoms and parenting satisfaction among a national sample of male Vietnam veterans. *Journal of Traumatic Stress, 17*, 311–315.

Savarese, V. W., Suvak, M. K., King, L. A., & King, D. W. (2001). Relationships among alcohol use, hyperarousal, and marital abuse and violence in Vietnam veterans. *Journal of Traumatic Stress, 14*, 717–732.

Shaw, D. M., Churchill, C. M., Noyes, R., & Loeffelholz, P. L. (1987). Criminal behavior and post-traumatic stress disorder in Vietnam veterans. *Comprehensive Psychiatry, 28*, 403–411.

Simonoff, E., Elander, J., Holmshaw, J., Pickles, A., Murray, R., & Rutter, M. (2004). Predictors of antisocial personality: Continuities from childhood to adult life. *British Journal of Psychiatry, 184*, 118–127.

Straus, M., & Gelles, R. (1990). How violent are American families? Estimates from the National Family Violence Resurvey and other studies. In M. A. Straus and R. G. Gelles (Eds.), *Physical violence in American families* (pp. 95–112). New Brunswick, NJ: Transaction.

Sundin, J., Fear, N. T., Iversen, A., Rona, R. J., & Wessely, S. (2010). PTSD after deployment to Iraq: Conflicting rates, conflicting claims. *Psychological Medicine, 40*, 367–382.

Taft, C. T., Kaloupek, D. G., Schumm, J. A., Marshall, A. D., Panuzio, J., King, D. W., et al. (2007). Posttraumatic stress disorder symptoms, physiological reactivity, alcohol problems, and aggression among military veterans. *Journal of Abnormal Psychology, 116*, 498–507.

Taft, C. T., Pless, A. P., Stalans, L. J., Koenen, K. C., King, L. A., & King, D. W. (2005). Risk factors for partner violence among a national sample of combat veterans. *Journal of Consulting and Clinical Psychology, 73*, 151–159.

Taft, C. T., Vogt, D. S., Marshall, A. D., Panuzio, J., & Niles, B. L. (2007). Aggression among combat veterans: Relationships with combat exposure and symptoms of posttraumatic stress disorder, dysphoria, and anxiety. *Journal of Traumatic Stress, 20*, 135–145.

Teten, A. L., Schumacher, J. A., Taft, C. T., Stanley, M. A., Kent, T. A., Bailey, S. D., et al. (2010). Intimate partner aggression perpetrated and sustained by male Afghanistan, Iraq, and Vietnam veterans with and without posttraumatic stress disorder. *Journal of Interpersonal Violence, 25*, 1612–1630.

Thomas, J. L., Wilk, J. E., Riviere, L. A., McGurk, D., Castro, C. A., & Hoge, C. W. (2010). Prevalence of mental health problems and functional impairment among active component and National Guard soldiers 3 and 12 months following combat in Iraq. *Archives of General Psychiatry, 67*, 614–623.

Unwin, C., Blatchley, N., Coker, W., Ferry, S., Hotopf, M., Hull, L., et al. (1999). Health of UK servicemen who served in Persian Gulf war. *Lancet, 353*, 169–178.

Vasterling, J. J., Proctor, S. P., Amoroso, P., Kane, R., Heeren, T., & White, R. F. (2006). Neuropsychological outcomes of army personnel following deployment to the Iraq war. *Journal of the American Medical Association, 296*, 519–529.

Vaughan, D. (2006). Demobilised and addicted to danger. *Today's Officer, Fall*, 20–24.

Waller, W. (1944). *The veteran comes back*. New York: Dryden Press.

Wessely, S., & Jones, E. (2004). Psychiatry and the lessons of Vietnam: What were they and are they still relevant? *War and Society, 22*, 89–103.

Woodhead, C., Rona, R. J., Iversen, A., MacManus, D., Hotopf, M., Dean, K., et al. (2010). Mental health and health service use among post-national service veterans: Results from the 2007 Adult Psychiatric Morbidity Survey of England. *Psychological Medicine,* Epub ahead of print.

Yager, T., Laufer, R., & Gallops, M. (1984). Some problems associated with war experience in men of the Vietnam generation. *Archives of General Psychiatry, 41,* 327–333.

Zoriic, Z., Karlovic, D., Buljan, D., & Maruic, S. (2003). Comorbid alcohol addiction increases aggression level in soldiers with combat-related post-traumatic stress disorder. *Nordic Journal of Psychiatry, 57,* 199–202.

PART VII

Presidential Address

12

Childhood Trauma, Psychopathology, and Violence

Disentangling Causes, Consequences, and Correlates

CATHY SPATZ WIDOM AND SALLY J. CZAJA

Since Kempe's (Kempe, Silverman, Steele, Droegemueller, & Silver, 1962) ground-breaking work called attention to the battered child syndrome, research designed to document the long-term consequences of child maltreatment has grown. Numerous studies using a variety of research designs have demonstrated relationships between early adverse childhood experiences and later psychological, behavioral, and health outcomes (Gilbert et al., 2009; Johnson, Cohen, Brown, Smailes, & Bernstein, 1999; Jonson-Reid, Drake, Kim, Porterfield, & Han, 2004; Kinard, 1999; Lansford et al., 2002; Leiter, 2007; Mullen, Martin, Anderson, Romans, & Herbison, 1996; Perez & Widom, 1994; Spataro, Mullen, Burgess, Wells, & Moss, 2004; Widom, DuMont, & Czaja, 2007; Yates, Carlson, & Egeland, 2008). Two outcomes associated with child maltreatment—post-traumatic stress disorder (PTSD) and violence—have received considerable attention, whereas there is sparse research that examines the interrelationships among child maltreatment, PTSD, and violence. Moreover, there has been general reluctance to use the term "cause" or to refer to causality in describing these relationships, despite the fact that many scholars and clinicians believe that certain types of childhood adversities—child maltreatment in particular—"cause" a particular disease outcome or form of psychopathology.

We obviously cannot randomly assign children to experimental and control conditions in order to determine whether child abuse and/or neglect cause certain outcomes. However, disentangling causal from simple correlational relationships will permit us to better design and target interventions with maltreated children. The goal of this chapter is to examine one form of childhood trauma (child abuse and neglect) and its relationship to psychopathology and violence and, in the process, to highlight some of the challenges that confront the field of child maltreatment research, and finally to consider whether these relationships might be causal or whether these associations represent co-occurrences that are likely to have origins in other risk factors.

Three general criteria have been used extensively in the fields of epidemiology and medicine to establish causal links between a variety of risk factors and diseases: association, direction of influence, and nonspuriousness. Evidence for association can be provided by any statistic that shows the degree of a relationship between two variables. To establish the direction of influence, one must demonstrate that a "cause" precedes its "effect," or at least that the direction of influence is from cause to effect. Finally, to address the issue of spuriousness, one must eliminate rival or competing hypotheses and demonstrate that no hidden factors account for the relationship between the variables. That is, one needs to show that the relationship is maintained when all extraneous variables are held constant.

In this chapter, we use traditional criteria for determining causality and apply these criteria to findings from a prospective cohort design study of the consequences of childhood abuse and/or neglect. We focus particularly on two outcomes—PTSD and violence—and have organized the chapter into several sections. First, we briefly summarize the bivariate literatures on child maltreatment, PTSD, and violence. Second, we describe challenges confronting researchers in the field of child maltreatment research and how these impede efforts to establish causality. Third, we briefly describe the study we are using to examine these issues. The next section addresses issues of *association* and focuses on whether child abuse and neglect (CAN) is associated with increased risk for trauma, PTSD, and violence. We then examine the *direction of influence*—that is, does CAN precede PTSD and violence, or is there a different temporal order? Following this discussion of directionality, we turn to the issue of competing hypotheses and examine whether the relationship between childhood trauma, PTSD, and violence persists after controlling for *alternative or rival explanations*. The final section of this chapter concludes with a brief summary of what we have learned from these analyses and calls attention to additional issues that are important to consider when attempting to disentangle these relationships

Brief Summary of Previous Literature: Primarily Bivariate

As noted above, there is considerable literature relating child maltreatment to subsequent outcomes. Here, we briefly summarize the literatures that focus primarily on bivariate relationships, that is, the relationships between child maltreatment and PTSD, child maltreatment and violence, and PTSD and violence.

Child Maltreatment and PTSD

Numerous cross-sectional studies have found relationships between retrospective reports of childhood abuse or childhood adversities and PTSD. For example, in the National Comorbidity Study (Kessler, Sonnega, Bromet, Hughes, & Nelson, 1995), women with PTSD reported rape and childhood sexual abuse as the most upsetting traumatic events ever experienced, and 7% to 8% of men and women with PTSD reported childhood physical abuse as the most upsetting trauma experienced. Breslau (2009; Breslau, Chilcoat, Kessler, & Davis, 1999) reported that the likelihood of developing PTSD increased as the number of experienced traumatic events increased.

Using a prospective cohorts design, Widom (1999) found that individuals with documented histories of childhood physical or sexual abuse or neglect were at increased risk for a lifetime diagnosis of PTSD when followed up and assessed at approximately age 29: 30.9% met the criteria for a lifetime diagnosis of PTSD, compared to 20.4% of a matched control group. Specifically, 37.5% of those with histories of sexual abuse, 32.7% of those with histories of physical abuse, and 30.6% of those with histories of neglect met lifetime criteria for PTSD.

Child Maltreatment and Violence

Several longitudinal studies using different designs have found that CAN increases a person's risk for violence. In an early paper on the "cycle of violence," Widom (1989b) reported that children with documented cases of child abuse and/or neglect were at increased risk of arrest for violent crime relative to a matched control group of nonabused and nonneglected children. Smith and Thornberry (1995) found that abused and neglected children had more self-reported and officially documented cases of violent and moderate delinquency than nonabused and nonneglected children, even after controlling for sex, race, and family structure. Another longitudinal study of boys in Pittsburgh found that abused and neglected boys were more likely to self-report violence and delinquency than nonmaltreated boys (Stouthamer-Loeber, Loeber, Homish, & Wei, 2001). Similarly, Lansford et al. (2007) reported that children who had been physically abused had significantly more court records of violent offenses than nonabused peers, even after controlling for a number of variables, including socioeconomic status.

PTSD and Violence

Research relating PTSD to violence (see Chapter 11 in this volume) has focused primarily on veterans, although there is at least one study of forensic mental inpatients who had committed serious violent and sexual crimes. Of these inpatients, 9 out of 27 (33%) were diagnosed with PTSD. Of the whole sample, those who had committed more violent crimes such as murder and manslaughter had more PTSD symptoms than other violent criminals, and violent criminals had more PTSD symptoms than sexual offenders (Gray et al., 2003). Papanastassiou,

Waldron, Boyle, and Chesterman (2004) studied a sample of mentally ill offenders who had committed homicide and found that 11 of 19 (58%) developed PTSD after their index offense and identified that offense as traumatic. Dutton, Hohnecker, Halle, and Burghardt (1994) found that battered women who had attempted to murder or successfully murdered their abusive spouse had more severe PTSD than a clinical sample of battered women with PTSD.

Challenges to Research on Child Maltreatment

In contrast to other fields, there are a number of major challenges confronting investigators in the field of child maltreatment research. First, this is a relatively new field of investigation. Second, there is no gold standard by which to determine whether child abuse or neglect has occurred. As Knutson and Heckenberg (2006) noted, "the field has not achieved a gold standard against which operational definitions of physical abuse and other forms of maltreatment can be judged" (p. 69). Similarly, in a discussion of neglect, Dubowitz (2006), a pediatrician, suggested that there might never be a single definition of neglect, given the multiplicity of purposes for its definition. For example, a pediatrician might have a rather low threshold for considering a situation as neglect, being primarily concerned with the health of the child. In contrast, a child protection service worker, bound and guided by state laws and limited agency resources, typically will have a higher threshold. Finally, a prosecutor might have the highest threshold for considering something neglect, pursuing only the most serious cases. For researchers, these varying definitions of maltreatment mean that the "maltreated" and/or "control" populations covered by different studies might not be comparable. Whereas nominal definitions are often similar, operational definitions frequently differ. We would not expect convergence in findings unless studies utilized the same or similar definitions. Third, mandatory child abuse reporting laws make researchers reluctant to examine these issues, fearing a loss of participants because of the sensitive nature of the issues and the impact of reporting. Fourth, studies primarily utilize cross–sectional designs, making it difficult to assess the direction of influence.

A fifth challenge is that information about childhood abuse is often based on retrospective self–reports, which are susceptible to a number of potential biases (Briere, 1992; Henry, Moffitt, Caspi, Langley, & Silva, 1994; Offer, Kaiz, Howard, & Bennett, 2000; Ross, 1989; Widom, 1988) and raise questions about the reliability and validity of the data as measures of childhood events (as opposed to measures of a person's current recollection of childhood events). People's retrospective reporting about their adverse childhood experiences is limited by how good their memory is, how they evaluate the experience when looking back on it, and whether they choose to disclose these experiences.

In addition, scholars have pointed out that information we remember from childhood might be heavily dependent on information told to us in childhood or later and/or constructed by a parent (Radke-Yarrow, Campbell, & Burton, 1970). For research purposes, it is difficult to determine whether a person is recalling the objective details of a particular experience or reconstructing details of what occurred based on other knowledge. One study of a large sample of 18-year-old youth who had been studied prospectively from birth found no evidence to support the validity of retrospective measures of subjective psychological states and processes, including recollections of childhood experiences (Henry et al., 1994). In another study, Offer et al. (2000) examined autobiographical memory in a longitudinal study of mentally healthy adolescent males who were then reinterviewed at approximately age 48. These authors found substantial differences between adult memories of adolescence and what was actually reported during adolescence, including about parental discipline.

A related problem in making inferences about the association between retrospectively assessed childhood maltreatment and later outcomes is recall bias (Raphael, 1987). The net effect of recall bias is to inflate measures of association by creating differential accuracy in reports of childhood experiences as a function of current (physical or psychological) health status. One recent example is provided by White, Widom, and Chen (2007), who found that current life status, including depression, drug problems, and life dissatisfaction, was related to adult retrospective reports of physical abuse for both men and women.

Finally, the lack of an appropriate comparison group is often a serious problem because much childhood victimization occurs in the context of multiproblem homes, and child abuse and/or neglect might be only one of the family's problems. The general effects of other family variables (such as poverty, unemployment, parental alcohol or drug problems, or other inadequate social and family functioning) need to be disentangled from the specific effects of childhood abuse or neglect. Controlling for other relevant variables is vital because a failure to take into account such family variables might result in the reporting of spurious relationships.

The Study

One needs to understand a bit about the design of this study in order to evaluate whether data from it can be used to address issues of causality. As mentioned earlier, the common cross-sectional design is limited in this respect. The design of this study differs in major ways from most of the research in the field. We utilized a specialized cohort design (Leventhal, 1982; Schulsinger, Mednick, & Knop, 1981) in which abused and neglected children were matched with nonabused and nonneglected children and followed prospectively into adulthood.

Because of the matching procedure, the subjects are assumed to differ only in the risk factor (that is, having experienced childhood sexual or physical abuse or neglect). Because it is not possible to assign subjects randomly to groups, the assumption of equivalency for the groups is an approximation. The control group might also differ from the abused and neglected individuals on other variables nested with abuse or neglect. Complete details of the study design and subject selection criteria have been published elsewhere (Widom, 1989a). Figure 12.1 provides an overview of the chronology and phases of the study.

Cases were drawn from the records of county juvenile and adult criminal courts in a metropolitan area in the Midwest during the years 1967 through 1971. Only court-substantiated cases of CAN were included. In order to avoid potential problems with ambiguity in the direction of causality and to ensure that the temporal sequence was clear (that is, child abuse or neglect preceded outcomes of interest), abuse and neglect cases were restricted to those in which the children were less than 12 years of age at the time of the abuse or neglect incident.

Physical abuse cases included injuries such as bruises, welts, burns, abrasions, lacerations, wounds, cuts, bone and skull fractures, and other evidence of physical injury. *Sexual abuse* charges varied from relatively nonspecific charges of "assault and battery with intent to gratify sexual desires" to more specific charges of "fondling or touching in an obscene manner," rape, sodomy, incest, and so forth. *Neglect* cases reflected a judgment that the parents' deficiencies in child care were beyond those found acceptable by community and professional standards at the time. These cases represented extreme failure to provide adequate food, clothing, shelter, and medical attention to children.

Years			Mean age
1967–1971	Court Substantiated Cases of Abuse and Neglect (N=908)	Matched Control (N=667)	6
1987–1988	Arrest records collected		26
1989	National death index (NDI) search		27
1989–1995	In-person interview (1,196)		29
1994	Arrest records & NDI search		33
2000–2002	In-person interviews (896)		40
2003–2005	Medical exam & interview (808)		41
2009–2010	Intergenerational transmission of neglect and abuse		47

Figure 12.1 Overview of the study.

A critical element of this design was the establishment of a comparison group, matched as closely as possible on the basis of sex, age, race, and approximate family socioeconomic status during the time period under study (1967 through 1971). To accomplish this matching, the sample of abuse and neglect cases was first divided into two groups on the basis of the children's age at the time of the abuse or neglect incident. Children who were *under school age* at the time of the abuse or neglect were matched with children of the same sex, race, date of birth (± one week), and hospital of birth through the use of county birth record information. For children of school age, records of more than 100 elementary schools for the same time period were used to find matches with children of the same sex, race, date of birth (± six months), class in the same elementary school during the years 1967 through 1971, and home address (within a five-block radius of the abused or neglected child, if possible). Overall, there were 667 matches (74%) for the abused and neglected children.

The first phase of this research involved an archival study in which the two groups (abuse/neglect and control) were identified and law enforcement records were searched in order to determine criminal histories (Widom, 1989b). In the second phase, we tracked and located these individuals and then conducted two-hour in-person interviews between 1989 and 1995 using a series of structured and semistructured questionnaires and rating scales and a standardized psychiatric assessment. On the basis of ethical and scientific reasons, the study involved an unusual component: the interviewers were kept blind to the purpose of the study, the inclusion of an abused and/or neglected group, and the participants' group membership. Similarly, participants were not told the purpose of the study; instead they were told that they had been selected to participate as part of a large group of individuals who grew up in the late 1960s and early 1970s.

As can be seen in Figure 12.1, 1,196 people were interviewed (76%) at the first follow-up interview (1989–1995), approximately 22 years after the childhood maltreatment experiences of the abuse/neglect group. In-person interviews were again conducted during 2000–2002, 2003–2005, and, most recently, 2009–2010.

Definitions of child abuse and neglect were based on legal criteria in existence in this Midwest county jurisdiction during the years 1967 to 1971. Psychiatric disorders were assessed during the 1989–1995 interviews by using the National Institute of Mental Health (NIMH) Diagnostic Interview Schedule (DIS) III-R (Robins, Helzer, Cottler, & Goldring, 1989) to make diagnoses according to the *Diagnostic and Statistical Manual of Mental Disorders* (3rd ed.) (*DSM-III-R:* American Psychiatric Association, 1987) for PTSD (Widom, 1999) as well as major depressive disorder (Widom et al., 2007), dysthymia, generalized anxiety disorder, antisocial personality disorder (Widom, 1998), and alcohol and drug abuse (Widom, Ireland, & Glynn, 1995; Widom, Weiler, & Cottler, 1999). The trauma assessment was based on information collected using the

Lifetime Trauma and Victimization History instrument, which was administered during the 2000–2002 interviews (see Widom, Czaja, & Dutton, 2008; Widom, Dutton, Czaja, & Dumont, 2005). To assess violence, we used information from official criminal histories (arrests for violence) and self-reports of violent behavior. Whether a person had a violent arrest was based on official juvenile and adult arrest data collected in 1987–1988 and again in 1994 from local, state, and federal law enforcement records. Arrests for violence included those for the following crimes and attempts: assault, battery, robbery, manslaughter, murder, rape, and burglary with injury. Self-reports of violence were based on responses to a seven–item measure (Wolfgang & Weiner, 1989) that asked participants whether they had ever hurt someone badly enough that that person required medical attention, threatened someone because he or she wouldn't give them money, used a weapon to threaten someone, forced someone to have sex with them, shot someone, attacked someone with the purpose of killing him or her, and/or used physical force to get money or drugs.

Establishing Causality

The first step in establishing causality is to determine whether there is an association between CAN and the outcomes—in this case, PTSD and violence. Table 12.1 demonstrates very clearly that CAN increases a person's risk of experiencing subsequent traumas and victimization experiences into adulthood. This relationship is demonstrated across a variety of traumatic experiences that include serious accidents, physical harm and assault, sexual assault, witnessed physical violence, kidnapping, and stalking. More than half of the maltreated children (52%) reported having been physically harmed in childhood, and more than one-third (36%) reported being physically abused, compared to 33% and 14%, respectively, of the matched controls. Similarly, a greater number of individuals with documented histories of maltreatment reported having experienced some form of unwanted (36%) or forced sex (19%), in comparison to 18% and 13% of the control group, respectively.

Not surprisingly, based on the documented official cases of CAN and the reported extensive histories of trauma and victimization experiences, we found that CAN increased risk for the development of PTSD (Widom, 1999). Almost a third (31%) of the abused and neglected group met the criteria for a *DSM-III-R* lifetime diagnosis of PTSD, compared to 20% of the matched controls (odds ratio [OR] = 1.75, 95% confidence interval = 1.2–2.3).

Childhood maltreatment also increased risk for the perpetration of violence (using both arrests and self-reports of violence as indicators). About a fifth (21%) of the abuse/neglect group had an arrest for violence through 1994, compared to 16% of the controls (OR = 1.44, 95% confidence interval = 1.07–1.95).

Table 12.1 Abused and Neglected Children Are at Increased Risk for Numerous Lifetime Traumas and Victimizations

Description	Abuse/Neglect (%)	Control (%)	Odds Ratio
Lived in war zone	6.8	3.3	2.16 (1.12–4.15)*
Serious accident	33.2	23.5	1.61 (1.20–2.17)**
Physically harmed	75.9	59.5	2.14 (1.61–2.85)***
Threatened with weapon	53.9	45.1	1.43 (1.09–1.86)**
Threatened face to face	58.6	49.6	1.43 (1.10–1.87)**
Assaulted with weapon	37.2	22.8	2.01 (1.49–2.71)***
Physically harmed as child	52.3	33.2	2.21 (1.68–2.91)***
Physically abused as child	36.0	13.7	3.56 (2.52–5.00)***
Coerced into unwanted sex	36.2	17.7	2.64 (1.92–3.62)***
Attempted forced sex	19.1	12.9	1.59 (1.10–2.31)**
Private parts touched	11.7	6.6	1.88 (1.16–3.04)**
Family/friend murdered	38.6	31.9	1.34 (1.02–1.78)*
Saw another person being sexually attacked	8.8	2.8	3.22 (1.64–6.34)***
Something stolen with force (mugging)	16.1	10.9	1.57 (1.06–2.34)*
Kidnapped	10.1	5.1	2.10 (1.23–3.59)**
Stalked	25.6	20.0	1.37 (1.00–1.89)*

*p < 0.05.
**p < 0.01.
***p < 0.001.
Source: Widom, C. S., Czaja, S. J., & Dutton, M. A. (2008). Childhood victimization and lifetime revictimization. *Child Abuse and Neglect, 32,* 785–796 (adapted from Table 1).

Self-reports of violence showed a similar pattern; almost a third (32%) of the abuse/neglect group reported having engaged in a violent act, compared to 23% of the controls (OR = 1.62, 95% confidence interval = 1.25–2.10). Thus, one must conclude that childhood abuse and neglect is associated with later perpetration of violence.

Because this chapter is focused on disentangling relationships among child maltreatment, PTSD, and violence, we looked at the co-occurrence of PTSD and violence (see Fig. 12.2). The stacked bars in Figure 12.2 show the proportions of the overall sample, the abuse/neglect group, and the control group with no PTSD or violence, PTSD only, violence only, and both PTSD and violence. Figure 12.2 shows that there are significantly more individuals with histories of childhood abuse and/or neglect who both have PTSD *and* are violent (16%) than there are

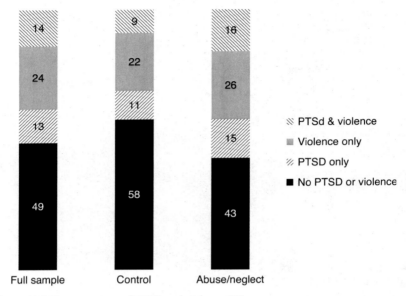

Figure 12.2 Co-occurrence of PTSD and violence (%).

among the matched controls without documented histories of abuse/neglect (9%). However, these findings also show that the co-occurrence of PSTD and violence appears in only 14% of the sample overall.

Figure 12.3 shows that the extent of lifetime trauma and victimization experiences reported by these three groups (those with no PTSD or violence, those with either PTSD or violence, and those with both PTSD and violence) differs considerably. Not surprisingly, all types of trauma and victimization experiences were more prevalent among individuals with PTSD or violence histories, and they were particularly prevalent among those with both.

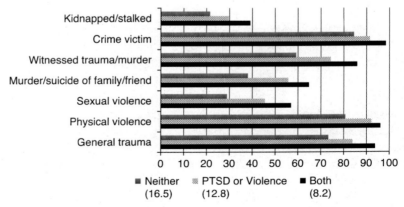

Figure 12.3 Lifetime traumas and victimization experience (%). The average number of traumas is presented in parentheses.

In sum, these findings provide support for the first criterion necessary in order to establish causality: association. CAN is associated with increased risk for trauma and PTSD, increased risk for violence, and increased risk for the co-occurrence of PTSD and violence. However, demonstrating associations among child abuse and/or neglect, PTSD, and violence is only the first step in the process of establishing a causal relationship. Associations are relatively easy to establish.

Now, we focus on the next two criteria for establishing causality (temporal sequence and eliminating competing hypotheses), but we also address issues of the measurement of key variables and recall bias, because these represent serious challenges to the field. To address each issue, we use data from our study and present the results of new analyses.

Temporal Sequence

The initial design of this study addressed concerns about issues of temporal sequence by selecting cases of child abuse and neglect that occurred before the child was 12 years old (that is, children were aged 0 to 11 at the time of the abuse and/or neglect incident). In earlier work, we reported that child maltreatment preceded arrests for delinquency in the vast majority of the sample (Widom, 1989a). It is more difficult to assume that the onset of PTSD followed the child maltreatment experience. Although we know the age of the child at the time of the abuse/neglect petition, there was no assessment of PTSD at that time. Therefore, in order to formally test whether the criterion of temporal sequence was met by these cases, we conducted hazard analyses to determine the sequencing of age of onset of PTSD and age of first arrest for violence.[1] The hazard rate is the potential for an event (abuse/neglect, onset of PTSD, or first arrest for violence) to happen in a year, given that the person has not experienced that event prior to that year. Figure 12.4 shows the hazard functions for age of onset of PTSD and first arrest for violence for the abuse/neglect group and controls. In general, the results of this analysis show that the abuse/neglect petition occurred before the age of onset of PTSD and the first arrest for violence, and that the abuse/neglect group had earlier ages of onset than the controls for both PTSD and violence.

In order to examine this issue more thoroughly (and following the heterogeneity argument presented by Breslau in Chapter 1), we also examined individual cases to determine the distribution of temporal order sequences. Several possible temporal sequences were examined (see Fig. 12.5), including the following: child abuse/neglect is *not* followed by PTSD or violence, child abuse/neglect precedes

---

[1] Age of onset of PTSD was based on information from the NIMH DIS-III-R administered during the 1989–1995 interviews. We do not have information about the age of onset of self-reported violence.

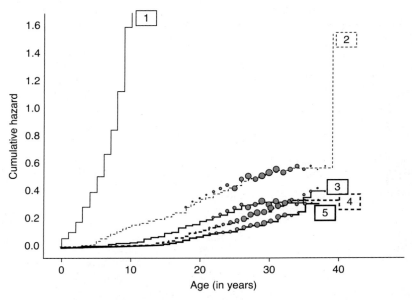

Figure 12.4 Hazard functions for PTSD and arrests for violence by group. Events: (1) age at petition: abuse/neglect; (2) onset PTSD: abuse/neglect; (3) onset PTSD: control; (4) onset violence: abuse/neglect; and (5) onset violence: control. The lines show the cumulative proportion of cases experiencing the event at each age. The hazard rate is the potential for an event (abuse/neglect, onset of PTSD, or first arrest for violence) to happen in a year given that the individual has not experienced it prior to that year. The circles represent the number of individuals who are censored or dropping out of the rate calculation as they reach a given year without experiencing the event.

PTSD, child abuse/neglect precedes violence, child abuse/neglect leads to PTSD which leads to violence, and child abuse/neglect leads to violence which leads to PTSD. Figure 12.5 shows that there is a great deal of heterogeneity in these temporal sequences. First, it should be noted that 30.6% of the overall group had none of the three experiences we are focusing on (childhood abuse/neglect, PTSD, or violence). Second, it is clear that individuals can develop PTSD and be arrested for violence without having a documented history of child abuse or neglect. Third, there is a small group of individuals who develop PTSD and are arrested for violence, and our data suggest that the more common sequence is from child abuse/neglect to PTSD to violence. Finally, it is clear that there is a substantial group of individuals with documented cases of child abuse/neglect (31.4%) who do not develop PTSD or have an arrest for violence.

Eliminating Competing Hypotheses

The next step in trying to disentangle causality from correlation is to rule out competing or alternative explanations of the relationships. Therefore, we conducted

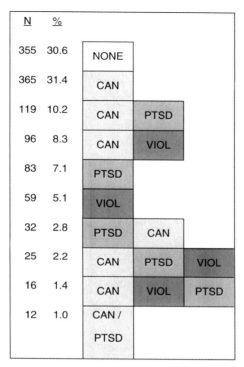

N	%			
355	30.6	NONE		
365	31.4	CAN		
119	10.2	CAN	PTSD	
96	8.3	CAN	VIOL	
83	7.1	PTSD		
59	5.1	VIOL		
32	2.8	PTSD	CAN	
25	2.2	CAN	PTSD	VIOL
16	1.4	CAN	VIOL	PTSD
12	1.0	CAN / PTSD		

Figure 12.5 Heterogeneity in temporal ordering. CAN = child abuse/neglect; PTSD = post-traumatic stress disorder; VIOL = violence; CAN/PTSD = both at the same time. Excludes two cases with two other patterns.

a series of regressions predicting PTSD, violence (self-report and arrests for violence), and both PTSD and violence, with several possible risk factors that might explain these relationships. Table 12.2 shows the results of these regression analyses; similar to the results of an earlier paper on PTSD (Widom, 1999), the impact of child abuse/neglect on PTSD alone, violence alone, and both PTSD and violence becomes nonsignificant with the introduction of these other risk factors. It is noteworthy that having *DSM-III-R* diagnoses of conduct disorder or alcohol or drug abuse and/or dependence predict all three outcomes (PTSD alone, violence alone, and both PTSD and violence), despite controlling for the other risk factors, suggesting that these other variables—conduct disorder or substance abuse problems—might be mediators explaining the link between CAN and violence and PTSD. However, in our examination of causality, these findings are the first that are *not* consistent with causal interpretations and suggest instead that child abuse/neglect might be a marker for other risk factors.

Table 12.2 Regressions Predicting PTSD, Violence, and Both PTSD and Violence

	Adjusted odds ratios		
	PTSD only	*Violence only*	*Both*
Abuse/neglect	1.28	1.18	1.21
Parent(s) arrested	1.48*	1.34	1.80**
Parent(s) alcohol or drug problem	1.11	1.09	1.35
Parent(s) on welfare	1.13	1.13	1.00
Large family (5+ kids)	1.06	1.44**	1.10
Conduct disorder	1.75***	3.83***	2.56***
Separated, divorced, or widowed	1.32	1.56**	1.50
No college degree	2.21*	1.49	1.74
Alcohol and/or drug diagnosis	2.45***	1.76***	2.22***

Note: All equations control for age, race/ethnicity, and sex. PTSD = post-traumatic stress disorder diagnosis.
***$p < 0.001$.
**$p < 0.01$.
*$p < 0.05$.

Measurement of Key Constructs

There is a dilemma in the field of child maltreatment regarding the best way to measure CAN, and this makes it particularly difficult to examine issues of causality. Obviously, it is critical that the measurement of this key construct (childhood maltreatment) has reliability and validity. One decision is whether to adopt a widely used instrument that might suffer problems of limited validity or an instrument with greater validity that is less commonly used. A second issue is how much time the researcher will devote to assessing these key constructs. There is tension between how much time the researcher "should" spend versus how much time he or she can or wants to spend. On the one hand, survey instruments have notable advantages such as relative ease of administration and scoring. On the other hand, the disadvantages of survey questions are that there are often only a few specific items, and items are often vague and ambiguous. In addition, answers often reflect a person's "cognitive appraisal of events," and, as discussed earlier in this chapter, there is considerable debate about the validity and reliability of retrospective reports of childhood experiences.

To illustrate some of these challenges to measuring child maltreatment, we examined the extent to which a person's self-reports of sexual abuse and physical abuse (Fig. 12.6) are stable and consistent over time or unstable and inconsistent. We use as the anchor of this analysis data on whether the person had a documented case of physical or sexual abuse (official) during the years 1967–1971 and self-reports during interviews that were conducted during 1989–1995 (see Widom and Morris [1997] and Widom and Shepard [1996] for details of the self-report measures) and again in 2000–2002 (Widom et al., 2005). The format of the self-report questions varied during the two interviews, but each interview used multiple questions to determine the presence or absence of a self-report of child abuse.

The top half of Figure 12.6 shows that about half (49%) of those with documented court cases of childhood sexual abuse were consistent over time, but that 29% did not report sexual abuse at either interview. Fifteen percent of those

Official Report 1967–1971	Interview 1 1989–1995	Interview 2 2000–2002	Percent
	Childhood sexual abuse		
Yes	Yes	Yes	49
Yes	Yes	No	15
Yes	No	Yes	8
Yes	No	No	29
No	Yes	Yes	10
No	Yes	No	6
No	No	Yes	4
No	No	No	80
	Childhood physical abuse		
Yes	Yes	Yes	72
Yes	Yes	No	11
Yes	No	Yes	9
Yes	No	No	8
No	Yes	Yes	23
No	Yes	No	17
No	No	Yes	17
No	No	No	43

Figure 12.6 Consistency of self-reports of childhood sexual and physical abuse over time in relation to official reports of childhood sexual and physical abuse.

with documented histories of sexual abuse self-reported sexual abuse at the first interview but then did not report it at the second interview. A smaller group (8%) reported no sexual abuse at the first interview but did report sexual abuse at the second interview. Among those without a documented history of sexual abuse (matched controls), fully 80% were consistent in not reporting a history of sexual abuse. Ten percent of the matched controls were consistent in reporting histories of childhood sexual abuse at both interviews, and a small portion were inconsistent, with a self-report of sexual abuse at one of the interviews but not both.

The bottom portion of Figure 12.6 shows that the majority (72%) of individuals with documented histories of childhood physical abuse were consistent over time, but that the remaining quarter of people either vacillated in their reports from time period to time period (20%) or did not report a history of physical abuse at all (8%). Among those without a documented history of childhood physical abuse (matched controls), less than half (43%) were consistent over time in not reporting physical abuse. However, about a quarter (23%) were consistent in reporting physical abuse over the two interviews. The remaining 34% of the controls were people who reported physical abuse at one interview but not at the other.

Thus, there is considerable inconsistency in self-reports of child abuse, the meaning of which is not currently known. However, these findings also suggest that cross-sectional studies represent only snapshots of a person's life that might vary with experiences or reappraisals of past events.

Recall Bias

We have already noted that most of the research in the area of child maltreatment is based on retrospective reports of child abuse/neglect in which the time lag might be only a few years (when adolescent samples are involved) or many years later (when adults are surveyed). In an earlier paper (Widom et al., 1999), we looked at the extent to which CAN increased the risk of having a lifetime *DSM-III-R* diagnosis of drug abuse and/or dependence using both the official records of abuse/neglect and retrospective reports of CAN. Our use of retrospective reports of child maltreatment from our first interview (conducted between 1989 and 1995) is similar to what occurs in a typical cross-sectional design in the field. That is, we assessed psychopathology (in this case, drug abuse) and a history of child maltreatment at the same point in time, when these individuals were approximately 29 years old.

In order to compare the findings based on the retrospective reports with those from our prospective study, we examined the extent to which individuals with documented histories of any form of abuse (physical or sexual) or neglect in our sample met the criteria for a lifetime *DSM-III-R* diagnosis of drug abuse and/or dependence. These two sets of results (Widom et al., 1999) are presented in Figure 12.7. Looking at the top part of the figure, it is very clear that the vast majority of individuals (75%) who have a lifetime diagnosis of drug abuse report having a history of child abuse or neglect. These retrospective (cross-sectional) results indicate a very strong relationship between childhood victimization and drug abuse and parallel what is found in the literature using cross-sectional designs.

The bottom portion of Figure 12.7 shows the results when we looked prospectively using documented cases of childhood abuse and neglect, followed these individuals into young adulthood, and assessed whether they met the criteria for a drug abuse diagnosis. The prospective findings are dramatically different from the cross-sectional ones: the percent of individuals with documented cases who have a lifetime diagnosis of drug abuse (35%) is almost identical to that of the matched control group (without histories of abuse/neglect) (34%). Thus, these two different sets of findings present a vastly different picture of the

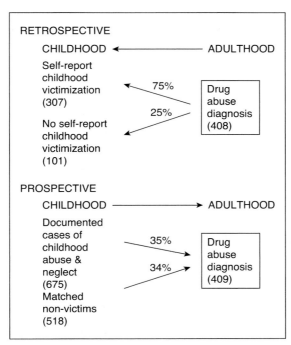

Figure 12.7 Comparison of retrospective and prospective views of the relationship between childhood abuse/neglect and *DSM-III-R* diagnosis of drug abuse and/or dependence at approximate age 29. Used with permission from Widom, C. S., Weiler, B. L., & Cottler, L. B. (1999). Childhood victimization and drug abuse: A comparison of prospective and retrospective findings. *Journal of Consulting and Clinical Psychology, 67*(6), 867–880.

relationship between childhood maltreatment and one particular form of psychopathology (drug abuse). As a researcher, one would prefer to find a consistent picture, regardless of the type of design. But these findings raise questions about the meaning of retrospective reports of child maltreatment in relation to psychopathology.

A related way to examine the validity of retrospective reports of child abuse/neglect is to ask whether there are any systematic biases associated with patterns of self-reports. To examine this issue, we again used retrospective self-reports of child abuse/neglect (yes/no) and official reports of child abuse/neglect (yes/no) to create four groups: No-No (No self-report/No official report), No-Yes (No self-report/Yes official report), Yes/No (Yes self-report/No official report), and Yes-Yes (Yes self-report/Yes official report). We would expect the people who have both an official report and self-report (the Yes-Yes group) to have the highest rates of psychopathology. Conversely, the people who are in the No-No group (neither a self-report nor an official report) should have the lowest rates of psychopathology. Furthermore, we might expect that people in the mixed groups (Yes-No or No-Yes) would have intermediate, but approximately equal, rates of psychopathology.

Figure 12.8 shows the extent to which the four groups meet the criteria for a lifetime *DSM-III-R* diagnosis of a variety of psychiatric disorders, including PTSD, alcohol or drug abuse and/or dependence, major depressive disorder, dysthymic disorder, generalized anxiety disorder, and antisocial personality disorder. Surprisingly, the results differed from the predictions above. People who self-reported having a history of abuse/neglect had the highest rates of psychopathology across all the disorders. For only two disorders (PTSD and dysthymia) was there an increase in risk associated with a documented history. For individuals with a documented history of child abuse/neglect who did not self-report a history (Yes-No group), the rates are the lowest for all forms of psychopathology assessed here, with the one exception of a diagnosis of antisocial personality disorder. Thus, these findings suggest that retrospective self-reports of childhood victimization are stronger "drivers" of rates of psychopathology than official reports and/or that people who have more problems in adulthood look back on childhood and report more problems.

Conclusions and Suggestions for Moving the Field Ahead

In this chapter, we have shown that child maltreatment increases risk for both PTSD and violence, but the results of our analyses indicate that we cannot rule out alternative competing hypotheses. There might be other factors driving these relationships, and we have suggested at least two (conduct disorder and substance abuse problems) that might be considered potential mediators. In addition, the extent of overlap among CAN, PTSD, and violence is relatively

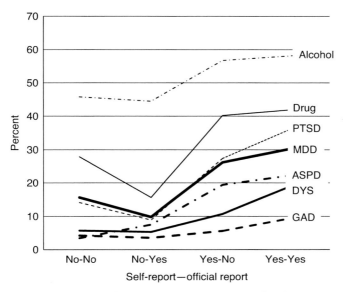

Figure 12.8 Prevalence of psychiatric disorders by merging official reports (Yes/No) and self-reports (Yes/No) of child abuse and neglect into four groups (*DSM-III-R* lifetime diagnoses.) Alcohol = alcohol abuse and/or dependence; ASPD = antisocial personality disorder; Drug = drug abuse and/or dependence; DYS = dysthymia; GAD = generalized anxiety disorder; MDD = major depressive disorder; PTSD = post-traumatic stress disorder.

small (14%) in this sample. Given the widespread assumptions and press coverage of individuals who are reported to have PTSD and have engaged in violent behaviors, these findings might be surprising. We believe these new findings suggest that these relationships are more complicated than previously thought. There is a small group of abused and neglected individuals who have these multiple problems and warrant special attention. However, many abused and neglected children do not develop PTSD or engage in violent behavior.

We believe that the field of child maltreatment research needs to engage in more research on some of the measurement issues raised here. But there remain additional challenges that we have not addressed here that make disentangling these relationships even more complex.

Age

Childhood victimization at one age might have different consequences than victimization at other ages. It has been hypothesized that the age and/or developmental period at which a child is maltreated might play an important role in future psychological functioning (Cicchetti & Lynch, 1995; Manly, Kim, Rogosch, & Cicchetti, 2001; Widom, 2000). In addition, some have argued that the earlier the maltreatment occurs in a child's life, the more likely it is that the child will fail to achieve important developmental milestones, and that this will put that child at greater risk for poor psychological functioning in later life (Aber, Allen, Carlson, & Cicchetti, 1989; Cicchetti, 1989; Wolfe, 1987). (This notion of "cascading consequences" is consistent with the presentation in Chapter 6). Keiley, Howe, Dodge, Bates, and Pettit (2001) found that the earlier children experienced physical maltreatment (i.e., prior to the age of 5), the more likely they were to experience adjustment problems in adolescence. Kaplow, Dodge, Amaya-Jackson, & Saxe (2005) reported that an earlier age of sexual abuse onset predicted higher levels of anxiety years later. Other researchers found that earlier age of the first report of maltreatment (0–8 years) was a predictor of poor daily living skills (English, Grahma, Litrownik, Everson, & Bangdiwala, 2005). In contrast, some researchers have theorized that younger children might be protected against many of the phenomena that would produce distress in older children (Maccoby, 1983). Thornberry, Ireland, and Smith (2001) found that individuals who were maltreated in adolescence (defined as ages 12 through 17) displayed more consistent negative consequences (e.g., delinquency) in late adolescence than youth who experienced maltreatment prior to age 12. Finally, Kaplow and Widom (2007) reported that an earlier onset of maltreatment (0–5 years) predicted more symptoms of anxiety and depression in adulthood, whereas a later onset of maltreatment (6–11 years) was predictive of more behavioral problems in adulthood. In sum, although the evidence is mixed for the role of age of onset of abuse, it is clear that age needs to be taken into account and that there might be different causal relationships depending on the age of the child at the time of the abuse or neglect and the type of outcome examined, or that the age of the child is related to the duration and type of abuse experience, and this might be confounded with outcomes.

Also, often omitted from discussions of the relationships among childhood trauma, psychopathology, and violence is the age of the person being studied. When the person of interest is a child, information is often based on a parent's report, and there is some literature suggesting that great care needs to be taken in interpreting parent's reports of child characteristics (Klaus, Mobilio, & King, 2009; Meiser-Stedman, Smith, Glucksman, Yule, & Dalgleish, 2007; Rothen et al., 2009; Stover, Hahn & Berkowitz, 2010). In contrast, when the person of interest is an adult, especially an older adult, one worries about the possibility that a person's life script has become solidified over time. Finally, with cross-sectional studies, by definition the results capture only what has happened in that person's life at that point in time. Experiences at a later point might change the developmental trajectory of the person in multiple ways.

Context Matters

One theoretical model that has become the basis for much contemporary thinking about child maltreatment is based on an ecological view of child development (Belsky, 1980; Bronfenbrenner, 1977). This approach emphasizes the importance of social context, considering the child in the context of the broader environment in which he or she functions. The child grows up and develops within the context of a family, but this perspective recognizes that children and families are embedded in a larger social system that includes communities, neighborhoods, and cultures. There is emerging evidence that the long-term impact of childhood trauma might depend on the larger context—the characteristics of the family or community in which the child lived at the time of the abuse or neglect experience (see Chapter 6). We argue that understanding the relationships among CAN, PTSD, and violence also requires the consideration of contextual variables.

One example is illustrated by the recent work on gene × environment interactions. In this volume, Sarah Jaffee (Chapter 3) discusses the role of genetics in understanding the consequences of child maltreatment. A number of studies have now reported that different levels of the gene for transcription of monoamine oxidase A (MAOA), a neurotransmitter related to emotion regulation, might protect against the effects of early childhood experiences in terms of risk for violent and antisocial behavior (Caspi et al., 2002). However, this effect might differ for white versus black maltreated children (Widom & Brzustowicz, 2006). As noted in the paper by Caspi et al., most of the work up to that point had studied samples of white males, but our study differed in its inclusion of males, females, blacks, and whites. Surprisingly, this study replicated the findings of earlier research (notably that of Caspi et al. [2002]) for whites but found that high levels of MAOA did not protect black abused and neglected children from the risk of antisocial and violent behavior.

Another example of how context matters for understanding the consequences of CAN is provided by an analysis of the neighborhoods in which these individuals reside in middle adulthood. It should be recalled that the abused and neglected children and controls in the current study were matched on childhood neighborhoods, schools, and hospitals of birth. Yet despite the fact that the children from both groups came from the same neighborhoods and went to the same schools in childhood, Figure 12.9 shows major differences in their descriptions of the neighborhoods they lived in when they were interviewed in middle adulthood. Individuals with histories of childhood abuse and neglect were living in neighborhoods with more negative characteristics and greater risk exposure. This differential context is important because it is likely that some of these characteristics (e.g., presence of people selling or distributing illegal drugs, drunks and drug addicts) might contribute to the development of some forms of

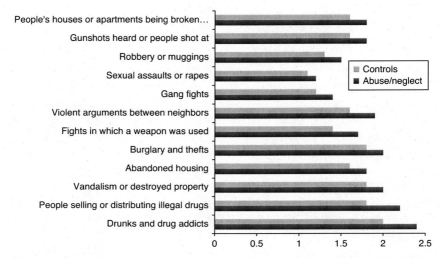

Figure 12.9 Participant reports of characteristics of their current neighborhood for abuse/neglect and control groups in middle adulthood (2000–2002). Horizontal bars represent the extent to which these characteristics were a problem in the person's current neighborhood, from "not at all" to "very much" on a scale of 0–4.

psychopathology, at least in terms of providing access to drugs and exposure to violence. It is also likely that there are differences in their adult neighborhoods in terms of resources, services, and opportunities for treatment.

Confounds

In trying to disentangle whether the relationships among childhood trauma, psychopathology, and violence represent causes, consequences, or correlates, it is necessary to take into account other characteristics or confounds. For example, child abuse/neglect has been shown to increase risk for deficits in IQ and reading ability (Perez & Widom, 1994). It is not known whether these deficits are the result of malnutrition experienced by neglected children, brain damage as a result of physical abuse, stress associated with these childhood traumas, or a function of lower parental IQ among those who maltreat children. One possibility is that these deficits place children at increased risk for subsequent psychopathology and might play a role in understanding the pathways from child abuse/neglect to these outcomes. However, if we exclude these children from our studies in order to reduce "noise," then what do we conclude? Eliminating these children leads to nonrepresentative samples.

Representativeness of Samples

Another challenge in child maltreatment research is assessing the representativeness of samples, particularly generalizing from a particular sample to the broader population. This is a concern when researchers use nonrepresentative, specialized, or convenience samples, including inpatients, clients in therapy groups, prisoners, college students, or members of health maintenance organizations. Researchers need to ask how maltreated individuals in these groups might differ from people who were abused or neglected in childhood but are not in such circumstances. Not all abused and neglected children end up in treatment for psychiatric or substance abuse problems; likewise, not all abused and neglected children are able to go to college. If the "survivors" are the ones who attend college or university and the nonsurvivors are those who end up in prison or hospitalized, then these characteristics need to be taken into account when interpreting findings (cf. Rind, Tromovitch, & Bauserman, 1998). This is one important advantage of prospective longitudinal studies, as they permit the researcher to follow groups of children into the future and document those who succeed as well as those who succumb, or to document trajectories of both groups along the way.

Concluding Comment

The bad news is that we in the field of child maltreatment research do face serious challenges. However, the good news is that we have come a long way from the early days of Kempe's classic paper on the battered child syndrome (Kempe et al., 1962). Hopefully, this chapter has shown that understanding the consequences of child abuse and neglect and determining whether child maltreatment *causes* certain outcomes is incredibly complicated. The relationships among child abuse and neglect, psychopathology, and violence are not deterministic and are not necessarily linear. To use Susser's (1991) criterion, child abuse and neglect do seem to "make a difference," but attributing causality in terms of outcomes remains a challenge.

Acknowledgments

This chapter is based on the presidential address delivered at the 2011 annual meeting of the American Psychopathological Association. The authors express appreciation to Helen Wadsworth Wilson for comments on an earlier draft of this manuscript and to members of the weekly lab meeting who provided feedback on arguments regarding causality.

Disclosure Statement

This research was supported in part by grants from the Eunice Kennedy Shriver National Institute of Child Health & Human Development (HD40774), NIMH

(MH49467 and MH58386), NIJ (86-IJ-CX-0033 and 89-IJ-CX-0007), NIDA (DA17842 and DA10060), NIAAA (AA09238 and AA11108), and the Doris Duke Charitable Foundation. Points of view are those of the authors and do not necessarily represent the position of the United States Department of Justice or National Institutes of Health.

References

Aber, J. L., Allen, J. P., Carlson, V., & Cicchetti, D. (Eds.). (1989). *The effects of maltreatment on development during early childhood: Recent studies and their theoretical, clinical, and policy implications.* New York: Cambridge University Press.

American Psychiatric Association (1987) *Diagnostic and Statistical Manual of Mental Disorders, Third Edition, Revised.* Washington, D.C.: American Psychiatric Association.

Belsky, J. (1980). Child maltreatment: An ecological integration. *American Psychologist, 35,* 320–335.

Breslau, N. (2009). The epidemiology of trauma, PTSD, and other posttrauma disorders. *Trauma Violence Abuse, 10*(3), 198–210.

Breslau, N., Chilcoat, H. D., Kessler, R. C., & Davis, G. C. (1999). Previous exposure to trauma and PTSD effects of subsequent trauma: Results from the Detroit area survey of trauma. *American Journal of Psychiatry, 156*(6), 902–907.

Briere, J. (1992). Methodological issues in the study of sexual abuse effects. *Journal of Consulting and Clinical Psychology, 60*(2), 196–203.

Bronfenbrenner, U. (1977). Toward an experimental ecology of human development. *American Psychologist, 32,* 513–531.

Caspi, A., McClay, J., Moffitt, T. E., Mill, J., Martin, J. L., Craig, I. W., et al. (2002). Role of genotype in the cycle of violence in maltreated children. *Science, 297*(5582), 851–854.

Cicchetti, D. (1989). How research on child maltreatment has informed the study of child development. In D. Cicchetti & V. Carlson (Eds.), *Child maltreatment* (pp. 377–431). Cambridge, UK: Cambridge University Press.

Cicchetti, D., & Lynch, M. (Eds.). (1995). *Failures in the expectable environment and their impact on individual development: The case of child maltreatment.* New York: Wiley.

Dubowitz, H. (2006). Defining child neglect. In M. M. Feerick, J. F. Knutson, P. K. Trickett, & S. M. Flanzer (Eds.), *Child abuse and neglect* (pp. 107–128). Baltimore, MD: Paul H. Brookes Publishing Co., Inc.

Dutton, M. A., Hohnecker, L. C., Halle, P. M., & Burghardt, K. J. (1994). Traumatic responses among battered women who kill. *Journal of Traumatic Stress, 7*(4), 549–564.

English, D. T., Graham, J. C., Litrownik, A. J., Everson, M. D., & Bangdiwala, S. I. (2005). Defining maltreatment based on chronicity: Are there differences in child outcomes? *Child Abuse and Neglect, 29*(5), 575–595.

Gilbert, R., Widom, C. S., Browne, K., Fergusson, D. M., Elspeth, W., & Janson, S. (2009). Child maltreatment 1 burden and consequences of child maltreatment in high-income countries. *Lancet, 373*(9657), 68–81.

Gray, N. S., Carman, N. G., Rogers, P., MacCulloch, M. J., Hayward, P., & Snowden, R. J. (2003). Post-traumatic stress disorder caused in mentally ill offenders by the committing of a serious violent or sexual offence. *Journal of Forensic Psychiatry & Psychology*, *14*(1), 27–43.

Henry, B., Moffitt, T. E., Caspi, A., Langley, J., & Silva, P. A. (1994). On the "remembrance of things past": A longitudinal evaluation of the retrospective method. *Psychological Assessment*, *6*(2), 92–101.

Johnson, J. J., Cohen, P., Brown, J., Smailes, E. M., & Bernstein, D. P. (1999). Childhood maltreatment increases risk for personality disorders during early adulthood. *Archives of General Psychiatry*, *56*, 600–606.

Jonson-Reid, M., Drake, B., Kim, J., Porterfield, S., & Han, L. (2004). A prospective analysis of the relationship between reported child maltreatment and special education eligibility among poor children. *Child Maltreatment*, *9*, 382–394.

Kaplow, J. B., Dodge, K. A., Amaya-Jackson, L., & Saxe, G. N. (2005). Pathways to PTSD Part II: Sexually abused children. *American Journal of Psychiatry*, *162*, 1305–1310.

Kaplow, J. B., & Widom, C. S. (2007). Age of onset of child maltreatment predicts long-term mental health outcomes. *Journal of Abnormal Psychology*, *116*, 176–187.

Keiley, M. K., Howe, T. R., Dodge, K. A., Bates, J. E., & Pettit, G. S. (2001). The timing of child physical maltreatment: A cross-domain growth analysis of impact on adolescent externalizing and internalizing problems. *Development and Psychopathology*, *13*, 891–912.

Kempe, C. H., Silverman, F. N., Steele, B. F., Droegemueller, W., & Silver, H. K. (1962). The battered-child syndrome. *Journal of the American Medical Association*, *181*(1), 17–24.

Kessler, R. C., Sonnega, A., Bromet, E., Hughes, M., & Nelson, C. B. (1995). Posttraumatic stress disorder in the National Comorbidity Survey. *Archives of General Psychiatry*, *52*(12), 1048–1060.

Kinard, E. M. (1999). Psychosocial resources and academic performance in abused children. *Children and Youth Services Review*, *21*, 351–376.

Klaus, N. M., Mobilio, A., & King, C. A. (2009). Parent-adolescent agreement concerning adolescents' suicidal thoughts and behaviors. *Journal of Clinical Child & Adolescent Psychology*, *38*, 245–255.

Knutson, J. F., & Heckenberg, D. (2006). Operationally defining physical abuse of children. In M. M. Feerick, J. F. Knutson, P. K. Trickett, & S. M. Flanzer (Eds.), *Child abuse and neglect* (pp. 69–106). Baltimore, MD: Paul H. Brookes Publishing Co, Inc.

Lansford, J. E., Dodge, K. A., Pettit, G. S., Bates, J. E., Crozier, J., & Kaplow, J. (2002). A 12-year prospective study of the long-term effects of early child physical maltreatment on psychological, behavioral, and academic problems in adolescence. *Archives of Pediatrics and Adolescent Medicine*, *156*, 824–830.

Lansford, J. E., Miller-Johnson, S., Berlin, L. J., Dodge, K. A., Bates, J. E., & Pettit, G. S. (2007). Early physical abuse and later violent delinquency: A prospective longitudinal study. *Child Maltreatment*, *12*, 233–245.

Leiter, J. (2007). School performance trajectories after the advent of reported maltreatment. *Children and Youth Services Review*, *29*, 363–382.

Leventhal, J. M. (1982). Research strategies and methodologic standards in studies of risk factors for child abuse. *Child Abuse and Neglect*, *6*, 113–123.

Maccoby, E. E. (1983). Social-emotional development and response to stressors. In M. Rutter & N. Garmezy (Eds.), *Stress, coping, and development in children*. New York: McGraw-Hill.

Manly, J. T., Kim, J. E., Rogosch, F. A., & Cicchetti, D. (2001). Dimensions of child maltreatment and children's adjustment: Contributions of developmental timing and subtype. *Development and Psychopathology, 13,* 759–782.

Meiser-Stedman, R., Smith, P., Glucksman, E., Yule, W., & Dalgleish, T. (2007). Parent and child agreement for acute stress disorder, post-traumatic stress disorder and other psychopathology in a prospective study of children and adolescents exposed to single-event trauma. *Journal of Abnormal Child Psychology, 35,* 191–201.

Mullen, P. E., Martin, J. L., Anderson, J. C., Romans, S. E., & Herbison, G. P. (1996). The long-term impact of the physical, emotional, and sexual abuse of children: A community study. *Child Abuse & Neglect, 20,* 7–21.

Offer, D., Kaiz, M., Howard, K. I., & Bennett, E. S. (2000). The altering of reported experiences. *Journal of the American Academy of Child & Adolescent Psychiatry, 39,* 735–742.

Papanastassiou, M., Waldron, G., Boyle, J., & Chesterman, L. P. (2004). Post-traumatic stress disorder in mentally ill perpetrators of homicide. *Journal of Forensic Psychiatry & Psychology, 15*(1), 66–75.

Perez, C. M., & Widom, C. S. (1994). Childhood victimization and longterm intellectual and academic outcomes. *Child Abuse and Neglect, 18*(8), 617–633.

Radke-Yarrow, M., Campbell, J. D., & Burton, R. V. (1970). Recollections of childhood: A study of the retrospective method. *Monographs of the Society for Research in Child Development, 35*(5), iii–iv + 83.

Raphael, K. G. (1987). Recall bias: A proposal for assessment and control. *International Journal of Epidemiology, 16*(2), 167–169.

Rind, B., Tromovitch, P., & Bauserman, R. (1998). A meta-analytic examination of assumed properties of child sexual abuse using college samples. *Psychological Bulletin, 124*(1), 22–53.

Robins, L. N., Helzer, J. E., Cottler, L. B., & Goldring, E. (1989). *National Institute of Mental Health Diagnostic Interview Schedule—Revised.* St. Louis, MO: Washington University.

Ross, M. (1989). Relation of implicit theories to the construction of personal histories. *Psychological Review, 96*(2), 341–357.

Rothen, S., Vandeleur, C. L., Lustenberger, Y., Jeanprêtre, N., Ayer, E., Gamma, F., et al. (2009). Parent-child agreement and prevalence estimates of diagnoses in childhood: Direct interview versus family history method. *International Journal of Methods in Psychiatric Research, 18,* 96–109.

Schulsinger, F., Mednick, S. A., & Knop, J. (1981). *Longitudinal research: Methods and uses in behavioral sciences.* Boston: Martinus Nijhoff.

Smith, C., & Thornberry, T. P. (1995). The relationship between childhood maltreatment and adolescent involvement in delinquency. *Criminology, 33,* 451–481.

Spataro, J., Mullen, P. E., Burgess, P. M., Wells, D. L., & Moss, S. A. (2004). Impact of child sexual abuse on mental health: Prospective study in males and females. *British Journal of Psychiatry, 184,* 416–421.

Stouthamer-Loeber, M., Loeber, R., Homish, D. L., & Wei, E. (2001). Maltreatment of boys and the development of disruptive and delinquent behavior. *Development and Psychopathology, 13,* 941–955.

Stover, C. S., Hahn, H., Im, J. J. Y., & Berkowitz, S. (2010). Agreement of parent and child reports of trauma exposure and symptoms in the early aftermath of a traumatic event. *Psychological Trauma: Theory, Research, Practice, and Policy, 2,* 159–168.

Susser, A. M. (1991). What is a cause and how do we know one? A grammar for pragmatic epidemiology. *American Journal of Epidemiology, 133,* 635–648.

Thornberry, T. P., Ireland, T. O., & Smith, C. A. (2001). The importance of timing: The varying impact of childhood and adolescent maltreatment on multiple problem outcomes. *Development and Psychopathology, 13*, 957–979.

White, H. R., Widom, C. S., & Chen, P.-H. (2007). Congruence between adolescents' self-reports and their adult retrospective reports regarding parental discipline practices during their adolescence. *Psychological Reports, 101*, 1079–1094.

Widom, C. S. (1988). Sampling biases and implications for child abuse research. *American Journal of Orthopsychiatry, 58*(2), 260–270.

Widom, C. S. (1989a). Child abuse, neglect and adult behavior: Research design and findings on criminality, violence, and child abuse. *American Journal of Orthopsychiatry, 59*, 355–367.

Widom, C. S. (1989b). The cycle of violence. *Science, 244*, 160–166.

Widom, C. S. (1998). Childhood victimization: Early adversity and subsequent psychopathology. In B. P. Dohrenwend (Ed.), *Adversity, stress, and psychopathology* (pp. 81–95). New York: Oxford University Press.

Widom, C. S. (1999). Posttraumatic stress disorder in abused and neglected children grown up. *American Journal of Psychiatry, 156*(8), 1223–1229.

Widom, C. S. (2000). Understanding the consequences of childhood victimization. In R. M. Reese (Ed.), *Treatment of child abuse* (pp. 339–361). Baltimore: The Johns Hopkins University Press.

Widom, C. S., & Brzustowicz, L. M. (2006). MAOA and the "cycle of violence": Childhood abuse and neglect, MAOA genotype, and risk for violent and antisocial behavior. *Biological Psychiatry, 60*(7), 684–689.

Widom, C. S., Czaja, S. J., & Dutton, M. A. (2008). Childhood victimization and lifetime revictimization. *Child Abuse & Neglect, 32*, 785–796.

Widom, C. S., DuMont, K., & Czaja, S. J. (2007). A prospective investigation of major depressive disorder and comorbidity in abused and neglected children grown up. *Archives of General Psychiatry, 64*(1), 49–56.

Widom, C. S., Dutton, M. A., Czaja, S. J., & Dumont, K. (2005). Development and validation of a new instrument to assess lifetime trauma and victimization history. *Journal of Traumatic Stress, 18*(5), 519–531.

Widom, C. S., Ireland, T., & Glynn, P. J. (1995). Alcohol abuse in abused and neglected children followed-up: Are they at increased risk? *Journal of Studies on Alcohol, 56*, 207–217.

Widom, C. S., & Morris, S. (1997). Accuracy of adult recollections of childhood victimization Part II: Childhood sexual abuse. *Psychological Assessment, 9*(1), 34–46.

Widom, C. S., & Shepard, R. L. (1996). Accuracy of adult recollections of childhood victimization: Part I: Childhood physical abuse. *Psychological Assessment, 8*(4), 412–421.

Widom, C. S., Weiler, B. L., & Cottler, L. B. (1999). Childhood victimization and drug abuse: A comparison of prospective and retrospective findings. *Journal of Consulting and Clinical Psychology, 67*(6), 867–880.

Wolfe, D. A. (1987). *Child abuse: Implications for child development and psychopathology.* Newbury Park, CA: Sage.

Wolfgang, M. E., & Weiner, N. (1989). Unpublished interview protocol: University of Pennsylvania Greater Philadelphia Area Study. Philadelphia: University of Pennsylvania.

Yates, T., Carlson, E., & Egeland, B. (2008). A prospective study of child maltreatment and self injurious behavior in a community sample. *Development and Psychopathology, 20*, 651–671.

Index

Note: Page numbers followed by *f* or *t* refer to figures or tables, respectively.

maternal, infant immune function and,
    198–200, 200*f*
maternal mental health and,
    196–97
maternal prenatal physiology and,
    197–98
Virginia Tech shooting, 171–72
vulnerability
    of adolescents, 143–45, 146
    of children, 143–45, 146

war, 169. *See also* adolescents; children
    First World War, 267
    Gulf War, 16, 17, 271

Second World War, 267
Vietnam War, 268, 269, 271
wheeze risk, 200–201
women, battered, 294
World Trade Center, 131, 136, 169, 171
worst event method, 7–8, 11

zone of impact, 161, 165–71
    problems within
        chronic living, 165
        physical health, 165
        psychological, 165
        PTSD within, 165, 168, 169
        resource loss within, 165